T0229901

AIDS, Rhetoric, and Medical Knowledge

This book examines the formation of scientific knowledge about the AIDS epidemic in the 1980s and shows the broader cultural assumptions on which this knowledge is grounded. Alex Preda highlights the metaphors, narratives, and classifications that framed scientific hypotheses about the nature of the infectious agent and its means of transmission and compares these arguments with those used in the scientific literature about SARS. Through detailed rhetorical analysis of biomedical publications, the author shows how scientific knowledge about epidemics is shaped by cultural narratives and categories of social thought.

Preda situates his analysis in the broader frame of the world risk society, where scientific knowledge is called upon to support and shape public policies regarding prevention and health maintenance, among others. But can these policies avoid the influence of cultural narratives and social classifications? This book shows how culture affects prevention and health policies as well as the ways in which scientific research is organized and funded.

Alex Preda holds a doctorate in sociology from the University of Bielefeld and received the 1998 dissertation prize of the Academic Society of Westfalia-Lippe. He has taught at the universities of Bielefeld and Konstanz, Germany. He is coeditor of *The Sociology of Financial Markets*.

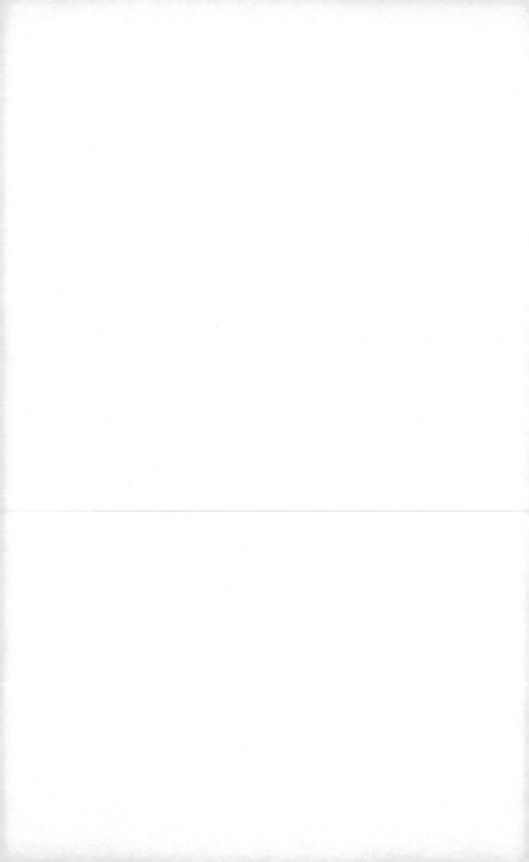

AIDS, Rhetoric, and Medical Knowledge

ALEX PREDA

University of Edinburgh

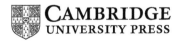
CAMBRIDGE
UNIVERSITY PRESS

CAMBRIDGE UNIVERSITY PRESS
Cambridge, New York, Melbourne, Madrid, Cape Town,
Singapore, São Paulo, Delhi, Mexico City

Cambridge University Press
The Edinburgh Building, Cambridge CB2 8RU, UK

Published in the United States of America by Cambridge University Press, New York

www.cambridge.org
Information on this title: www.cambridge.org/9780521837705

First published 2005

A catalogue record for this publication is available from the British Library

Library of Congress Cataloguing in Publication Data
Preda, Alex, 1960–
    AIDS, rhetoric, and medical knowledge / Alex Preda.
        p.   cm.
    Includes bibliographical references and index.
    ISBN 0-521-83770-7
    1. AIDS (Disease) – Social aspects.   2. Social medicine.   3. Rhetoric.
4. Medicine – Language.   I. Title.
    RA643.8.P737   2004
    362.196'9792 – dc22   2004045757

ISBN 978-0-521-83770-5 Hardback

For Roxana and Dante

vi·rus (vīrəs), *n.*, *pl.* **-rus·es. 1.** an infectious agent, esp. any of a group of ultramicroscopic, infectious agents that reproduce only in living cells [...] **5.** a corrupting influence on morals or the intellect; poison [...]

> (Webster's Encyclopedic Unabridged Dictionary of the English Language)

SIR, [...] AIDS appeared out of the blue a few years ago and, apart from causing immunodeficiency, it has been responsible for two other syndromes – the "minimum publishable unit syndrome" (MPUS) and the "how many authors can I cram onto one paper syndrome" (HMACICOOPS). These syndromes may well be responsible for as many deaths as AIDS itself. Many important medical papers must have been squeezed out by the interminable reporting of AIDS, and, more importantly, a great deal of useful and potentially more beneficial research has not been founded or carried out because so many scientists have jumped on the AIDS bandwagon knowing that most of their work, whatever the results, will be published in reputable journals, which seem to be AIDS struck. [...] It is this sort of publication that has encouraged MPUS and HMACICOOPS to such an extent that they threaten to strangle our journals and stop good work being done or published. It is time journals of international repute took a stand and stamped these malignant syndromes out.

> (A. R. Mellersh, "AIDS and Authors," *The Lancet* 11/8393, July 7, 1984, p. 41)

Contents

Acknowledgments

This book has been in the making for some time. As is the case with projects that grow over the years, it has benefited from the input of many people and from many intellectual exchanges. In the project stage, it was like a small planet that gained mass, shape, and momentum from the various intellectual forces with which I interacted. These forces were situated on different orbits: some were more distant, playing a role in the context of my work; others were nearer, exerting a direct influence on it. On a more distant orbit, two people have made the creation of this book possible. Hans Ulrich Gumbrecht many years ago placed a bet on a very uncertain outcome when he awarded me a doctoral fellowship in the Graduate School of Communication, which he was leading at the University of Siegen. This book now exists because of his bet. Sepp Gumbrecht is known for encouraging young, unknown students and for his willingness to take a risk with them. It is only fitting, then, to acknowledge my debt to him in a book about the rhetoric of risk. K. Ludwig Pfeiffer encouraged and supported me during my first years of study at the Graduate School. Above all, the emphasis on interdisciplinary study, and the openness and dialogue systematically promoted by Sepp and Ludwig as the School's first directors, have shaped my belief in the conversation of scholars from the social sciences and the humanities, a belief which I hope this book mirrors clearly.

A third scholar from whom I have greatly benefited, directly and indirectly, is Franz-Xaver Kaufmann: his encouragement, trust, and willingness to accept research interests different from his own made possible the continuation of my work at the University of Bielefeld.

On a very near orbit, I have strongly benefited from being the student and collaborator of Karin Knorr Cetina at the University of Bielefeld and the University of Konstanz. Karin, I cannot even begin to recount here all that I have learned from you regarding research methods and sociological perspective. You too placed a bet, and I hope it has paid off.

The arguments presented in this book were developed in many intellectual exchanges with the members of the laboratory studies group at the University of Bielefeld. It is fitting to pay tribute here to the special intellectual atmosphere and dynamic exchanges in the weekly meetings of this group in the second half of the 1990s. I must single out Karin, Stefan Hirschauer, Jens Lachmund, and Klaus Amman as partners in conversations, and sometimes even in friendly disputes. Stefan, Jens, and Klaus took a keen interest in my work and never spared their criticism, as good friends do: thank you.

From a geographical distance, Steven Epstein read parts of the text and shared his work with me: thank you, Steve.

Alia Winters and Ed Parsons, my editors at Cambridge University Press, have valued my book project and supported it. Special thanks go here to Alia, who provided many useful observations for the final version of the manuscript.

Patricia Skorge gave me invaluable assistance in improving the style of this book and patiently accepted many requests for help on short notice. She is a true professional and has done a wonderful job. Ann Marie Schroeder also helped in solving many problems in the production of the final version of this manuscript.

Last, but not least, Roxana constantly encouraged me in the writing process and provided moral support throughout. Dante, our son, developed a late, yet unexpectedly strong interest in my having written a book. It is to them that I owe my greatest debt.

Abbreviations

AIM	Annals of Internal Medicine
AJDC	American Journal of Diseases in Children
AJE	American Journal of Epidemiology
AJPH	American Journal of Public Health
EID	Emerging Infectious Diseases
JAHC	Journal of Adolescent Health Care
JAMA	Journal of the American Medical Association
JP	Journal of Pediatrics
JSTD	Journal of Sexually Transmitted Diseases
MMWR	Morbidity and Mortality Weekly Report
NEJM	New England Journal of Medicine

Introduction

AIDS and Scientific Knowledge

Brightly colored condoms, arranged in the shape of bicycles, eyeglasses, or flowers: part of an extensive campaign against the AIDS risk, these have been a common sight on billboards in Germany for several years now. An advertising spot presented on the Arte television channel (which defines itself as the cultural television channel of Europe) calls on viewers to "fight together." The spots on German television (distributed by both private and public channels) are about "not giving AIDS a chance." At the beginning of December, the major television and radio stations, advertising companies, and the press reminded the public not only about Christmas and family values, but also about risks, being safe, and not giving viruses any chance to spread. Since December 1st was declared World AIDS Day, the AIDS risk has been featured regularly in the media in the pre-Christmas period. Not that this topic is completely absent from the media in the first eleven months of the year; in fact, the opposite is true. The activities around December 1st are simply an extra reminder to be vigilant, keep up the fight, and not give this deadly enemy any opportunity. And fight it the populace must because these risks seem now to be almost everywhere.

The media have alerted people to "contamination risk," "occupational risk," "technological risk," and "Third World risk." In the 1990s, cases of patient–physician or patient–dentist contamination (Stine 1993, p. 418), and blood bank and organ transplant contamination – to name only a few of the situations highlighted by the media in

Western Europe and the United States – gained prominence.[1] The rapid spread of AIDS in underdeveloped and developing countries has also been a major topic. Issues such as "risk factors" and "risk behavior," along with the latest epidemiological trends and "risk groups," old and new, have received media attention. With the advent of a number of epidemiological models, there has been a globalization of "AIDS risk" as well (Mane and Aggleton 2001, p. 23; Maticka-Tyndale 2001); since the end of the 1980s, the AIDS risk topics featured in the press and on radio and television have multiplied and diversified. This public presence of AIDS has been amplified by its being made a subject for novels, plays, docu-fictions, Hollywood-style and French existentialist movies, television medical drama series, votive painting, and avant-garde artworks, among other things (Treichler 1993; Miller 1992).

Reports and articles about "risk behavior" and "factors" in various parts of the world are not a rarity. Tourists and travelers are warned about them when traveling to some region with a "risk pattern." Host countries, when not adopting concrete legislation, are thinking aloud about screening the risks tourists might bring in with them. In 1994, when the organizers of the Tenth International AIDS Conference in Yokohama announced in their preliminary programs[2] that nobody coming to Yokohama to discuss risk reduction (among other topics) would be denied a visa because of his seropositive status, they implicitly asserted that the exceptional character of the occasion legitimated an exceptional, temporary suspension of risk screening.[3]

Health institutions have been confronted with the topic of "AIDS risk" from the beginning: the reaction to this challenge has been to enact measures for preventing, screening, coping with, controlling, or minimizing risks. This implies, among other things, increasing the knowledge of various social groups about AIDS risk; inducing overall

---

[1] Cases of dentist–patient contamination have been much publicized in the United States, whereas the theme of blood bank contamination seems to be a European one; the most prominent cases were recorded in France at the end of the 1980s and in Germany in 1993–4. Both events enjoyed a large amount of publicity and have been debated in courts of law.

[2] See, for example, the Advance Program of the Conference, p. 41; also, www.aidsinfobbs.org/periodicals/atn/1993/187.05. Downloaded on May 13, 2004.

[3] According to reports in German newspapers (Tageszeitung, August 6, 1994, pp. 1, 3; Frankfurter Allgemeine Zeitung, August 6, 1994, p. 7) there were attempts on the part of the organizers to forbid seropositive conference participants from entering Japan.

behavioral changes supposed to be risk-reductive; increasing the knowledge of public health institutions about individual and collective risks; systematically monitoring these risks in one form or another; preparing healthcare institutions to meet future challenges, according to knowledge about risk; and modifying other policies (concerning insurance and immigration, for example) according to the same knowledge. This broad spectrum of risk-reduction policies has been implemented in many countries.

Many social studies of AIDS operate with and have a concept of "risk" at their core: they describe individual and collective risks, analyze their avoidance, or examine social and behavioral "risk factors." "AIDS risk" has also become an important topic for health economics and for calculating the present and future costs of medical care, research, and drug development. Social security institutions, insurance firms, as well as courts of law, have been confronted with the relationship between AIDS risk on the one hand, and responsibility, care, partnership, and general human rights on the other.

At perhaps a deeper level, "AIDS risk" continues to be a topic for biomedical research. In its basic and applied aspects, research is oriented according to certain criteria of "risk persons," "risk groups," "behavior," and the like. Drug design and clinical trials, as well as clinical and epidemiological studies, constantly operate with notions of risk: at their core is the effort to construct trial groups as homogeneously as possible according to risk criteria. Especially in the United States, this has generated much criticism from activist organizations; counter-trials have become part of an alternative expert culture (Arno and Feiden 1993; Epstein 1992, 1996).

AIDS risk is then a topic for (1) clinical and epidemiological research; (2) applied pharmaceutical research; (3) public and health policy; (4) politics, economics, ethics, and law; (5) the social sciences; (6) the media; and (7) the arts and entertainment industries. What these approaches have in common, in spite of their diversity, is the assumption that notions such as "AIDS risk," "risk factors," "risk behavior," "risk groups," and "populations at risk" can be understood because they are ultimately grounded in a body of expert medical knowledge about AIDS. In other words, this body of knowledge about the syndrome, its modes of transmission, and the nature of the infectious agent is taken as reliable ground for specifying other aspects and implications of "risk." "AIDS risk" as an issue for expert, scientific knowledge precedes particular (political, juridical, economic) redefinitions of risk. Scientific knowledge determines what "risk" is and what it is not, and how it can be assessed in its various aspects.

The relation of precedence is understood as a logical as well as an empirical–historical one. Its empirical–historical dimension is given by "AIDS risk" initially appearing as a medical issue. Its logical dimension is that "AIDS risk" as a medical topic is necessarily prior to its being a topic for health, insurance, or legal policies. It is hardly imaginable that "AIDS risk" would be referred to without appealing in some way to scientific knowledge. Even mid-1980s televangelists preaching that AIDS was the wrath of God visited upon sinners took care to legitimate their statements by constantly referring to this knowledge (Patton 1985; Treichler 1988b). References to expert knowledge and the experts' presence are constant features of the media's handling of the issue. The idea that this knowledge is a necessary condition (in both the logical and the empirical sense) for analyzing particular aspects of AIDS risk can also be found in historical accounts (e.g., Grmek 1990), as well as in many social studies. They all refer to expert knowledge not only as a source of authority and legitimation but also as the epistemic condition for "AIDS risk."

Scientific Knowledge and Rhetoric

At the center of this book lies the relationship between rhetoric and scientific knowledge about AIDS. In this, I depart from the thesis of AIDS as a "full blown medical and cultural phenomenon" (Sturken 1997, p. 147), which implies that these two aspects are completely separate and brush against each other only at their fringes. I examine here their entanglement at the core of scientific knowledge. There are several social sites where scientific knowledge about AIDS is produced: research institutions, laboratories, clinics, operating theaters, and treatment centers. Moreover, as Steven Epstein (1996) has shown, social movements and alternative organizations are large, significant sites of knowledge production. The study will concentrate on only one such site, one which does not even appear in the previous enumeration; indeed, it does not appear to be a site at all: or, if it is one, then it is very, very flat. It seems to lack the richness, depth, and complexity of the lab, the clinic, and the operating theater, and the vigor, determination, and commitment of social movements. It consists of a thousand disparate pieces which circulate constantly, continuously appearing and disappearing in all sorts of places. This site consists of expert articles on AIDS in medical journals; they are what form the core of what is known as medical AIDS discourse. (That a text can be and is a social site is argued at length in the pages to come.)

Seeing journal articles as knowledge-producing social sites may appear paradoxical; after all, a (scientific) text is ultimately merely a vehicle for expressing knowledge produced elsewhere, a means for transmitting knowledge, not an engine that constitutes it. In expressing knowledge, texts may rearrange and reconfigure it according to the logic of literary representation and the canons and conventions of scientific prose (e.g., Gross 1999; Prelli 1989; Knorr 1981). Textual resources, the nature of which is ultimately rhetorical (Fish 1989, pp. 472–3), can perhaps persuade (which is in itself bad enough) but cannot produce knowledge. In other words, a (scientific) text can (more or less successfully) convey its knowledge content to the reader by using rhetorical devices – i.e., it can persuade the reader that something is the case, but its task ends there. Instruments of persuasion may have different forms: coherence and rigor in textual organization and an apparent minimum of rhetoric (as is common in scientific texts) are only two examples of rhetorical strategies. However, such texts remain no more than instruments for transmitting something, or to put it more colloquially, for selling some knowledge content to the reader.

Moreover, isn't rhetoric (that of scientific texts included) contingent upon the skills of the author and, therefore individual, fluctuating, and non-standardizable? Does it not, ultimately, belong to the realm of the literary critic, and exclusively so? To make matters even worse, what about the rhetoric of this text? Isn't it proof of what Woolgar and Pawluch (1985) would call ontological gerrymandering, when a text claims to have something sociologically relevant to assert about the textual (i.e., rhetorical) production of knowledge by pretending not to have any rhetoric – or, if it has, that it is just an innocent means of conveying some external knowledge?

In setting myself the aim of looking more closely at "AIDS risk" in this book, I was confronted with the ways in which rhetoric appears to insinuate itself parasitically into scientific knowledge. For if rhetoric

is supposed to not have any place in scientific texts, yet invariably in-
sinuates itself into them, how else can it be regarded than as a parasite
that lives and feeds on the knowledge content it helps convey to readers? It may successfully persuade skeptical readers; the usual scientific
rhetoric of clarity and rigorousness may help convey the message better, but it is still a parasite. Worse still, in this light, do (scientific) texts
not actually start to look like parasites on the activities through which
scientific knowledge is produced? Do they not live on the richness and
complexity of the local production of (scientific) knowledge? If there
is something to be said about this, then texts are not the place to look:
they may say something about communicating, about transporting this
knowledge, about making it available to the public – but not about its
production. In the flatness of a (scientific) text, one is confronted with
the rhetoric that lives and feeds on the knowledge content and therefore
should be rigorously separated from it, but how?

I argue that:

1. Texts are not to be viewed as flat, thin conveyors of knowledge,
   but rather as social "dispositives" (Derrida 1972a, p. 359).
2. Rhetoric is not the (more or less sophisticated) form of the knowledge content, meant only to persuade the reader that something
   is the case, but a social practice producing knowledge.

Arguments contesting the parasitic position of rhetoric with respect
to the authorial intention and to content are not new: they have almost become commonplace in the fields of literary studies (De Man
1983; Fish 1989), historiography (White 1985, 1987), anthropology
(Geertz 1988), and economics (McCloskey 1998, 1990, 1994). Arguments about the conceptual primacy of writing and texts for the social
constitution of meaning are also commonplace in so-called deconstruc-
tivist philosophy (e.g., Derrida 1972a,b, 1979; Sarup 1988; Norris
1990). In the field of sociology, the idea that texts should be viewed as
social dispositives and rhetoric as a social practice is a matter of debate and dissension. More recently, Actor-Network Theory (ANT) has
argued that texts act as "immutable mobiles" (Latour 1999), transporting knowledge across various contexts and disentangling it from local
practices. The sociology of knowledge and science has shown the double (local and textual) embeddedness of scientific knowledge (Knorr
1981; Latour and Woolgar 1986), its reconfiguration according to the

logic of literary representation (Woolgar 1988; Potter 1988), as well as the role played by rhetoric in the constitution of scientific knowledge (Prelli 1989; Gross 1996; Gragson and Selzer 1993; Berkenkotter and Huckin 1995; Ceccarelli 2001; Fahnestock 1999; Halliday and Martin 1993; Montgomery 1996; Myers 1990; Swales 1990). The arguments for rhetoric as a social practice are presented and detailed throughout the study not in a purely theoretical fashion but by means of examining the concrete historical constitution of scientific knowledge about AIDS.

The first argument is this: what would appear to be nothing more than strategies of argumentation actually played a constitutive role with respect to the primary knowledge about the nature of the infectious agent, its means of transmission, and its causal role in the Acquired Immunodeficiency Syndrome. In other words, social representations of "risk" are intrinsic to this knowledge. This means that both the conditions under which it becomes possible to speak about a new syndrome and the concrete forms taken by the scientific knowledge about the syndrome, its causal agent, and its modes of transmission were generated by representations of risk. They played a central part in making the Acquired Immunodeficiency Syndrome *the* Acquired Immunodeficiency Syndrome – that is, a condition under which old, familiar diseases became new, complex, previously unseen diseases. Moreover, they were central in shaping knowledge about the nature of the infectious agent: something coming out of the environment, a behaviorally determined agent, a gender- or genetically determined predisposition, or a mixture of all of these. Later on, when it was debated whether the French or the American retrovirus was the causal agent, these representations were at the core of the two sides' arguments: both vigorously contended that theirs was the etiological agent because it fit patterns of risk. In shaping medical knowledge about the retrovirus, its effects, and its means of transmission, risk representations also constituted an order of knowledge from which they themselves emerged as secondary and derived, and as feeding on the essential medical knowledge about the syndrome. Risk representations emerged as dependent on whether the causal agent is environmentally or sexually transmitted, spatial location, gender particularities, and membership in certain population segments – i.e., on factors derived from knowledge about the causal agent and how it is transmitted, which, in turn, were constituted by "risk."

Scientific Knowledge and the World Risk Society

Scientific representations of risk become fully relevant only if we consider them against the broader picture of the world risk society. In the past decade, the notion of risk society has attained a visibility comparable to that attained by the concept of "postmodern society" in the 1980s; intellectual fashions aside, this notion helps us better understand the broader significance and consequences of scientific knowledge about risk.

The sociological concept of risk is usually understood in opposition to the notions of uncertainty and danger. Whereas uncertainty designates lack of valid knowledge about a present or future event, risk implies a set of procedures and techniques through which valid, albeit probabilistic knowledge about the event in question is obtained. Risk emerges when social actors are able to compute the probability of a (natural or social) event, as, for example, when social organizations compute the probability of a technological failure and forecast its consequences (as in the case of electricity grid failures) or compute the rate of spread of infectious diseases (SARS is a good example here).

Analogously, at a basic level the notion of danger presupposes an undesirable (natural or social) event occurring with a lack of social knowledge about its causes, concrete shape, and consequences. By contrast, risk implies a set of tools and procedures through which knowledge about the causes, shapes, consequences, and means of prevention of undesirable events is gained. In both pairs (risk/uncertainty and risk/danger), the concept of risk is grounded in tools and procedures through which unknown events are made into an object of analysis and valid expert knowledge is gained. This body of knowledge enables social actors and institutions to devise paths of action, maintain trust, make decisions, and prevent or reduce the consequences of undesirable events.

It follows, then, that expert scientific knowledge plays a central role with respect to risk. At the macro-social level, however, the picture becomes more complicated. Roughly speaking, we encounter two main theories about how risk works at this level: a systemic approach promoted mainly by Ulrich Beck (1992), Scott Lash (2000), and Niklas Luhmann (1990), and an anthropological one promoted by

Mary Douglas (1992a, 1985) and Aaron Wildawksy (Douglas and Wildawsky 1982).

Beck's argument is that processes of social modernization (individualization, industrialization, the penetration of technology into all spheres of social life, and the expansion of capitalist exchanges) bring with them not only benefits, but also undesirable effects (e.g., technological failures, epidemics, economic recession, and environmental destruction). Once these are recognized, science is called upon to analyze them and devise countermeasures. Scientific knowledge lies at the core of modernization processes, and the solutions it provides are inescapably scientific: analysis and knowledge will be used to counteract the undesirable effects of modernization. But there is no guarantee that these measures designed to counteract risks will not, in turn, have undesirable side effects. This, in fact, happens in many cases. The social consequences, argues Beck, are manifold: late modern societies learn that total indemnity from risks is impossible. They have to reflect constantly upon the social consequences of the decisions taken at the collective, institutional, and individual level; risk society implies then a stage of advanced modernization, where society "disenchants and then dissolves its own taken-for-granted premises" (Beck, Bonss, and Lau 2003, p. 3).

Another consequence is that risk groups occupy a prominent place in the social fabric: they are defined by their exposure to undesirable events *and* by their means for reducing exposure (Scott 2000, p. 35). This is evident in the process of biomedicalization, among others, where the health state of individuals is comprehensively monitored on a mass level with the help of standardized risk-assessment tools (Clarke et al. 2003, p. 172).

Yet another consequence is that, due to globalization processes, risk society becomes world risk society: undesirable events can no longer be geographically contained but rather unfold on a planetary scale. Epidemics such as SARS (which surfaced simultaneously in several cities on two continents) and AIDS are cases in point.

There are, however, still more implications: developed societies learn that the total management of undesirable effects is impossible, but in this process they are confronted with the fears and anxieties of their citizens. A major social institution that should alleviate fears and restore trust is science itself, because undesirable effects cannot be managed without scientific expertise. The increased need for expertise in all domains of social life gives rise to a class of "professionals of representation, simultaneously oriented towards their constituency (social reality, the citizenry) and their professional rivals (fellow scientists and politicians)" (Pels 2000, p. 7). Several levels of dialogue have to be maintained in the social management of risks: a dialogue among experts/scientists, as well as dialogues between the general public and scientists, and between policy makers and scientists. In many cases, group interests intervene in this dialogue and can shape it in decisive ways (Brint 1994, p. 18).

The maintenance of social order also requires trust in social institutions, which in turn requires the ability of these institutions to account for events. This implies, among other things, that responsibility is assumed and blame is ascribed. The notion of risk intervenes in this process: Niklas Luhmann (1990, pp. 10, 23; see also Nelkin and Gilman 1988) argues that causes of undesirable events can be attributed either to one's own social institutions (and they become risks) or to external entities (natural and supra-natural forces, external enemies, and radically different societies), in which case they become dangers. "Risk" is not only a tool for assessing the probability of undesirable events, but also a device for attributing responsibility, maintaining trust, and ensuring social order.

In a similar line of argumentation, Mary Douglas (1967) sees risk as a cultural component of social order: social cohesion, she argues, is determined by the degree of internal and external cohesion of social groups, among other things, as well as by the categories with which these groups operate. In making use of categories such as pure/impure, safe/unsafe, social groups establish paths of individual and collective action and, at the same time, trace the boundaries of their social world. From this perspective, risk appears as one of the categories with the help of which social actors make sense of their world: it is used for defining responsibility, placing blame, establishing accountability, and maintaining trust. At the same time, risk is a device with the help of which fundamental distinctions between society and nature are established: we talk about risks generated in our own society, but we talk about dangers coming from nature or from other societies perceived as radically different (e.g., in the case of terrorism).

Ultimately, risk appears as irreducible to a set of technical procedures for estimating the probability and harm degree of events: "*it is cultural perception and definition that constitute risk*" (Beck 2000, p. 213; emphasis in original).

There are several important implications here: the first is the distinction between scientific knowledge and cultural definitions of risk. According to this distinction, scientific knowledge is influenced in its interests, but *not* in its substance, by cultural perceptions of risk. These may orient the focus of research, whereas the content of scientific knowledge is determined by other factors.

The second implication derives from the the first: because society is constrained to reflect upon the risks it generates and scientific knowledge is distinct and separated from broader cultural perceptions, experts must enter into a dialogue with a concerned public to find effective ways of preventing and/or avoiding risks. This dialogue is an intrinsic feature of reflexive modernization: examples here are the dialogue between AIDS experts and alternative AIDS organizations (Epstein 1996), between experts and environmental groups, and between nuclear scientists and concerned farmers (Wynne 1996). Such dialogue requires a "public understanding of science" (see, e.g., Locke 2002), that is, social groups that acquire a relevant amount of expert knowledge and efficiently translate their own viewpoints into the language of science.

A third and even larger implication concerns democracy itself: if scientific expertise plays such a prominent role in all domains of social life, to what extent is the democratic decision-making process influenced by it? Several authors have recently argued that "technical democracy" (Callon, Lascoumes, and Barthe 2001) or "expert democracy" (Turner 2003), with scientific expertise at its core, raise important problems with regard to transparency, dialogue, civil society, and participation in policy-making.

With respect to the topic examined here, these implications can be specified as follows:

1. Can we maintain a sharp distinction between scientific knowledge about AIDS and cultural representations of risk?
2. To what extent is this knowledge influenced in its very substance by cultural representations of risk?
3. How do such representations work and what is their effect?

4. What are the practical consequences of (2) and (3) for the organization of AIDS research, prevention, and treatment policies?
5. What are the challenges posed to the "expert democracy" by
   scientific knowledge of AIDS?

Seen in this perspective, an examination of the ties between scientific knowledge and "AIDS risk" has deep implications, addressing the
possibility of an informed dialogue, the participation of the public in
policy-making, and the nature of the "knowledge society" itself. In
Chapter 7, I discuss these implications in more detail. For now, I turn
to how "AIDS risk" works with regard to scientific knowledge.

What Is "AIDS Risk?"

(1) At the first, basic level, "risk" can be regarded as a rhetorical device
aimed at enhancing authors' illocutionary force (Austin 1970, pp. 235–
52). This is what emerges if we look at the usual opening or closing
sequences of a medical paper on AIDS. Many opening sentences say
something like, "In this paper, we study the risk of transmission . . . ," or
"We report [the occurrence of *x*] in a risk population. . . . " Closing sequences repeat the pattern in a somewhat changed form: "The findings
support the view that risk of transmission . . . ," or "The study of this
risk population shows that. . . . " In these cases, the illocutionary force
of "reporting *x*" or "studying *y*" is enhanced by "risk": one reports or
studies this or that not for its own sake but because of risk. In other
words, "risk" is a tool or device by which a text formulates claims
about its epistemic intentions and assertions, and about its position
with respect to other texts.

(2) At a further level, "risk" can be seen as a classifying device:
it establishes limits (i.e., categories) within which a certain form of
pneumonia or skin cancer is to be seen as "normal" or "usual." It also
establishes by whom a retrovirus can be sexually transmitted, and how.
One and the same form of pneumonia or skin cancer can be classified
with the help of "risk" as unusual, problematic, previously unseen,
or as seen in a category where it is not possible for it to be seen otherwise. Risk defines the domain of the possible, traces its limits, and
shapes a pattern of knowledge. As such, "risk" produces categories of
everyday medical practice and of everyday life. These categories are

constitutive for the patients' identities, how they account for infection, and the physicians' management of the syndrome. One example is the classification of risk subjects through medical interview practices, in which the interviewees ascribe themselves to a category that is taken for granted by virtue of the operation of ascribing. Another example is that of AIDS patients' self-classification in everyday life, as belonging to a clear-cut risk category, and their continuous identification with that category, even if their personal circumstances are much more complex (Carricaburu and Pierret 1992). Another example is that patients classified as belonging to a risk category are more ready to accept (and in some cases even expect) a diagnosis of HIV infection. Patients with similar symptoms who perceive themselves as non-risk are much more reluctant to accept such a diagnosis.

More generally, "risk" is a device that classifies and reclassifies diseases as seen/unseen, usual/unusual. It is generated by the work of ascribing different meanings to these diseases according to the social categories to which they are assigned. The figure of "risk" plays an instrumental role in the construction of AIDS as a phenomenon in its own right and acts as a negotiating device with respect to its definition. Moreover, the syndrome has varying meanings depending on the risk categories to which it is ascribed. Because "risk" is a device for defining the disease and classifying its forms, it can be seen as a set of classificatory operations *and* their outcomes.

(3) At a deeper level, "risk" acts as a device for producing causality from and through agency. This may seem paradoxical, because causality and agency are mutually exclusive: the retrovirus entering the bloodstream and attaching itself to the surface of CD4+ cells, reproducing itself in these cells and exhausting them, and so forth, cannot be represented as having purposeful agency. But it is agency, presented in terms of risk, that makes possible the construction of various forms of natural causality: descriptions of natural events leading to infection and to the syndrome (even when given in the language of protein strings and biochemical reactions) are embedded in discourses about agency. The natural history of the causal agent is produced from the social history of the patient. For example, the (biochemical) description of the way in which amyl nitrites may affect the immune system and lead to immunodeficiency is made possible by, and grounded in, a discourse about the risk agency of people belonging to some urban

subcultures – people who sleep little, spend a good deal of time in discotheques, and have excessive amounts of sex, exhausting their bodies to the point where the amyl nitrites consumed interact with parts of a weakened immune system whose cells have been partially depleted. Another example: the (physiochemical) description of how the HI-virus is passed from women to men (a medical mystery for a very long time) is tied to narratives about uncircumcised African men, whose long foreskins covering the penile shaft oversensitize the penile glans and are a medium for infections. These narratives are complemented by those about tribal traditions forbidding circumcision, which are encountered in exactly those places where infection with HIV is at its highest. Representations of social agency frame the physiological discourse about the HI-virus entering the body; the latter, in turn, confirms and legitimates the social risk.

(4) "Risk" is a device that accounts for the order it produces and for the construction of natural causality through agency. In an order of knowledge with heterogeneous categories (homosexuals, Haitians, African men, prostitutes, female sexual partners, drug users, infants, blood parts recipients), each risk category defines itself via difference (homosexuals are non-Haitians, non-Africans, non-infants) and by reference to the classification system.

Another device is provided by the narratives on how the infectious agent was transmitted from one risk category to another: from primates carrying the virus to Africans, then from the latter to Haitians working in Zaire, from Haitians to homosexuals, from them to drug users, then to female sexual partners, to infants, prostitutes, and so on.

A third mechanism is that of constructing a past for the present – by showing, for instance, that risk had already been there for a long time. This is illustrated by the post hoc (and ad hoc) proofs of antibodies to varieties of HIV in blood probes from various risk categories, collected well before the first reports on the syndrome. Another illustration for the case in point is the reinterpretation of clinical files of persons deceased in the 1960s and the 1970s as being actually indicative of an AIDS diagnosis.

A fourth device is the reconstruction of social agency from relations of natural causality: of the heterosexual male risk as derived from the retrovirus entering the body through the oversensitized penile glans, or of the homosexual male risk as derived from the single-cell lining of the rectum. From this perspective, "risk" appears not as a result of etiologic and epidemiologic models of disease, but rather as a device that plays a role in the construction of these models, enabling the representation of (1) disease origins and (2) etiologic agents.

(5) "Risk" also appears as a device for producing the future from present orders of knowledge and the corresponding relations of natural causality. The common acceptance of risk as the computable probability of something occurring in the future occurs at this level. In the present context, however, the question is a more complex one. It can be formulated as follows: how does it become possible to produce computable probabilities from heterogeneous social categories? Under which conditions are these categories invested with forecasting power? For example, how does it become possible to compare "quantities" of risk of Kaposi's sarcoma in homosexuals and in the general population, starting from the premise that Kaposi's sarcoma is so rare, so problematic, that it is not even seen in the general population? How does it become possible to compute the "quantity" of risk of AIDS in the general population, under the premise that AIDS risk is actually category-specific? The answer requires taking into account the devices by which "quantities" of risk are produced from qualitatively different risk categories, as well as the ways in which these "quantities" of risk (re)produce qualities of risk. The construction of risk-in-the-future implies several transformations of distinct risk qualities into "quantities" and the reworking of "quantities" into distinct qualities. It implies, moreover, a "normal" risk – expressed in the statistical figures showing how many sexual contacts, what age, what geographical location, and which gender constitute the norm of being at risk of getting the HI-virus. It implies wiping out accidents, individual idiosyncrasies, and so forth, in favor of figures showing what it means to be a person normally at-risk, with which everyone can be compared. The future can be produced from the present because of the work done by "risk."

The representation of AIDS risk as a computable probability rests on this classificatory system, which allows the transformation of heterogeneous categories into "quantities." Conversely, risk as a quantity reinforces the categories of the system. Consequently, "risk" should be regarded neither as a natural fact mirrored by the expert discourse, nor as a simple corollary of medical knowledge about the infectious agent. It is, rather, a complex, multilayered result of classification

operations, a device for producing classifications, a strategy for setting up etiologic models, a device for providing the syndrome with a
cluster of meanings, and a concrete quality resulting from quantifying
and amalgamating various other qualities.

These different dimensions might give the impression that rhetorical practices of risk are graded from the simplest to the most complex,
and that, accordingly, the simplest would matter less than the more
sophisticated ones. In this perspective, risk as an illocutionary force
in asserting epistemic claims is less important than the device producing causality through agency. This might also give the impression that
only at the simplest level does risk act as a rhetorical device, whereas
at more complex levels it is not rhetoric anymore. My argument is
that all these dimensions of "AIDS risk" are imbricated, reciprocally
reinforcing and (re)producing each other. In textual practices, they can
never be regarded as distinct from one another.

One might think that "AIDS risk" is nothing but another piece of
fiction or a fantasy, something that exists at best in the flat world of
texts; given the death toll from AIDS, this view seems curious at the
very least. My argument is that "AIDS risk" is a rhetorical (and therefore social) practice, and as such it is neither a product of authors'
imaginations nor an ideological instrument; it is something very real,
and it has consequences, but its order of reality is not constituted according to a clear-cut distinction between soft and hard worlds that
never mingle. It is the rhetorical practice of "AIDS risk" that constitutes
the system of knowledge we have about the syndrome, its etiological
agent, and its modes of transmission. It is this practice that generates
the concrete, lived definitions of risk subject, the self, her means of
protection, and her relationships to other subjects and to animate and
inanimate objects. But in constituting the system of medical knowledge,
this practice seems to withdraw to a marginal position, appearing as
something derived from hard-won scientific concepts. Showing how it
unfolds therefore means showing the moments through which it both
co-constitutes the system of medical knowledge and withdraws to its
present position.

In this case one could ask: where is this practice to be retrieved
from? Is it to be recovered from the history of medical concepts about
the Acquired Immunodeficiency Syndrome, from gradual progress in
this area? Or is it to be recovered from the passage from a "primitive"

to an "enlightened" stage in the mid-1980s, as historians of medicine argue? Showing how this textual practice unfolds presupposes examining the genealogy (Foucault 1966, 1989) of scientific knowledge about AIDS, with which it is coextensive. This examination is based not on the assumption of something being produced by external forces, but on that of collocation of producer and products. At the same time, it presupposes examining the body of scientific knowledge by questioning its claims of unity and homogeneity, and its inconsistencies, contradictions, and fragmentation. It presupposes inquiring how the rhetorical practices of "risk" are reproduced in various discourses which run parallel or in opposite directions, intersect each other, or stand in mutual contradiction. In other words, this practice reproduces itself not as the simple repetition of the same statements; rather, it unfolds in a variety of discourses, simultaneously performing different movements.

The expression "medical AIDS discourse" presupposes that there is a unitary body of medical knowledge about the syndrome, knowledge that has evolved from the simpler hypotheses (or the astonishment) of the beginning, along more or less straight paths, up to today's sophisticated standpoint. This is indeed the position adopted by historians of AIDS, as well as by many social scientists (Treichler 1988a,b, 1992; Patton 1990; Seidel 1992): as more became known about the retrovirus and its means of transmission, the risks of different categories became better known, so that we can tell today what puts a woman at risk, or a heterosexual man, a man from Kinshasa, or an infant in Milan. There is indeed little doubt that considerable progress has been made in medical research on AIDS in the past twenty years. But take the risk category of women: a closer look reveals that in the 1980s there were several discourses on "female sexual partners," "spouses," "mothers," "prostitutes," and "African women," which ran in parallel and sustained different, indeed conflicting epistemic claims about the retrovirus and the ways it was transmitted. Each of these discourses actually contradicts the others: a spouse having sexual intercourse only with her husband (and getting the retrovirus from him) cannot transmit it further. Hence, transmission from female to male is not possible. Or, if she can transmit it, this happens through "household contacts," in which case the nature of the retrovirus must be revised. Prostitutes are "reservoirs" of the retrovirus: males get it through direct contact with the semen of other males, deposited in the vagina. Therefore, transmission from female to male is actually nothing but disguised male-to-male transmission. African women have frequent sexual intercourse, and the retrovirus is transmitted through vaginal secretions to their partners; therefore, female-to-male transmission is possible.

The discourses on "infants and AIDS" are necessarily distinct: there is one on infants as such, and one on infants as "Haitians" or "Africans," offspring of "high-risk households." This dual perception made "pediatric AIDS" what it is – i.e., distinct from other, well known pediatric immunodeficiency syndromes. Or take the representations of Kaposi's sarcoma (KS), which are central in making the Acquired Immunodeficiency Syndrome a new and problematic disease: we encounter a representation of KS in homosexual men as radically different from the African KS, which legitimates the skin cancer as a previously unseen sign of an immunodeficiency. We also encounter a representation of KS in homosexual men (and not only) as identical with the African KS, which legitimates the African origins of AIDS. Further, the African KS is old and new, endemic and epidemic at the same time, according to whether or not it is an argument for the human T-lymphotropic virus III being the causal agent of AIDS. What is generally termed the "medical AIDS discourse" emerges on closer inspection, I submit, as a variety of representations and narratives crossing, overlapping, and contradicting each other.

At the same time, I argue that theses and views on the causal agent and its transmission that are regarded as valid today were produced in these manifold discourses, transferred between them, modified, and abandoned or taken up again. One example is that of sexually transmitted diseases, widely regarded today as a major risk factor (if not *the* risk factor) for the Acquired Immunodeficiency Syndrome (in fact, every major medical conference on AIDS is a conference on AIDS and sexually transmitted diseases, or STDs). The view that STDs are the major risk factor was formulated in the first medical papers on the syndrome, which related it to STD agents causing immune deficiencies. Later on, STDs as a risk factor reappeared in a discourse that made them features of risky environments, or consequences of risky lifestyles; they became something that may accidentally accompany immune deficiencies. In turn, these retroviruses (HTLV-III, LAV) were represented as the causal agents of the syndrome by virtue of being similar to STD agents. STDs (and their agents) opened the gates through which the retroviruses (this time not STD-like) entered the body and the bloodstream (through sores or abrasions). Sexually transmitted diseases were thus reinterpreted several times according to their specific discursive context.

One objection could be raised here: it may well be that the "medical AIDS discourse" is actually made up of heterogeneous threads running in different directions. But what actually counts is the way in which they are made sense of in particular contexts by medical practitioners, bound by their particular, locally determined practices. In other words, what counts is the way in which texts are read in particular contexts and how this reading process is related to significant aspects of local medical practices. It may well be that there were some medical papers arguing that semen carrying HIV is deposited in prostitutes' vaginas like sediments, but the problem is: what difference does that make with respect to local medical practices? Does this influence the practice of the clinician; are these discourses disseminated in the broader medical world; do they have consequences? Because if they do not, we are again left with a flat world of texts having little to do with the real world. This possible objection contains several aspects: the first pertains to the audience of medical papers. It amounts to asking: are medical journal articles really widely read in the community? Isn't the readership restricted instead to a small circle of researchers? Or, to put it more radically: is there a readership at all? The second objection, which is more complex, puts the reading process in opposition to the supposed primacy of texts. Readers filter through their own intentionality what texts have to offer; they interpret, select, adapt, reject, and provide texts with new meanings. In short, reading implies a set of operations on texts which the latter cannot control; otherwise, it would mean that from the outset a text already contains all its readers' intentions and therefore all possible interpretations. Such a state contradicts the conditions of possibility of a text. As there is no reason to believe that medical practitioners are not readers in this sense, it follows that medical texts as such have less sociological relevance than the process of reading.

A third, no less important objection, concerns the real impact of medical articles on how physicians and other medical practitioners act toward their patients and families. There is mounting evidence (which I discuss in the following chapters) that the rhetorical categories of the medical AIDS discourse do have real consequences for diagnosis, prevention, counseling, and health policies.

Medical journal papers on AIDS do matter, in the sense that they have a readership that goes beyond a small circle of specialists. Evidence for this claim is provided by, among other things, the fact that more than a decade ago some of the major European AIDS non-governmental organizations (NGOs) set up reference departments to translate papers published by the leading medical journals in the field. These translations are distributed to medical practitioners. The same is done in Western Europe by governmental organizations (such as the German Federal Center for Health Education); specialized journals of abstracts and databases (to be found in several European countries) do the same for professionals and lay people alike. This situation is to be found, for example, in France and Germany, where nationwide organizations such as AIDES and Deutsche AIDS-Hilfe systematically translate medical journal articles and distribute them to practitioners.

Concerning the supposed primacy of the text vs. reading, the following should be said here:

(1) The text is the necessary prerequisite for the constitution of reading; reading as such is no more an abstract, universal process than there is an abstract, universal text.

(2) (Scientific) texts do not and cannot include all readers' interpretations. But they provide limits of possibility. In other words, texts trace the limits of what can be an object of debate, approval, contestation, development, selection, interpretation, and transformation through reading (Prelli 1989). They provide the inter-subjective social world with typifications (Bazerman 1994, p. 28). Take, for example, the medical texts about transmission of HIV through "household contact." Aiming initially at explaining how infants and children have become infected, they focused later on saliva and tears as media of transmission or as an alternative to the sexual transmission between spouses. Medical papers about "household contacts" elicited a considerable amount of reader response in the form of letters addressed to journal editors. (This leaves aside other forms of reader response, such as the hysteria of the media and public about contamination through saliva, tears, and sweat, which was manifest in the mid-1980s.) The responses of researchers and medical practitioners commented upon medical journal articles, contested them, provided empirical evidence

for and against them, and singled out and commented on certain paragraphs, and so forth; a very large spectrum of interpretations was expressed by the "letters to the editor" concerning the transmission of HIV through "household contact." But all these reactions started from the assumption that "household contact" is a topic of discussion, something that can be talked about. That such a topic does not appear natural or self-evident is shown by subsequent debates about the retrovirus being at the same time characteristic of a sexually transmitted disease and transmissible only with the help of other sexually transmitted diseases.

(3) One of my previous arguments was about the difficulties of distinguishing clearly between the products of a social practice and this very practice located in those products. The argument about reader response vs. text actually puts into opposition something characterized as a (social) activity – reading – and something presented as a product – text. From this opposition, the argument leads to the conclusion that a product cannot have conceptual or empirical primacy over the activity. But if one goes beyond this opposition (which is itself a rhetorical device), there are no grounds for postulating a radical difference between textual practices and reading practices. In fact, they are the same kind of social practice located in the products of the practice, only these products are not identical. Reader responses may take many forms, only one of which is producing even more texts ("letters to the editor" are a case in point). A text may be read in many ways: it may be transformed, denied, accepted, deconstructed, and so forth, in the process of reading. But all readings are made possible by the reader being able to organize her response, whatever form this may take, on the basis of her participation in a social practice.

This does not imply that there is a kind of Machiavellian machine somewhere determining our total amount of knowledge or that there is something like "The Machine." It does not imply that all texts, or all reader' responses ultimately embody some kind of invariant mechanism (or deep structure) of knowledge. Rhetorical practices cannot be absolutely identical, because: (1) They are collocated with their products, so we can recover only the rhetorical practice of a certain discourse, not *the rhetorical practice*. (2) When (re)producing, rhetorical practices change shape. They are thus not really like machines (which one expects to function approximately in the same way regardless of conditions), but rather like viruses. They are dead out-side the discourses they inhabit. They can only reproduce in these very discourses, multiplying them (and thereby multiplying themselves) in a non-identical fashion. In attempting to trace the rhetorical practice of "AIDS risk," I do not claim that *the* ultimate machine (rhetorical prac-tices being unlike machines), or *the* ultimate risk definition, has been recovered, but only that a specific rhetorical practice, producing a spe-cific body of knowledge, has been traced. (The question of whether the rhetorical practice of risk appears in this study only as a dead specimen under the microscope or rather is alive and multiplying is examined in Chapter 7.)

AIDS Risk and History

In recent years, historians of medicine and cultural analysts have looked at how "AIDS risk" was turned into a biomedical topic. Historical studies distinguish three phases:

(1) The first runs from mid-1981 to 1986 and is characterized by the use of a group-oriented concept of risk, which distinguished be-tween, on the one hand, geographically, socially, and culturally defined groups who were susceptible to the risk of infection, and on the other hand, the rest, who were regarded as being safe (Berridge 1992a,b; Berridge and Strong 1991; Strong and Berridge 1990; Oppenheimer 1988; Treichler 1988a). Vulnerability to the infectious agent was ex-clusively related to belonging to such a "risk group," which in turn was defined through lifestyle. Hemophiliacs were an exception: they were presented as being at risk not because of their lifestyle but because their safe lifestyle had been destroyed. The "lifestyle" of hemophiliacs was presented in the biomedical discourse as a result of medical and technological advances that made self-administered transfusions and storage of blood parts possible; the hemophiliac identity was largely presented as a biomedical creation. Carricaburu and Pierret's field study of hemophiliacs living with HIV in France (1992, pp. 97–121) showed that they too perceive themselves as a product of biomedicine. Histo-rians and community activists took a critical stand with respect to the way risk was defined in this phase, arguing that it left children, women, and heterosexuals out (although such cases had already been signaled) and that it produced a discriminating and stigmatizing notion of risk, which was much exploited by the media.

(2) In the second phase, which began around 1986 and lasted until the early 1990s, the notion of "risk group" was replaced by that of "risk behavior." The transition to this new perspective was made possible by the identification of the human immunodeficiency virus in 1983.[4] Risk was understood primarily as an individual attribute: the vulnerability to infection was attributed to individual behaviors, and safety did not come from belonging to the right group or population but from the behavior one adopted. This change of perspective is regarded as having enabled a larger and more complex definition of risk, which included women, heterosexuals, and infants. At the same time, it allowed differentiated patterns of risk. However, because it was behavior-oriented, it could not account for cases of infection where behavior did not seem to play a major role, as in children, infants born with the virus, or hemophiliacs. This is why such cases were defined as being dependent on the risk behavior of another person: the mother, as in the case of infants, or a blood donor, as in the case of hemophiliacs. The cases of hemophiliacs infected with HIV as a consequence of blood parts transfusions were what led to the topic of institutional and technological risk in the biomedical discourse, that is, to the debate over whether permeability to infection can still be ascribed to a group or to certain kinds of behavior, or whether it has become an intrinsic feature of medical institutions.[5]

(3) A third phase in the definition of risk started in the early 1990s: its core feature is the emphasis on the Third World and on institutional aspects of risk. These aspects consist mainly of the professional or occupational risk of medical personnel, the risk of the patient of becoming infected during interaction with medical personnel, as well as the intrinsic institutional risk posed by blood banks. Some of these topics were already present in the biomedical discourse in the mid-1980s (such as the risk of medical personnel becoming infected during

---

[4] It was named human T-lymphotropic virus III, lymphadenopathy-associated virus, or both, until 1988 (Rawling 1994).

[5] AIDS-related institutional risk is a complex topic which is not addressed here. It has, however, only recently gained prominence in Europe and the US, so one has to differentiate between representations of institutional risk for Western and Eastern Europe. The topic of AIDS risk has diversified since the end of the 1980s and has come to include features of occupational, institutional, technical, and behavioral risk. As this study is mainly concerned with the role played by the rhetoric of risk in the medical construction of the syndrome, topics such as institutional or occupational risk are not followed here in detail.

interaction with patients) but rose to prominence at the beginning of the 1990s. Historians usually distinguish neatly between these phases (Oppenheimer 1988, pp. 280–1, 1992) and evaluate the passage from a group- to a behavior-oriented definition of risk (or, as they put it, from "lifestyle" to a "transmissible agent") positively, in view of the diminished social stigma effects. This passage had a positive effect on the political discourse and on health policy, directly influencing the adoption of more realistic and efficient prevention measures. It is thus argued that a behavior-oriented concept of risk does not lead to the stigmatization of social groups or lifestyles and that it enables a more direct and person-centered prevention approach, as well as better epidemiological estimates.

A closer look at the way historians of medicine talk about "AIDS risk" reveals that they identify (1) a conceptual break and (2) a scientific advance in the transition from a group-oriented to a behavior-oriented concept, made possible by previous advances in identifying the nature of the infectious agent and its modes of transmission. After an initial phase of scientific confusion and puzzlement, biomedical progress took its normal course. Commenting on the impact made by the identification of HIV and subsequent blood tests, Gerald Oppenheimer claims that they led to a double shift: from the epidemiological to the biological definition of disease, and from group to behavioral risk (the latter becoming full-blown with the advent of heterosexual risk):

Standardized blood tests thus initially provided a biological justification for the previously defined high-risk groups. At the same time, antibody testing could determine which individuals within the risk groups were seropositive and which were not. As a result, group membership and carrier status could theoretically be separated. Given the logic of the biological model, moreover, the concept of high-risk group membership should actually have withered away, and been replaced by the notion of *high-risk activities* that made infection more likely (italics in original). Despite this logic, a shift in emphasis from "status" to "act" did not occur until "mainstream" heterosexuals were targeted as a population at risk. (Oppenheimer 1992, p. 64)

"Risk" appears here as the consequence of biomedical knowledge about natural facts such as the infectious agent and the corresponding means of transmission. This state of knowledge determined which concept of risk was adopted. Consequently, the status of "AIDS risk" is relativized with respect to the advancement of medical knowledge about the nature of the infectious agent, its effects, and its means of transmission.

What strikes the reader of medical journals is that the syndrome, in spite of being signaled and discussed in the medical press against a background of longstanding, well established medical knowledge, was reported as being completely new, mysterious, and highly problematic. The whole story began with epidemiological reports about opportunistic infections (a skin cancer and a form of pneumonia) which had been known and described since the 1870s and the 1930s, respectively. And yet, they were presented as very new, problematic, rare, and indeed as previously unseen. There had been research on retroviruses since the beginning of the 1970s, and on human retroviruses since the mid-1970s. Still, it took more than two years to identify the infectious agent of AIDS as a human retrovirus. This process was related to a conflict in the medical world and later led to a political agreement between the presidents of France and the US about which researcher identified what retrovirus (Rawling 1994, p. 343; Grmek 1990). Furthermore, AZT (azidothymidine), one of the main drugs used in AIDS therapy, had been developed in the mid-1960s and had therefore been known for a long time (Arno and Feiden 1993, p. 247). It has been used in AIDS therapy only since 1987.

Medical historians argue that it was exactly this frame of established medical knowledge about the retroviruses and the immune system, along with the advances in lab analysis techniques that have made possible the identification and description of such a complex syndrome as AIDS (Grmek 1990; Oppenheimer 1988, 1992). Professional struggles between epidemiologists and "bench" scientists over the definitions of the syndrome (Oppenheimer 1992, p. 75), along with stereotypes, the power of epidemiological tradition, previous criticisms of the CDC (Centers for Disease Control and Prevention), and too rigid an orientation toward the hepatitis B model were responsible for delays. When it comes to discussing the knowledge background against which the first opportunistic infections (and with them, the syndrome) were presented as new, mysterious, and problematic, historians embrace the orthodox viewpoint that they really were very new, mysterious, and problematic. Unanswered remains the question of why heterosexual cases of *Pneumocystis* pneumonia and other opportunistic infections were concomitantly reported and ignored.

Other unexplained issues are why risk groups such as "Haitians" were maintained as a medical AIDS category for so long, although this was obviously absurd; and why groups such as women and infants, in spite of being reported on very early, were acknowledged as being at risk only later. The same questions apply for the "Africans," a category that survived "Haitians" in the statistics, although both were ethnically defined. These developments have been explained in terms of a racist bias in the medical knowledge (Chirimuuta and Chirimuuta 1989) or different medical beliefs about the relationships between ethnic groups and homosexuality. Others have branded such explanations simplistic, claiming that they do not take into account the complexity of medical knowledge of AIDS (Patton 1990).

The notion of "risk groups" is seen in two ways: (1) as an early error, due to lack of sufficient knowledge about the nature of the syndrome, its action, and its transmission (Grmek 1990); (2) as actually quite useful, because it provided medical knowledge with a heuristic instrument for building up conjectures about the nature of the infectious agent and making "the epidemic potentially less frightening by making it appear more likely that the disease would eventually be understood and controlled" (Oppenheimer 1992, p. 52). The consensus is that "risk groups" were in operation until the mid-1980s, being abandoned afterwards in favor of "risk behavior" and "risk factors."

A closer look at "risk groups" and "risk behavior" reveals that there is no point of rupture at which the first was replaced by the second leading to a radical change in the understanding of AIDS risk. Rather, "risk groups," "risk factors," "risk behaviors," "cofactors," and "high and low risk" were used simultaneously and continuously from the first articles published on the topic of unexplainable opportunistic infections. The empirical evidence speaks rather for a cluster of these notions operating together rather than for them replacing one another; therefore, the idea of a conceptual break should be reexamined.

AIDS-related medical and biological research have come to the attention of cultural critics and sociologists (e.g., Treichler 1988a,b, 1992, 1999; Patton 1990; Epstein 1988, 1996) who have asked concrete questions about the status of risk groups and the meanings surrounding the syndrome. Their initial question was: "how was it possible that x and not y has been presented as a risk category, and how was this accomplished?" One of these questions is why women and infants at risk of contracting AIDS, in spite of being signaled and described by several clinical papers relatively early, were given the status of risk categories much later than others (Treichler 1988a,b); other questions have concerned the discursive background against which homosexuals have come to be represented as the main risk group for AIDS (Epstein 1988). The answers have focused primarily on gender-oriented features of the biomedical discourse and on differences in the biomedical representation of the male and female body. Thus, Steven Epstein has argued that in the 1970s homosexuality had already been represented as a medical condition and as a lifestyle conducive to contracting sexually transmitted diseases. This discursive repertoire provided the basis for representing homosexuals as the AIDS risk group par excellence, and it supported the thesis of AIDS as a variety of sexually transmitted disease. Paula Treichler's arguments have focused on the systematic representation of women and infants as secondary categories that cannot achieve a risk status of their own, being derived from the main risk categories. Thus, between 1981 and 1985, women and infants were ascribed risk status only insofar as they stood for another category: as spouses of bisexuals, sexual partners, or children of intravenous drug users, Haitians, and Africans. This regime led to the paradoxical situation of signaling and describing cases of women and infants and at the same time neglecting the fact that they might be at risk. Although valuable, these approaches have been concerned only with certain partial aspects of the role played by risk in the construction of the syndrome, emphasizing above all the gender-oriented distinctions which led to some categories being presented as being at risk while others were ignored.

Discourse and Speech Acts

The present study does not argue for either a break or continuity in the medical history of "AIDS risk," or for or against "good" or "bad" medical knowledge. It examines "aberrations" in a larger context, as intrinsic to the economy of discourse and to its specific rationality. It also questions the paradoxical character of this economy, in which diseases are at the same time old and new, problematic and unproblematic.

The following issues are examined here: (1) how "risk" generates the possibility of a discourse about a new immune deficiency syndrome;

(2) the relationship between "risk" and the representations/definitions of the syndrome; (3) the role "risk" plays in the construction of etiologic and epidemiological models; (4) and (5) the conditions under which "risk" is made possible as a forecasting instrument and as a computable probability; and (6) how "risk" provides the syndrome with context-bound, heterogeneous meanings.

Up to this point, I have liberally used terms such as "discourse" and "rhetoric"; the time has come to introduce some specifications. This task is made even more difficult by the plethora of definitions and conceptualizations produced in the past twenty-five years (e.g., Bowers and Inei 1993; Fairclough 1992; Van Dijk 1993; Dillon 1986; Fuller 1993; Gusfield 1976; Hak 1989; Nash 1989; Peters 1990). It is not my aim here to provide an overview of all these notions and approaches. However, the following specifications necessarily focus on those that are relevant to my analysis. Some of these conceptualizations have extended the notion of discourse to any kind of linguistic exchange, be it written or oral; some have argued that because discourse is the general domain of the production and circulation of rule-governed statements it need not be speech-based. This broad definition includes visual artifacts in the sphere of discourse, and textual ones (Mills 1997, p. 9).

Another, perhaps more productive approach is to define discourse not by its object, but by its operations. Michel Pêcheux (1990, pp. 297–9), in the footsteps of Mikhail Bakhtin, conceives discourses as sets of practical operations (called "machines") that structure social experience through utterances. These operations relate primarily to one another and not to a given, external reality. They are located in their products (texts and images) and are understood as collections and networks of practices (Lay, Gurak, Gravon, and Myntti 2000, p. 7; Fairclough 2001, p. 236). These networks can expand in various directions; as a consequence, the products of the "discursive machine" do not need to be logically consistent and coherent. Rather, they are flexible and adaptive enough to generate contradictory yet related texts, according to circumstances. In a similar vein, Ron Scollon (2001, p. 6) puts forward the view that discourses can be best conceived as social actions embedded in networks of practical doings and sayings (see also Schatzki 1996, p. 99). Another related argument has been recently formulated by literary and legal scholars engaged in debates about violent and hate speech (e.g., Butler 1997; MacKinnon 1993; Douglas 1995). They argue that speech cannot be conceived as a mere medium for communicating abstract ideas; the act of communicating is a form of conduct (hence, of social action) that enacts the message (Butler 1997, p. 351).

In this perspective, discourses and practices are mutually constitutive (Scollon 2001, p. 162) without being linearly linked to each other. Rather, these linkages are shaped differently at various points in the network, and they can be shifted around. Concretely, this means that we should conceive of texts as configurations of "frozen" social action that incorporate knowledge and cognitive skills and require at the same time certain kinds of knowledge and skills from human actors. Human actors and texts are positioned in a cognitive network, which enables the circulation, justification, acceptance, and practical use of knowledge. Pêcheux's and Scollon's arguments are similar to those of Bruno Latour (1988), who argued that scientists mobilize networks of texts (journal articles and other publications), along with laboratory artifacts, to support their knowledge claims. These networks of texts, generated by sets of highly flexible and adaptive operations, achieve in time a life of their own. What, then, do these operations look like?

One answer has come from the rhetoric of science. Over the past two decades, it has become relevant for sociology mainly via two channels: (1) the sociology and philosophy of (scientific) knowledge, and (2) theories of social practice as an alternative to structuralist and functionalist theories of social action (e.g., Schatzki, Knorr-Cetina, and von Savigny 2001). Since the end of the 1970s, the new sociology of knowledge and science (e.g., Latour and Woolgar 1986; Knorr 1981; Woolgar 1988; Ashmore 1989) has questioned the traditional assumptions that there is a clear distinction between the content of a scientific theory (its logical structure) and the form in which it is expressed (its rhetoric as a literary genre) and that although the second is socially produced, the first is immune to interests, power, persuasion, or other social influences.

It was argued instead that (scientific) knowledge is intrinsically conditioned by the linguistic frames that make it possible for it to exist as expressed knowledge. Therefore, we are confronted with a double embeddedness of knowledge – in local practices (of the lab, the corporation, the clinic, and so forth) and in the context provided by scientific discourses and embodied by scientific texts, journal articles, conferences, and symposia. Relevant in this respect are also conversations and debates between scientists (e.g., Lachmund and Stollberg 1992; Prior 1992). They show that making knowledge public actually implies complex (language-determined) processes of producing, negotiating, and legitimating what can be accepted as scientific knowledge. If we take scientific texts at their face value – that is, as pieces of writing – we can see that stylistic features, conventions, canons, rhetorical devices, argumentation structures, and metaphors leave an imprint on the knowledge content of scientific papers (Woolgar 1988; Bazerman 1988, 1989, 1994). The traditional distinction between content and form does not appear to be clear-cut anymore. Aspects of scientific texts considered to be purely formal and without relevance to content are now seen as socially legitimated ways of producing knowledge and socially informed writing techniques. They are inseparable from knowledge content. On the one hand, they are intrinsic to producing this content as written knowledge (and therefore as quintessentially scientific). On the other hand, they operate by selecting what is expressed (and expressible) scientific knowledge and what is not.

A related approach (also known as rhetoric of science) has been to show how shared conventions, semantics, and rhetorical devices form a web that makes the social reproduction of knowledge possible (e.g., Prelli 1989; Gross 1999; Pera 1994; Berkenkotter and Huckin 1995; Fahnestock 1999; Halliday and Martin 1993; Maasen and Weingart 2000; Swales 1990; Urban and Silverstein 1996). Because these elements are intrinsic to making knowledge public and thereby legitimizing it, they show the historical and social boundaries within which scientific knowledge can be (re)produced. A further direction of research[6] can be described as focusing on particular cases to show

---

[6] It should be said here that in the past decade discourse analysis has become a large and complex field that embraces several subdirections, which differ substantially in the methods they use, as well as in the empirical material they analyze. At the same time, discourse analysis has not been confined to the sociology of scientific knowledge; it is also largely practiced in media and communication studies and in the sociology of literature, and it has made its way into policy studies too. Outside the field of sociology, it has been largely used in literary studies and linguistics; many analytical techniques have been developed in these fields.

in detail how rhetorical, semantic, and stylistic techniques act as devices for producing legitimate knowledge (Potter, Wetherell, and Chitty 1991; Ceccarelli 2001; Gragson and Selzer 1993; Myers 1991; Sauer 1996).

The critique of the traditional distinction between content and form of knowledge has been accompanied by empirical studies from disciplines such as historiography (White 1973; De Certeau 1988), anthropology (Geertz 1988), and economics (McCloskey 1998; Mirowski 1994), showing that historical, anthropological, or economic knowledge cannot be distinguished from the ways it is expressed, and that apparently peripheral aspects (such as rhetoric) lie at their core.

These developments have been paralleled by theories of social practices[7] as an alternative to the concept of social action. Theories of social action[8] draw a clear distinction between the subject(s) of (social) action and its object(s) (Lemert 1990, p. 238): social action in elementary form is seen as the reciprocal tuning of (black box) beliefs and information held by subjects so that they can successfully (i.e., according to criteria of success) perform together a set of operations upon an inert object (Elster 1986, p. 12). Criteria and rules (of rationality) determine both the tuning operations (which need not necessarily be harmonious) and those performed upon the object. In this perspective, there is little or nothing to be said about texts, nor about rhetoric or language. Texts can be of sociological interest at best in the sociology of literature, and even then only as objects upon which some action is performed (by the author or by the readers). They are only conveyors of information and/or intentions. Information is seen as those elements hidden behind the rhetorical surface of a text and achieving a one-to-one correspondence with reality: statistical figures in an economics text, for example, are the information about the real phenomena of, say, prices or inflation (as a conceptual construct which manages somehow both to condense economic reality and to achieve a one-to-one correspondence with it). Similarly, a text can provide information about many aspects of reality, if not about all of them. It is simply an instrument

---

[7] An overview of these is provided by Stephen Turner (1994).

[8] See for example Gary Becker's (1986) account of social action from the viewpoint of rational choice.

(or a kind of information warehouse) used in the process of tuning the beliefs and information of social actors.

The character of texts as (more or less inert) objects or instruments is closely linked both to the distinction between their form (means of persuasion) and their content (information, intention), and to the capacity of the said content for establishing a one-to-one correspondence with external reality. What makes a text an object of (social) action is its capacity to store information (or intention) retrievable by actors, who can act on the grounds of the established correspondence with reality. The form–content distinction implies that there are various forces at work in a text, some of which are concentrated on the informational or intentional content, others on the form. These forces can coexist in various combinations in a text and are like those at work in oral speech.

But the notion of force itself, which is social and institutional in character, subverts the distinction between informational content and form. There are many situations – systematically explored by John Langshaw Austin (1976 [1962], 1970) in his speech act theory – where forces directed at the form of speech manage to achieve social actions by themselves. Austin argued that, at least in certain situations, utterances can be seen as forms of social action: they change the social setting in which they occur significantly and lastingly (e.g., when baptizing a child, making a will, or making a bet). Performing the utterance *is* performing the respective social action. Hence, performative utterances, such as bets or baptismal formulas, have to be distinguished from constative ones, which merely describe states of fact. Whereas constative utterances may be considered true or false, performative ones are felicitous or not, according to whether they successfully change the social setting in which they are formulated. This actually means that social reality can somehow (or in some cases) be changed by the inner force of language – which calls into question its role as simply a transparent medium in reproducing reality.

In this perspective, utterances can be characterized by three types of forces at work in them: locutionary, illocutionary, and perlocutionary forces (Austin 1976 [1962], pp. 101–2). They are present (in various degrees) in every speech act: whereas the locutionary force refers to concrete, context-bound production (uttering an intelligible sentence), the illocutionary force designates the intention of the speaker in formulating that utterance (advising, asking, ordering, requiring, and so forth). In turn, the perlocutionary force designates the impact of an utterance on the hearer/reader (making her do something, inducing a reaction to the utterance). The perlocutionary force of speech acts is the rhetorical force by which the audience is persuaded that the world changes as a consequence of their being performed (and by which they therefore change the world). Austin saw distinguishing between these three kinds of forces as a means of deepening the distinction between constative and performative utterances. One of the consequences is that the correspondences between content elements of a text and external reality cannot be given or automatically ensured; rather, they are the result of forces at work in both oral speech and texts. Although Austin argued that constative utterances can be seen as short-circuited performatives, he explained their performative character as stemming from their illocutionary force (Austin 1970). In the tradition of Ferdinand de Saussure (1959 [1916], p. 24), who privileged oral speech over written language, Austin (and many of his followers) focused his analysis on spoken utterances. However, there was never an explicit argument that written utterances cannot be analyzed as speech acts; in fact, we encounter many examples of written speech acts (such as wills, decrees, and contracts) in everyday life.

John Searle (1970, p. 25), in his development of speech act theory, argued that the distinction between constative and performative utterances is relative and context-bound: "propositional acts cannot occur alone; that is, one cannot just refer and predicate without making an assertion or asking a question or performing some other illocutionary acts." Searle (1979, pp. 12–16) distinguishes five types of illocutionary acts: assertives, directives, commissives, expressives, and declarations. From the perspective of scientific journal articles, assertive, commissive, and declarative illocutionary acts are especially interesting. Assertive speech acts commit the speaker to something being the case: scientific hypotheses, as well as scientific statements, belong to this class. Commissives commit the speaker to a future course of action: when they establish a program of research by stating that certain domains require further inquiry, for example, scientists employ commissive speech acts. The successful performance of declarative speech acts guarantees that the propositional content corresponds to the world: this is what happens, for example, when scientists declare having performed an experiment or a measurement. The question is whether these speech acts systematically have perlocutionary force too: because if they do, then rhetoric becomes an intrinsic feature of scientific writing.

The Sociological Inquiry of Scientific Texts

Texts as objects of sociological inquiry are very often legitimated with respect to the reading process. This process is socially determined and as such has sociological relevance (in the sense that, for example, one may look at the way in which medical experts "read" AIDS risk and at the social consequences of this reading); nevertheless, texts are not social processes but objects or "props," obtaining their meaning only through the socially organized activity of interpretation (e.g., De Vault 1990). A skilled reader can disentangle and rearrange the knowledge expressed in a text, ignoring persuasion devices. The premises of this opposition, first elaborated in literary theories of reader response (e.g., Iser 1993; Fish 1989), are that there are some fundamental distinctions between the readers' activities of interpreting, on the one hand, and texts, on the other: (1) the ontological distinction between a social activity and the tools it employs; (2) the epistemic distinction between the reader's (and reading's) own rationality (stripping knowledge of all adornments) and the type of rationality texts obey (putting the best possible persuasion devices to work to convince the reader). In the worst case, the reader can turn the text's own persuasion devices against textual and authorial intentions, to reach the conclusion that the text will always be betrayed by its own rhetoric, which regularly fails to persuade completely (De Man 1978, 1983). Moreover, the reader's rationality is not only opposed to that of the text, as in a kind of strategic game, but also superior to it. The reader will always be able to separate the knowledge content of a (scientific) text from its persuasion devices.

Consequently: (1) texts are of little relevance as objects of sociological study; and (2) therefore not much can be said about the social production of medical knowledge on AIDS starting from these premises. Even if we accept that in medical papers knowledge claims depend on particular persuasion devices, this would mean nothing more than that medical knowledge is (re)arranged according to a textual logic of persuasion, being produced according to other contextual rationalities, and that skilled expert readers will disentangle this knowledge anyway, rearranging it according to their own interests.

The counterargument is that the rules of knowing cannot be separated from the rules of persuasion. Just take the literary conventions of scientific papers, which begin with the textual arrangement in clearcut sections claiming to perform the reconstruction of how knowledge was produced in the clinic or laboratory: which cases were observed, what was seen, what methods were used, which results the lab analyses arrived at, whether or not therapy had an effect, and finally, what conclusions can be drawn from this long process of gaining knowledge. These conventions are continuous with those of the speech mode, requiring one to let the facts speak for themselves, facts which almost beg observation from the researcher. The author either (1) disappears behind the acting facts, (2) becomes an instrument these use for the purpose of letting themselves be observed, measured, and analyzed, or (3) intervenes in the direct speech mode as an entity of the same order as the facts. The order of human actors and phenomena is reversed; humans are arranged in a scientific paper according to the logic of phenomena, and not the other way around. According to these conventions, the textual logic claims to reproduce what it presents as the logic of the laboratory, but at the same time it brackets it out. In this textual arrangement, there is no place for statements about wondering about, say, laboratory results, but only about how things went logically from case observation to diagnosis, analysis, therapy, monitoring, more analysis, and so forth, to conclusions. By claiming to perform only the reproduction of an external logic of knowledge production, conventions of textual arrangement and speech mode in fact claim, paradoxically enough, to be only conventions and are thus taken as non-conventions, that is, as having a necessary character. They say: look, it is only a convention to arrange a medical paper like this; it is only done to show how these conclusions about a new form of Kaposi's sarcoma were obtained. They elicit the answer: well, if they say they are conventions, then they aren't, because they necessarily reflect this compelling logic.

Furthermore, there are the literary canons specific to scientific papers: the catalog of formulas acknowledged as authentic and legitimate for opening, framing, and ending medical papers. In short, authors use these canons for establishing a field of possible knowledge claims and for positioning their own claims within it, for example. When stating what has been previously published on a certain topic, a paper generates both precedence for its own epistemic claims and positions itself in a knowledge frame: it claims continuity, difference, contradiction, or novelty.

Rules of stasis (Prelli 1989) set out the issue to be argued or debated. In this sense, they are neither simple conventions of scientific writing, recognizable as such by the community, nor a set of explicit rules separable from the issues they have built up, such as kit assembly instructions; they are set out in the work of building up the issues. In setting out what is talked about, argumentation rules also set out how it is to be talked about, tracing both the limits of valid discourse and the limits of a valid modus operandi for a discourse. Argumentation strategies unfold around the issues set up by stasis rules: they both develop and supplement them with new ones. Arguing for or against an issue at stake does not challenge the rules of persuasion that validate the discourse, but rather reproduces them.

The consequences of the above arguments are that (1) rhetoric becomes a form of social action, (2) the idea of performance is seen as central to understanding this kind of action, and (3) language is an indispensable tool with the help of which social actors perform actions. This means that conveying information can never be separated from rhetoric and the means of expression by which this is achieved, and there is no way of showing (or deciding) that these very means of expression do not have a hand in producing information and/or intention. This is also valid for texts with an apparent lack of rhetoric (or minimal rhetoric), such as scientific ones. When rhetoric is understood to be means and techniques of expression, as the performance of linguistic (textual) expression, there is hardly a text that does not perform. The performative character of a text goes well beyond conventions and rules related to a specific (literary or non-literary) genre (Bakhtin 1986; Berkenkotter and Huckin 1995, p. 3; Swales 1990, p. 46). And if what is written and how it is written cannot be completely separated, texts are not simple informational warehouses. Rather, they are signifying, knowledge-producing practices[9] (Derrida 1972b, p. 124).

---

[9] Derrida (1972b, p. 363) repeatedly refers to texts as spectacles or as scenes that perform themselves, thus stressing their character as social practices. A related approach is the Actor-Network Theory developed by Michel Callon (1986, 1991), Bruno Latour (1988), and John Law (1986).

In this perspective, a (scientific) text can no longer be conceived as an inert object, a transparent medium that conveys knowledge about reality, or a simple rearrangement of the authors' claims according to the conventions of a literary genre. It appears rather as a social practice, and it not only traces the limits of possibility for speaking[10] but also provides the tools for doing so – the modalities and techniques of expression that allow one to speak about the world.

Another consequence is that rhetoric does not appear peripheral with respect to knowledge, or as impeding on it, but rather as a condition and a set of tools for producing knowledge. The rhetoric of a (scientific) text is not simply a device for convincing an incredulous audience, something added to the content or the message to be conveyed, or a simple rearrangement of facts so as to sound more convincing. It is both the space in which such facts have to be meaningfully performed (i.e., constituted) and the tools for performing them.

Overview of the Book

In a certain sense, the perspective adopted here is an historical one: the medical knowledge of AIDS is examined in its historical unfolding, and references are made to the background of historical knowledge against which the medical explanations of AIDS changed. However, this study does not set out to write another history of the medical advances in the field of AIDS, to be added to those already in existence. Therefore, it has to operate on two levels: one is that of what is medically asserted about the Acquired Immunodeficiency Syndrome – its causes, means of transmission, risk factors, and risk populations; the other is the level of how this is done – how these complex medical assertions are performed and how they come to express what they express.

Recovering the rhetorical practices that produce medical knowledge from the manifold theses, explanatory models, representations, and narratives implies looking not only at what is being said and written but also at how it is being said. This is the second level on which the

---

[10] This is the sense Foucault gives to his notion of discourse and discursive practices, characterized as the definition of a legitimate perspective for the subject of knowledge and the fixing of norms for building up concepts and theories (Foucault 1989, pp. 9–10).

study operates: I examine the movements of a large variety of medical representations and narratives and the specific practices through which they are constituted with respect to risk. The reader is thus provided with a double perspective: that of a network of models, representations, and narratives, on the one hand; on the other hand, the level of rhetorical practices producing them. Because the two are collocated, the study does not contain distinct chapters for each level but intends to recover the second from the first; however, shifts between these two levels are marked by different analytical techniques.

I examine here medical journal articles on the Acquired Immunodeficiency Syndrome from mid-1981 to 1989. Since the first report on "Pneumocystis pneumonia – Los Angeles" in the June 5, 1981 issue of the *Morbidity and Mortality Weekly Report* (a date which has now gone down in history), a vast amount of medical literature has been published on the topic. The number of papers on AIDS in medical journals alone increased ninefold between 1983 and 1988. A considerable share of them have been published in a relatively small number of select medical journals, considered to publish at the cutting edge of medical research. Thus, in 1983, 29% of the medical papers on AIDS worldwide were published by five journals, considered by media analysts and practitioners to be the most prestigious and influential in the field of medicine. At the end of the 1980s, this share came to represent about 10%, which, on a world scale, is nevertheless considerable. In analyzing these articles, I also take into account medical papers published by other journals ("pediatric AIDS" was a topic largely debated in pediatric journals at the end of the 1980s, for instance). In the first half of the same decade, pediatric AIDS papers were written mostly by the same researchers who regularly published in the most prestigious journals, so the body of expert knowledge has, for this period and in this regard, a relatively high degree of homogeneity.

There are now several international journals devoted exclusively to AIDS. The international journal database for medical literature, MedLine,[11] shows for the keyword "Acquired Immunodeficiency

---

[11] Unfortunately, MedLine provides no information about the articles published in 1981 and 1982, but judging by the general trend, it is to be assumed that the share of the five journals was even larger then. During my documentation, I could not find any medical

TABLE I. *Share of Five Leading Scientific Journals Among the Articles on the Acquired Immunodeficiency Syndrome Published Worldwide Between 1983 and 1989 (as Registered by MedLine)*

	1983	1984	1985	1986	1987	1988	1989
Medical articles on the Acquired Immunodeficiency Syndrome published worldwide	655	1139	1686	2563	3704	5794	5354
Share of the five journals	191 29.1%	256 22.4%	363 21.5%	412 16%	512 13.8%	558 9.6%	461 8.6%

Note: The five journals are: *The Lancet, New England Journal of Medicine, Journal of the American Medical Association, the Annals of Internal Medicine,* and *Science.*

Syndrome" that the number of medical articles published on this topic grew from 655 in 1983 to 5,354 in 1989 (the timespan of this study extends from 1981 to 1989). Until 1986, five journals had a considerable share of the total number of published articles (see Table 1). Although this share has diminished over the years (the number of articles published by them grew at a slower rate than the total number worldwide), it is to be assumed that these articles have essentially shaped the medical discourse about AIDS and risk, even if only because in the first years they represented almost one-third of the medical articles on AIDS published worldwide.

Because this is a qualitative study done from a historical perspective, not all medical papers published on AIDS between 1981 and now have been taken into account. To have a data set that is as homogeneous as possible, two criteria of selection have been chosen. The first was to select those medical journals which have published articles on AIDS from the beginning – that is, from mid-1981, when the appearance of a new and problematic disease was signaled in medical papers – and which have continued to publish on the topic until now. The second

papers published in other journals with international circulation in the second half of 1981. Notable exceptions were the reports published by *Morbidity and Mortality Weekly Report.*

criterion was the scientific prestige of the journals – their circulation figures and international repute. Although there are a great number of medical journals, few of them have a large international circulation and corresponding prestige, and the most prestigious are published in English. Some have published papers on AIDS from its beginnings and have constantly attracted an international authorship. Papers on AIDS from authors based in widely different countries have been published here. Interestingly enough, Luc Montagnier and his French team chose to publish their paper on the infectious agent of AIDS (then named lymphadenopathy-associated virus) in *Science* (May 20, 1983, 220, pp. 868–71), a U.S.-based journal, and not in a French one. The articles examined here come from *The Lancet*, the *Journal of the American Medical Association*, the *New England Journal of Medicine*, *Science*, the *Annals of Internal Medicine*, the *American Journal of Epidemiology*, and the *American Journal of Diseases in Children*, along with the weekly bulletin of the Centers for Disease Control and Prevention in Atlanta, Georgia *Morbidity and Mortality Weekly Report*.

I also examine letters, editorial pieces, and comments published in *Nature*, another highly prestigious journal. *Nature*, however, did not publish clinical or epidemiological articles on AIDS in the early 1980s (it published articles on the genetic structure of HIV after 1983). Compared with *Science, Nature* published more features, but less scientific articles between 1983 and 1989. During this period, *Science* published a total of 335 features and *Nature* a total of 420 features. The percentage of scientific articles published by *Science* was 37.6% of this total; the share of scientific articles among *Nature's* features was 10.71%. In 1983, for example, *Nature* did not publish any scientific article about AIDS, while *Science* published 6. During 1984, 25 scientific articles were published in *Science*, while *Nature* published only 5. *Science* reached a peak in 1986 with 27 articles (*Nature*: 3 articles). *Nature* had its peak in 1988 with 13 articles (*Science*: 23 articles). The articles published by *Science* included clinical and epidemiological analyses, while *Nature* focused on virology, molecular genetics, and the biochemistry of HIV. Due to these facts, I did not include *Nature* in Table 1.

Popular science accounts, as well as articles written by science journalists for newspapers and weekly magazines have not been taken into consideration, because they pose special problems with regard to the analysis (for such an analysis, see Sturken 1997, p. 220; Albert

1986; Lupton 1993; Lupton, McCarthy, and Chapman 1995; Tulloch and Chapman 1992; Baker 1986; Champagne 1991; Grover 1992; Herzlich and Pierret 1989; Jones 1992; Nelkin 1991; Sherry 1993). Interviews and media features on AIDS have also been left aside; they too require a separate analysis (see, as an example, Dobrovolskij 1997). In their analysis of how medical expertise on AIDS is represented in the media ("model of the thought-collective of the AIDS-world"), Horton and Aggleton (1989, p. 74) situate journal science (on AIDS) at the center of a radius whose circles are (in this order): handbook science; medical tabloids; textbook science; popular science journals; newspapers/magazines/television; talk social/gatherings/jokes. They assert that the center of medical knowledge production is located in the medical journals, each further step implying a series of transformations of the content and expression of knowledge. This would mean that medical knowledge as it is found in handbooks or in popular science journals has a different character from that of "journal science;" they are related yet different discourses.

As shown by Kinsella (1989, pp. 87, 259), the practices of science journalism and of writing popular science features rely heavily on constantly monitoring what professional science journals publish; most of these features are written by either compiling professional articles or interviewing their authors, thus reworking the topics of the articles. Since the 1970s, these journals – perceived as the most prestigious in the biomedical field (they also have the largest circulations) – have moreover secured a kind of monopoly: they are the exclusive sources from which news agencies can buy biomedical news. They reject submitted manuscripts that have already been thematized as news, thus deterring attempts to circumvent them. Clinicians' accounts, as well as publishing practices, ascribe a major role to both these journals and the articles they publish on AIDS topics. Historically, they were the first to publish articles on the immune deficiency syndrome in autumn 1981,[12] and although the number of AIDS-related articles has grown exponentially ever since, these journals have maintained a prominent

[12] The first reports on "unexplainable" cases of *Pneumocystis carinii* pneumonia and Kaposi's sarcoma were published in May 1981 by *Morbidity and Mortality Weekly Report*, followed by articles in the *New England Journal of Medicine* and *The Lancet* in August and September 1981.

place. From this perspective, it can be argued that the articles they published, along with the stands taken by the American Academy of Sciences (which are mostly written by the same authors), the CDC bulletins, and conference papers, form a relevant data set for examining the textual production of medical knowledge on AIDS and risk.

Clinicians' recollections about the beginnings of AIDS have not been taken into account, because recollections about the past tend to reprocess events somewhat, selecting and reinterpreting them. Interviews with clinicians from one of Germany's largest AIDS research clinics about their perception of medical journals' prestige and influence revealed that they considered some of the journals used in this study the most prestigious in their field (clinical medicine) and as most important for their work. Although they said they did not intend to submit papers for publication in these top international journals, they constantly read them because the most important clinical descriptions of AIDS were published there. They perceived papers published by these journals as being addressed to a readership like themselves (i.e., working in large therapy and research units, with a central position in the field); they described clinical journals of national or regional circulation as mainly addressing a readership of individual medical practices or smaller research units. Although it was clear that clinicians related the importance of international journals to the perceived prestige of their unit, it was also clear that they constantly monitor them. As one of them put it, these journals were the only places to find clinical studies of AIDS in children and women. That clinicians ascribe great importance to these journals is to be seen not as a new phenomenon, but rather as an index of the central position they have held in the field of medical knowledge on AIDS over the years.

Chapter 1 focuses on the rhetorical devices by which different classifications of the same diseases produced a new, unusual, and mysterious syndrome. Chapter 2 examines the paradoxical economy of risk categories and formulates answers to the question of why women and infants were not deemed risk categories, whereas "Haitians" were, somewhat incomprehensibly, maintained as a risk category for a long time. It shows how risk reemerged from this process as a very concrete entity and how the Acquired Immunodeficiency Syndrome's seemingly unambiguous, universal signification breaks down into a variety of particular, context-bound meanings, depending on what is seen as "risk."

Chapter 3 examines the role played by "risk" in the various representations of the causal agent and shows how etiological models were shaped by discourses on risky human agency. Chapter 4 examines how the thesis of a sole human retrovirus was constructed and imposed by arranging and rearranging "risks"; it also looks more closely at the role played by risk in the articles published by Drs. Gallo and Montagnier and shows how risk-related rhetorical strategies were used by both parties in their debates. Chapter 5 looks at how means of transmission and epidemiological models accounting for the origins of the virus were rhetorically determined. "AIDS risk" as a set of computable probabilities, a currently common view among epidemiologists (and social scientists), is the focus of Chapter 6. The question here is not to see whether there is some better statistical procedure of computing risk, but to examine what conditions make such computations possible. I show the rhetorical transformations by which heterogeneous qualities become quantities, which in turn reinforce and reproduce distinct qualities of risk. Chapter 6 also provides the reader with a short translation study, which shows the successive transformations from journal article to journal article by which a precise quantity of risk came to be produced from qualities and was then asserted, legitimized, and passed over as taken for granted.

Finally, Chapter 7 reviews the arguments about the relationship between rhetorical practices and scientific knowledge. I argue that rhetorical practices have concrete, important consequences for how research, prevention policies, diagnosis, and treatment are conceived. I also examine the question of the "expert democracy," i.e., of the conditions under which a genuine dialogue between expert knowledge and concerned social groups can take place in the public sphere.

Since the end of the 1980s, one trend in social studies of science has been reflexivism (Woolgar 1988; Knorr-Cetina 1999): because sociological texts are themselves a social enterprise, the ways they are produced do not radically differ from those in which knowledge is produced in other scientific disciplines. Hence, reflection is necessary to bring one's own production devices to the surface.

One of the possible dangers of the present book is ontological gerrymandering: that is, claiming that rhetorical practices produce knowledge and at the same time acting as if this book were devoid of any rhetorical turns and devices that might affect, soil, or unnecessarily

adorn the message it conveys to the reader. The reader has undoubt-
edly seen by now that even this introduction has used a considerable
number of such strategies, and she probably thinks that this is not all.
It is not my aim to proceed in a reflexive manner here, by unveiling my
own rhetoric in the very process of analyzing that of the medical AIDS
discourses. Rather, I bracket out reflection on my own strategies. But
let the reader be warned that such strategies are used here.

I

Making Up the Rules of Seeing

Opportunistic Infections and the New Syndrome

The Rhetoric of a New Syndrome

From a medical viewpoint, AIDS (Acquired Immunodeficiency Syndrome) is described as a syndrome manifested by a state of immunosuppression, due to the infection with varieties of the human immunodeficiency virus[1] (Stine 1993, p. 35). This means that there is no single disease involved, but that the state of immune deficiency allows various infectious agents to enter the body; subsequently, infections and various diseases develop. The immune deficiency also allows for organisms already present in the body that might otherwise remain harmless to get out of control and proliferate. In this sense, rather than being regarded as a single homogeneous disease, AIDS is seen as a condition of the human body in which the immune system can control neither the organisms already present in the body nor the ones that enter it. The agent that induces this condition of the immune system is now medically described as a human retrovirus (with several varieties) that, once in the body, binds itself to the surface of certain cells of the immune system (CD4+ cells), inhabits them for a while, and then begins to reproduce itself there, using the genetic material of the cells. The reproduction process consumes the cells and weakens the immune system to the point where it collapses.

[1] The official definitions of the syndrome (formulated by the Centers for Disease Control and Prevention and by the World Health Organization) have been revised several times and are periodically updated.

The first infections historically documented in relationship to this condition of the immune system (and hence to HIV) were *Pneumocystis carinii* pneumonia (PCP) and Kaposi's sarcoma (KS).[2] They were documented by reports published in June and July 1981, respectively, in *Morbidity and Mortality Weekly Report* (*MMWR*), which is the weekly bulletin of the Centers for Disease Control and Prevention in Atlanta, Georgia.[3] *Pneumocystis carinii* pneumonia is medically characterized as a form of pneumonia due to a microorganism present in the lungs. It was signaled and described before World War II and has remained in the catalogued repertoire of lung diseases ever since. Kaposi's sarcoma is characterized as a form of skin cancer, predominantly affecting the limbs. It was described by a Viennese physician in the 1870s and bears his name; it is now part of the standard repertoire of diseases studied by dermatologists. Both had thus been known for a long time in the international medical community.

Historical reconstructions of AIDS usually begin by stating that in mid-1981 the Centers for Disease Control and Prevention in Atlanta signaled inexplicable cases of a rare form of pneumonia (*Pneumocystis* pneumonia) and of a rare skin cancer (Kaposi's sarcoma) in their weekly bulletin *Morbidity and Mortality Weekly Report*; the cases were clustered in Los Angeles and New York.[4] These unexplainable phenomena, which were signaled with increasing intensity, led to the discovery and description of an underlying immune deficiency, which was named the Acquired Immunodeficiency Syndrome at the beginning of 1982. From this point onward, the story is well known.

---

[2] Medical reconstructions published after 1981 have claimed to describe the Acquired Immunodeficiency Syndrome in clinical cases seen before 1981 and tried to push back the first cases of AIDS as far as the 1950s. Initially, these reconstructions relied on reinterpreting clinical descriptions from hospital files. After 1983, when the human immunodeficiency virus was identified and described (as HTLV-III and/or LAV), reconstructions relied on analyzing serum and tissue samples, stored in a frozen state, from various parts of the world. The beginning is considered here to be the time of the first reports of infections and diseases explicitly related to an immune deficiency and considered as new and unexplainable – i.e., June 1981.

[3] "*Pneumocystis* Pneumonia – Los Angeles." *MMWR*, June 5, 1981, 30/21, pp. 250–1; "Kaposi's sarcoma and *Pneumocystis* Pneumonia Among Homosexual Men – New York City and California." *MMWR*, July 3, 1981, 30/25, pp. 305–7.

[4] The reconstruction of the "mysterious beginnings" in a historical flashback has also become a common rhetorical figure in cultural studies on AIDS (see, for example, Treichler 1988a, p. 197) as well as in journalistic accounts (Shilts 1987).

Scientific discoveries such as the discovery of a new disease exert a fascination not only on the scientific community and the lay public, but also on social scientists. For the first, discovery is the main drive and the ultimate goal. For the lay public, it is often accompanied by the promise of curing illnesses and improving people's lives. For social scientists, scientific discoveries are the domain where the role, influence, and limitations of social factors – such as interests, resources, and relationships – can be perhaps best examined.

That such factors play a role in discovery making has not been contested; the question is whether scientific discoveries are evaluated, acknowledged, and accepted by the scientific community according to universal standards of rationality or according to the resources, influence, and social relationships of the scientists themselves. The positivist tradition has solved this problem by distinguishing between the context of discovery and the context of justification. Whereas the former is messy (involving serendipity, accident, resources, interests, and the like), the latter is determined by rigorous criteria of universal applicability.

This distinction has been contested by sociologists and historians of science alike who argue that, in practice, the two contexts are indistinguishable: justification takes place in the process of discovery itself (e.g., Nickles 1992, p. 89; Hacking 1996, p. 51). Consequently, justification is not exclusively determined by logical criteria; factors such as interests, resources, and networks of relationships play a considerable role (Stump 1996, p. 445). We may construct an abstract, normative model of justification, entirely grounded in criteria of rationality, but the practice of scientific justification does not fit this model. The conceptual argument against the normative model is that empirical data are not sufficient by themselves for deciding to reject (that is, to justify) the discovery claim (e.g., Bourdieu 2001, p. 45; Nickles 1992, p. 105; Lynch 1992, p. 255n40). This is shown by numerous empirical studies of scientific discoveries (e.g., Pickering 1995; Latour 1988): social factors can never be eliminated from the context of justification.

Are then rhetorical practices among these factors? There are two lines of argument here, one coming from the philosophy of science; the other one, from the sociology of science. According to the first, writing scientific papers is an intrinsic part of the research process. Therefore, the persuasion devices and argumentative strategies used in scientific articles are part and parcel of the scientific discovery process. If the context of discovery cannot be separated from the context of justification, it follows that rhetoric does play a part in the justification of scientific discoveries (Nickles 1992, pp. 93, 96). Claims of discovery have to be presented to the scientific community and made plausible. This presentation (usually in scientific articles) belongs to the process of justification and is grounded in rhetoric: we can hardly imagine a presentation aimed at convincing the scientific community that does not employ any persuasion devices (Gieryn 1999, p. 188).

The second line of argumentation is that the fate of scientific discoveries – including their status as discoveries – is decided by the ability of scientists to mobilize heterogeneous resources to support their claims. These resources include not only social relationships but also laboratory instruments, experimental probes, and scientific articles (e.g., Latour 1999, pp. 99, 102). Scientists mobilize rhetorical resources, among others, in announcing their discoveries. These resources are especially important: journal articles, for example, circulate more quickly than laboratory probes and reach a larger audience. These articles diffuse discovery claims throughout the community and help build support for them. In other words, resources such as these standardize truth and discovery claims and make them portable – that is, transferable across various contexts (Nickles 1995, p. 160). Other scientists begin to see the same things in the same way: they acknowledge not only one's own results, but also the accompanying argumentation strategies. Rhetorical practices are thus an intrinsic part of scientific discoveries (see, e.g., Atkinson, Batchelor, and Parsons 1997, p. 121).

With respect to the case examined here, I look first at the rhetorical practices of discovering a new immune deficiency. The first questions that arise are: what was so unexplainable about a skin cancer form known since the 1870s? How did a known form of pneumonia come to be a mystery? Let us consider how the said forms of pneumonia (*Pneumocystis carinii*) and skin cancer (Kaposi's sarcoma) were signaled, presented, and discussed from mid-1981 up to the end of 1982. Historians of medicine regard these articles as being decisive for the biomedical community (Grmek 1990; Oppenheimer 1988, 1992), because (1) they pointed out the singularity of these forms of infection and cancer, thus indicating that they were the manifestation of a new disease; (2) they brought together two apparently disparate infections, stating that both *Pneumocystis* pneumonia and Kaposi's sarcoma (i.e., a form of pneumonia and a skin cancer) had a common cause; (3) they assessed the risk related to this new disease; and (4) they formulated the hypothesis of an immune deficiency as the underlying cause of the opportunistic infections.

The Cognitive Rules of the Unseen: The Unusual Opportunistic Infections

For comparison, here is how a case of *Pneumocystis carinii* pneumonia was described in a clinical report in April 1981, two months before the first new and unusual cases were signaled; the case was a patient with Cushing's syndrome, and it was reported because the association between this form of pneumonia and the syndrome had not been previously seen. The introduction of the report presents the disease as follows:

Pneumocystis carinii pneumonia as a complication of steroid therapy in immunocompromised patients has been well documented. However, pneumonia in the presence of endogenous hypercorticolism from Cushing's syndrome has not been previously reported. We report here a patient with Cushing's syndrome from bilateral adrenal hyperplasia in whom pneumocystis pneumonia developed. (*AIM*, April 1981, 94/4-1, p. 488)

First, the definition of *Pneumocystis* pneumonia determines its meaning: this pneumonia form is a well documented complication of steroid therapy in immunocompromised patients. The introduction has already framed the field in which the meaning of pneumonia and the knowledge claims of the paper can take shape. The claim is not to present something new or unseen, but to provide new documentation about a disease that is well known. The following paragraphs describe the clinical and laboratory findings and assert *Pneumocystis* pneumonia as the cause of the patient's death. The discussion section concludes that "*Pneumocystis carinii* pneumonia, probably as a complication of the endogenous hypercorticolism in Cushing's syndrome, is an infection such patients may develop" (*AIM*, April 1981, 94/4-1, p. 489). This frames the claims of the paper as conservative: by using hedging expressions such as "probably" and "may" after the accurate quantitative description of lab and clinical findings, the paper seeks to convey an image of "scientific reserve"; in fact, however, the conclusion creates the opposite effect – that of strongly reasserting what the introduction has stated. Apart from specific rhetorical figures, the overall textual strategy is to be low-key about something presented as unproblematic and part of established knowledge.

Another report on therapy for PCP in children, published a year earlier, presented a more differentiated picture:

Pneumocystis carinii, a ubiquitous protozoan organism that may reside symbiotically in the respiratory system of man and animals, develops pathogenic potential in immunosuppressed patients. This group includes patients with cancer undergoing chemotherapy or radiation therapy and patients receiving immunosuppressives for a variety of disease states. In addition, several malnourished or congenitally immunodeficient patients may have a rapidly progressive and often fatal interstitial pneumonitis owing to this protozoan. Only rarely is PCP found in normal, healthy individuals. (*AJDC*, January 1980, 134/1, p. 35)

The disease is defined here not on the level of studies and reports documenting it, but on that of the infectious agent, which is "ubiquitous" and "resides symbiotically" in humans and animals. PCP gets its meaning from categories such as "patients with cancer undergoing immunotherapy," "patients receiving immunosuppressives," "severely malnourished," "congenitally immunodeficient," as well as from the "normal healthy individuals," which undermines any attempt at clear-cut categories.

By contrast, the first reports on the AIDS-related *Pneumocystis* pneumonia present us with a much more complicated and contradictory picture: what was hitherto reported as "ubiquitous infection" (*NEJM*, December 10, 1981, 305/24, p. 1431), as frequent among people suffering from malnutrition, and as "frequently seen in patients having undergone immunosuppressive therapy," is now "highly unusual" and "uncommon." In opening its editorial note (which came immediately after the case descriptions), the first report from *Morbidity and Mortality Weekly Report* stated that:

Pneumocystis pneumonia in the United States is almost exclusively limited to severely immunosuppressed patients. The occurrence of pneumocystosis in these previously healthy individuals without a clinically apparent underlying immunodeficiency is unusual. (*MMWR*, June 5, 1981, 30/21, p. 251)

Apparently, a definition not unlike the preceding ones is used this time to make completely dissimilar claims and to frame PCP differently. A second look reveals significant divergences, however. The report on the Cushing syndrome–related pneumonia framed its claims by stating that pneumonia as a complication of immunosuppression is well known. This report establishes a frame for *Pneumocystis* pneumonia, which the reported cases do not fit. (Remember that the case of Cushing's syndrome also did not fit the "seen," but it was treated differently.) Because they do not fit the frame, cases are predicated as "unusual." They are an impossible possibility. This is achieved by a classification that provides the meaning of *Pneumocystis* pneumonia and its conditions of possibility: its relevant categories are those of "severely immunosuppressed patients" and "previously healthy individuals." The catachresis of "almost exclusively limited" gives PCP a paradoxical meaning: if it is exclusively limited, it is "seen," "well known," etc. But it is only "almost," which negates this very status. In this frame, infection and patients are incompatible with each other; this incompatibility makes the phenomenon "unusual." Similar strategies were used by other clinical articles too; thus, one article used the category of "normal adult" as incompatible with that of "immunocompromised host" to build a classification of PCP from which unusualness is derived (*JAMA*, April 2, 1982, 247/13, pp. 1860–1).[5] Other studies first acknowledged PCP as a relatively common disease and then classified it as common or uncommon according to population categories. A clinical report opened by stating the usualness of PCP; immediately thereafter, it characterized it as unusual, thus providing an even stronger frame for making this form of pneumonia epistemically problematic:

Pneumocystis carinii is an ubiquitous organism that infects human beings by a respiratory route. The organism appears to be relatively avirulent, since it rarely if ever causes disease in immunologically competent persons. In North America, almost all cases have occurred in patients who have had diagnoses of primary congenital immunodeficiencies or who have received immunosuppressive chemotherapy for malignant neoplastic disease or organ transplantation. Despite the rarity of *P. carinii* pneumonia in previously healthy persons, we

---

[5] See also *The Lancet*, December 12, 1981, II/8259, p. 1339, where a letter to the editor about PCP opens with the short statement that "*Pneumocystis* pneumonia almost invariably affects the immunosuppressed."

recently recognized 11 cases of this disease in young men with no previous history to suggest immunologic dysfunction. All 11 men were drug abusers or homosexuals or both. (*NEJM*, December 10, 1981, 305/24, p. 1431)

The opening assertion characterizes PCP as a respiratory disease caused by a "ubiquitous organism," which is avirulent (if it is so ubiquitous, one would assume that it is avirulent; but it is only "relatively avirulent"). The necessary condition of this predicament is the category of "immunologically competent persons." The next sentence provides the categories relevant for PCP as disease: people with congenital immunodeficiencies and recipients of chemotherapy or organ transplants. Here, PCP appears as usual; the unusualness comes from giving the disease a new meaning, incompatible to these categories, and from redefining a category according to this incompatible meaning. The rarity of PCP in healthy persons is contrasted with the eleven recognized cases, reclassified as "drug abusers," "homosexuals," and "both." The incompatibility that generates unusualness was clearly expressed by another report. After characterizing the "outbreak of *P. carinii* pneumonia" as "highly unusual," it provided the disease with a classification that made it unusual:

Although *P. carinii* causes several hundred cases of severe pneumonia in the United States annually, these cases were previously found almost exclusively in patients whose immunity was severely compromised by underlying disease, immunosuppressive therapy, or both. (*NEJM*, January 28, 1982, 306/4, p. 250)

Classifications of PCP constantly appeared in the first medical articles in this area; the theme was developed in an almost symphonic manner, to allow for the construction of "risk groups" and of an explanatory model:

P. carinii pneumonia is usually a disease of persons with previously recognized immunosuppressive disorders. In adults, pneumocystis is usually associated with hematologic neoplasia or organ transplantation, although the widespread use of immunosuppressive therapy (especially corticosteroids) has facilitated its occurrence in patients with a wide range of malignant neoplastic and inflammatory diseases. In children, pneumocystosis has also been associated with primary congenital immunodeficiency syndromes and protein-calorie malnutrition. (*NEJM*, December 10, 1981, 305/24, p. 1436)

The article continues with a description of PCP among infants and small children from Eastern Europe, as well as among adult Asian refugees. The theme appears again toward the end of the section:

Serologic data and limited autopsy studies suggested that pneumocystis is an ubiquitous organism to which many people are exposed in early life. Studies in animals have demonstrated that murine transmission can occur through a respiratory route. Nursery epidemics in economically disadvantaged regions and clusters of cases of *Pneumocystis* pneumonia among oncology patients at three separate hospitals have suggested that person-to-person spread does occur, probably by a respiratory route, and that normal, healthy persons can serve as vectors. (*NEJM*, December 10, 1981, 305/24, p. 1437)

The appearance of *Pneumocystis* pneumonia in persons from New York and Los Angeles (the five originating Los Angeles cases are discussed after "Asian refugees") is treated in a classificatory system, which makes it possible to speak about this form of pneumonia. PCP is something seen in certain social categories; the meaning of what is seen depends on each category. In an apparently paradoxical way, an immunodeficiency-related, unusual PCP is made possible by the incompatibility of these categories. Remember that immune deficiency was also presented as underlying the usual PCP. After discussing various forms of cellular immunity, the article stated that the eleven cases had "profound defects in the cell-mediated immune response," and "perhaps, given sufficient time, all [the patients] would have had a recognizable disease that caused their immunosuppression" (*NEJM*, December 10, 1981, 305/24, p. 1437). The explanatory model of an immunosuppression underlying the unusual PCP does not emerge from a simple analogy with the usual PCP (such an analogy might read as follows: because until now all usual cases of PCP were associated with immunosuppression, the unusual and new ones must be associated with that too). The incompatibilities asserted here are hardly reconcilable with an analogical explanation.

Instead, the explanation is made possible by building up incompatible categories. The unusualness and newness of PCP does not exclude explanatory models (though one cannot easily explain new and unusual phenomena); rather, it makes them possible. This is the frame into which "risk" makes its way, reinforcing the classification

provided and functioning as a name-giving device for the categories
newly introduced. It makes sense to write of risk for patients from Los
Angeles and New York only in this system, which puts them into several categories: "young men with no history to suggest immunologic
dysfunction," "drug abusers, homosexuals, or both," – at any rate,
people totally different from patients who have undergone immunosuppressive therapy, or undernourished people, or Asian refugees. At
the same time, "risk" appears here as a device for epistemic insight
and reconfiguration. The explicit argument for the "risk groups" is
formulated in closing the "discussion" section:

Since homosexuals are suddenly contracting a variety of opportunistic fun-
gal, viral and mycobacterial infections, it seems unlikely that this outbreak
has been due exclusively to a new virulent or resistant strain of pneumocystis.
This outbreak was more probably related to the immunologic consequences
of some unknown process. The high mortality rate also seems more likely
to have been due to the immunologic lesion than to virulence or resistance
of the specific organism or to peculiarities of clinical management. This outbreak of community-acquired P. carinii pneumonia among young male homosexuals and drug abusers raises questions about increased exposure to
pneumocystis as well as about the prevalence and origin of abnormal cellular responses in these populations. (NEJM, December 10, 1981, 305/24,
p. 1437)

Pneumocystis pneumonia is presented as (1) self-referential
("community-acquired") and thus not compatible with the given classification, (2) due to exposure to the same agent (old Pneumocystis
carinii), and (3) correlated with an immune deficiency. In turn, this
cannot be like the known, PCP-associated immune suppressions. This
is confusing, because the newly created categories are presented as resulting from the unusual PCP being and at the same time not being like
the usual PCP. The correlation between exposure to the Pneumocystis
agent and cellular immune problems emerges as a consequence of the
classificatory system, not as its criterion. "Risk" reinforces these categories and is justified by them. Moreover, it presupposes their continuous transformation: from "eleven patients" to healthy "young men,"
and then to "drug abusers or homosexuals or both," who are finally
inscribed in the order of disease.

The Unusual Kaposi's Sarcoma

Kaposi's sarcoma had also been well described and reported since the 1870s. In 1980, it was described in medical papers as having a "feasible and highly satisfactory" management (*Cancer*, 45/3, p. 427). Management of KS was characterized as "well reviewed." Kaposi's sarcoma was defined as follows:

(It) has been classified into three clinical forms: 1) a nodular, non-destructive type (the commonest); 2) a locally aggressive type; and 3) a generalized form. The first type represented 68% in one Ugandan study of 112 patients and is by far the most common in American studies. In our series of 14 patients, reported here after vinblastine therapy, 9 had this type, 2 had the locally aggressive and 2 had a generalized form. In our overall series of 37 patients, the overwhelming majority also had the nodular, non-destructive type of disease. (*Cancer*, 45/3, p. 429)

The classification providing the meaning for KS in turn depends on regional and national studies: they show concretely what "commonest" means and establish a remainder that is uncommon. The generalized form of KS is presented as neither problematic nor unusual, but rather as what remains after the first categories have been subtracted.

Another medical paper dating from the same year characterized KS as "extremely common in equatorial Africa among all ages, but in America it usually affects men primarily of Jewish and Italian descent over the age of 60 years" (*Cancer*, 1980, 45/4, p. 684). It stated that "an association between racial origin and Kaposi's sarcoma in North America has been shown. Of our 60 patients, 27 were of Jewish descent, 24 were of Italian origin, 2 were from other peri-Mediterranean regions, 2 were of Scandinavian descent, 2 were of Portuguese origin, and 2 were born in the United States but did not know their origins" (p. 685). This shows the impossibility of establishing a meaning for KS based on geographical or racial categories: these are sometimes shown as Jewish, sometimes as Italian, peri-Mediterranean (whatever this may mean), Scandinavian, or "unknown."

In the articles discussed here, KS was presented as usually or normally seen in totally heterogeneous population categories, such as "Ashkenazi Jews" (who come from Eastern Europe) or populations "from around the Mediterranean." A German medical treatise on AIDS-related diseases, published in 1991 and intended for practicing clinicians, presented Kaposi's sarcoma as "affecting in the first place older men from Southeastern Europe. It affects especially men from the Danube Delta or Italy."[6]

The "problematic" cases of Kaposi's sarcoma were presented in a rhetorical key, very similar to that of PCP: it was stated that Kaposi's sarcoma is "unusual," "rare," and "uncommon" and that it had been frequently seen in older men and in males from the Mediterranean area. The distinction between common and uncommon operated here on the grounds of contrasting something that had been seen in the past with the same thing as seen in the present, and of introducing a classification (based on the diagnosis of KS) between older men/males from around the Mediterranean and New York men:

> Kaposi's sarcoma is rare in the United States, where the annual incidence is 0.021–0.061 per 100 000 population. In North America and Europe, this disease commonly presents as tumors of the lower extremities, and the clinical picture is that of a localized disease with an indolent cure. Most patients are in their seventh decade. This form of the disease is commonest among Ashkenazi Jews and those of Mediterranean origin, and especially in men. The incidence of Kaposi's sarcoma in African Blacks residing in an endemic region is much higher than among Blacks and Caucasians in North America and Europe. (*The Lancet*, September 19, 1981, II/8247, p. 598)

This classification is decisive for the presentation of the clinical cases. The statement about the rarity of Kaposi's sarcoma in the general population is at the same time specified and negated by the statement that it actually occurs in categories such as older Ashkenazi Jews, older persons of Mediterranean origin (with men as a subcategory), and Africans. The opening (1) establishes a classification that provides KS with a meaning, (2) states the commonness of KS on the grounds of this classification, and (3) declares its rarity by putting the abstract population category side by side with the established ones. The study ends by "suggesting that the homosexual population may have an

---

[6] See Jäger, H. (ed.). 1991. *AIDS and HIV Infections. Diagnosis, Clinical Symptoms, and Treatment. A Handbook and Atlas for Clinics and Medical Practices* [*AIDS und HIV-Infektionen: Diagnostik, Klinik, Behandlung. Handbuch und Atlas für Klinik und Praxis*], Landberg: Ecomed, IV–1, p. 1.

increased risk of Kaposi's sarcoma" (*The Lancet*, September 19, 1981, II/8247, p. 600). The novelty and unusualness do not derive from the diagnosis itself (which is similar to that of the African variety of KS), but from the classification. When speaking of the "increased risk of Kaposi's sarcoma in homosexual men," this ambivalent formulation – which simultaneously suggests that the risk was already there and that it is new – gains its meaning and justification from the classification. New York–dwelling homosexual men are presented as a new category with respect to the old ones and therefore as being at an "increased risk"; at the same time, the figure of risk consolidates the classification and makes it appear valid:

The eight patients with Kaposi's sarcoma reported here have several distinctive unusual features. Their median age was 34 years at the time of diagnosis, instead of the seventh decade as in other series. The generalized distribution of their skin lesions, the presence of lesions on the head and neck, and the absence of predominantly lower extremity involvement is atypical of the form of Kaposi's sarcoma encountered in North America and Europe. [...] This rapid clinical course closely resembles that of the lymphadenopathic form of Kaposi's sarcoma seen in Africa. The etiology and pathogenesis of Kaposi's sarcoma is unknown. Several mechanisms have been proposed for the development of this tumor – the effects of an oncogenic virus, an immunosuppressed state resulting in impaired tumor surveillance, or a combination of both. Observations supporting immunosuppression as the underlying factor are the high incidence of Kaposi's sarcoma in renal transplant recipients and in patients receiving corticosteroids or cytotoxic drugs, and the anergy and depressed cellular immune function in patients with this tumor. Of interest is the observation that a considerable proportion of patients in whom Kaposi's sarcoma develops after organ transplantation have visceral involvement similar to that seen in our patients. [...] We do not know of reports of an increased risk of Kaposi's sarcoma in homosexuals. Furthermore, there have been no studies of immune function in this population. (*The Lancet*, September 19, 1981, II/8247, pp. 599–600)

KS in "homosexuals" is compared to both the African variety, which is "atypical for North America and Europe" and "unusual and distinctive," and to renal transplant recipients, in order to argue for an underlying immunosuppression. The meanings of Kaposi's sarcoma and the immune suppression depend on these categories. KS is presented as either usual or unusual, as a new skin cancer form arising from immune suppression, or a well-managed disease. Here again, in an apparently paradoxical way, unusualness makes possible the thesis of immunosuppression. "Increased risk of Kaposi's sarcoma in homosexuals" is asserted in an epistemic mode ("we do not know of reports"), in conjunction with "there have been no studies of immune function in this population." "Risk" is a device by which the paradoxical status of unusualness/usualness is maintained as such: new categories are similar and at the same time dissimilar to the old ones. Risk brings epistemic insight and legitimates the reconfiguration of the disease: KS and PCP are now to be found in the old categories, *but also* in new ones.

In both cases, classifications create an epistemic frame for speaking/writing of PCP and/or KS. They provide the possibility for formulating explanatory models about the role of the immunosuppression. Thus, a discursive mode that showed how to write about PCP and KS and that was by no means restricted to the articles analyzed here, was produced.[7] Without exception, the first reports and articles referred to the classification of Kaposi's sarcoma as providing the framework in which the thesis of underlying immunosuppression can be argued. Many of them used the strategy of opening the article with classifications, which were then repeated in the "discussion" or "comment" sections – where the immunosuppression thesis was asserted. Invariably, all of them used the word "unusual" to assert the immune deficiency thesis as the "unusual" usual. This mode was widely used in reporting other opportunistic and viral infections, as well as for asserting that an immune deficiency underlay them. Infections and diseases were introduced according to the scheme usual/unusual, seen/unseen, whereby their meaning was established according to risk categories.

The structure of the argument is: it was usual that we see a and b in x and y, but now we have an unusual situation, because we have seen a and b in z. This changes the meaning of a and b. Henceforth, it becomes usual that we see a and b in x, y, and z, but this remains unusual. (See also Figure 1.)

In clinical reports on other infections, the immunosuppression thesis was also supported by classification schemes. Thus, a report on herpes simplex lesions (bearing the title "Severe Acquired Immunodeficiency in Male Homosexuals, Manifested by Chronic Perianal Ulcerative Herpes Simplex Lesions") stated that:

---

[7] See also *JAMA*, March 26, 1982, 247/12, pp. 1739–41; *The Lancet*, July 17, 1982, II/8290, p. 125; *NEJM*, December 10, 1981, 305/24, p. 1466.

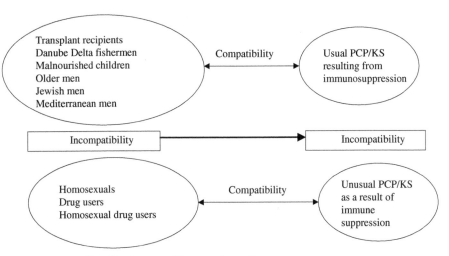

FIGURE 1. Classifications and "unusualness."

Chronic ulcerating lesions caused by herpes simplex viruses (HSV) are unusual even in patients with severe immunologic defects. These lesions occur in advanced lymphoproliferative disease, after immunosuppression for organ transplantation, during treatment with high doses of corticosteroids, and in certain primary immunodeficiency disorders. In four previously healthy homosexual men we found chronic perianal ulcers infected with HSV. (*NEJM*, December 10, 1981, 305/24, p. 1439)

The classification leads directly to the thesis of an underlying immune deficiency:

Ulcerative lesions caused by HSV are observed only in patients with severe deficient immunity associated with another underlying disease. That four patients [. . .] have been previously immunocompromised [. . .] suggests that some factor in all the patients was operative. The fact that they were homosexual men was striking. Reports of Kaposi's sarcoma and opportunistic infections similar to those that we observed [. . .] suggest that they are part of a nationwide epidemic of immune deficiency among male homosexuals. (*NEJM*, December 10, 1981, 305/24, p. 1441)

A double classification is used to make the immune deficiency both the underlying cause of herpes simplex lesions and a "nationwide epidemic." On the one hand, the reported cases are classified as not having immune defects, although an immune defect is asserted as the underlying cause. On the other hand, they are declared to belong to a

newly created category with respect to immune deficiency, which justifies speaking of a nationwide epidemic. Los Angeles cases of infection
with mycobacteria were later reported in a similar manner:

Although mycobacterial infection occurs more commonly in immunocompromised patients than in immunologically intact patients, it remains only an
occasional event even in these susceptible hosts. [...] *Mycobacterium avium
intracellulare* most commonly causes chronic, slowly progressive pulmonary
disease in middle-aged men and, heretofore, has rarely caused disseminated infection. Human pulmonary infections have been most commonly described in
the southeastern part of the United States. No accurate estimate of the prevalence of MAC infections is available, although skin test surveys suggest that
inapparent infection is common and varies geographically within the United
States. (*JAMA*, December 10, 1982, 248/22, p. 2982)

   Again, what infection with *Mycobacterium avium intracellulare* and
the underlying immune deficiency are is determined by the classificatory frame. In this perspective, the categories of "homosexual men" or
"drug abusers" are complex rhetorical constructions, which continually process four, five, or six "patients" to "otherwise healthy adults,"
"previously normal," "without a history of immunosuppression," and
then to "homosexual" and "drug abusers." With respect to the reported diseases, they are treated first as beyond the possible (they
cannot have these infections, cancer forms, and so forth) and afterward introduced to the classification as "striking" and "extraordinary"
(*JAMA*, December 10, 1982, 248/22, pp. 2980, 2982) – in short, as
the category from which all these opportunistic infections and diseases
receive their new meaning. A comment published in 1983 in the journal
Nature (302, p. 749) characterized the disease as "unusually uncommon" in groups such as IV drug users, their sexual partners, hemophiliacs, Haitians, and (of course) "male homosexuals." This litotes (unusually uncommon) is what makes the syndrome "disturbing...either
new or newly recognized"; the immune deficiency is new because it is
seen in these categories, and it is seen only here because it is new.

Classification as an Epistemic Practice

In view of all of the previous discussion, can we still say that risk categories appeared as determined by new and unusual diseases? Rather,
the opposite appears to be true. Classification operations produced "a

set of boxes…into which things can be put to do then some kind of work" (Bowker and Star 1999, p. 10). That is, they produced categories according to which a set of laboratory results, or a clinical diagnosis, could do different kinds of work. They could confirm a given knowledge frame, or (as in the cases discussed here) they could signal novelty and unusualness, redirecting the production of medical knowledge. These categories can be seen as sets of instructions (Berg 1997, p. 52) for reducing epistemic uncertainties: they provided medical practitioners with rules for seeing things. They established paths of action and traced the horizon of knowledge. As Émile Durkheim (1965 [1915], p. 172) put it, classificatory systems "have possibilities of extension which go far beyond the circle of objects which we know, either from direct experience or from resemblance." These possibilities, as I show in Chapter 2, played a key role with respect to how the medical knowledge of AIDS unfolded.

Murray and Payne (1989, pp. 26–8), among others, have argued that the AIDS risk groups have a tautological character, admitting only those cases that were selected on the grounds of a group definition. In this sense, it can be said that the meaning of *Pneumocystis* pneumonia, Kaposi's sarcoma, mycobacterium infections, and so forth, is redefined according to the new category, as the new and unseen pneumonia form, the unusual Kaposi's sarcoma, and the striking and extraordinary mycobacterium infection. Accordingly, the underlying immune deficiency receives the same meaning of new, unexplained, formerly unseen – as something very specific to the category to which it is ascribed. In this system, the meanings of opportunistic infections, of their underlying cause, and of the new categories are mutually reinforcing: the opportunistic infections are striking because the new categories are extraordinary, and the latter are extraordinary because the opportunistic infections are striking. Opportunistic infections and their underlying immune deficiency are new and old at the same time: this makes them recognizable and describable as what they are – Kaposi's sarcoma and *Pneumocystis* pneumonia.

But does such a classificatory system have real consequences? Does it leave its mark on the ways in which medical practitioners and patients (inter)act? According to Mary Douglas (1967, 1992a), "risk" must not necessarily be conceived primarily in terms of the probability calculus; rather, "AIDS risk" has to be understood as the result of a system

of classifications by which participants in a culture situate themselves
with respect to the representations of disease. At the same time, it is a
tool that enables actors to (re)produce and enforce their own identities
in this system. Douglas uses this notion of risk to develop her own
classificatory system, in which the ascription of social identities leads
to different notions of risk (1992a, p. 106). Her aim is to show the gap
that appears between the actors' classifications and the "natural fact"
of risk.

In his turn, Marcel Calvez (1990, pp. 43–58) has emphasized the
ways in which clinicians, paramedics, patients, and their social contacts (including relatives) use "AIDS risk" to generate classifications
reproducing (1) an order of disease that rigorously differentiates between "safe" and "dangerous" and (2) a social order of interactions
(closely related to (1)) between medical staff and patients, patients and
their social contacts, and medical staff and social contacts. In this way,
"risk" becomes an instrument for making sense of infections in an
orderly way and for identifying the actors' positions in this order, as
well as for creating and enforcing an interaction order closely related
to that of disease. In this perspective, it makes little sense to speak
of risk as a kind of probability calculus because it is used mainly as
a present-oriented, and not as a future-oriented, category. The actors
in the clinic make use of "risk" not to evaluate their future behaviors, and even less to compute probabilistic outcomes, but to construct
present-oriented classifications with respect to the disease – classifications in which they identify themselves as having varying degrees of
safety. The future is, thus, constructed through (re)producing classifications and categories of the present. Cultural differences in the ways
actors make sense of risk appear to be due no longer to the exoticism of
marginal or "tropical" cultures, but rather to the various ways in which
actors identify themselves and others when relating to this order of
disease.

Moreover, knowledge about AIDS risk used by actors to position
themselves with respect to disease representations is neither exclusively
derived from medical expert knowledge nor "natural." Rather, the actors in the clinic use medical knowledge to produce "risk" and then use
the latter as a tool for ordering and legitimizing their medical knowledge: they assemble the order of their social world using "risk" as a

cultural tool. Calvez stresses that the (re)production of medical knowledge generates a social order in the clinic, in the patients' family environment, and in relations with the outside world.

In the cases examined here, what "risk" designates is the paradoxical situation of using a classification to give meaning to diseases that cannot be represented without such a classificatory system. The meanings of the opportunistic infections crystallize in a system of categorial differences, where the categories are presented not only as mutually exclusive, but also as incompatible – as pertaining to different orders of possibility. "Risk" serves here as the rhetorical device that results from and at the same time allows for introducing a new order and contrasting it with the old one: the Kaposi's sarcoma of the "men from around the Mediterranean" (or that of "Africans") is incompatible with the KS of "homosexuals." Were it not for this system of differences, "risk" would lose its meaning. If, say, KS can be gotten by Jews, Italians, Scandinavians, Danube Delta fishermen, homosexuals, Africans, heterosexuals, women, and "others" alike, where's the risk? The social order of risk makes it possible to make the epistemic claims of the discourse more striking: the reported insights are about a new and extraordinary phenomenon. In this sense, "risk" is also a device by which knowledge claims are made relevant: insight into the new opportunistic diseases and underlying immune deficiency is new and important because the social categories of disease are new and striking. In turn, these new categories are made possible by the system of differences between old and new PCP and KS, respectively. Almost every report discussed here ends by referring to risk categories, to its own newness, and to the necessity of answering "tantalizing questions" and investigating further.[8] This shows that classification practices relying on social representations of risk operate not only on the fringes of medical knowledge, or exclusively among lay actors, but also at the very core of biomedical knowledge, enabling the management of problematic epistemic situations and the constitution of new knowledge domains.

---

[8] See *NEJM*, December 10, 1981, 305/24, pp. 1437, 1467 and January 28, 1982, 306/4, p. 252; *The Lancet*, September 19, 1981, II/8247, p. 600 and September 26, 1981, II/8248, p. 688; *MMWR*, June 4, 1982, 31/21, p. 278.

Classification and Scientific Discovery

What is the relevance of classification practices for the sociology of scientific discoveries? First, classification practices highlight scientific communication as an intrinsic part of the discovery process. Journal articles are not a neutral medium through which discoveries are made known to the scientific community. Scientific articles set out the cognitive framework in which something can be seen as a discovery; they establish rules for representing scientific objects as known or unknown, usual or unusual.

Second, articles play a role in rhetorical replication. As sociologists of science have pointed out, a key aspect for the success of scientific discoveries is the replication of experimental results in different laboratories (e.g., Gieryn 1999, p. 184; Collins 1992). Experimental replication serves as a powerful tool in the validation of scientific discoveries: it presupposes that other scientists obtain the same results when conducting the same procedure, under the same conditions, with the same instruments and tools, in a similar laboratory setting. When the results of experiments are reproduced in different laboratories by different scientists, the community becomes convinced about the procedural and substantial soundness of the discovery.

Although it is doubtlessly important, I argue that the replication of experimental results is not the only kind of replication involved in the justification of scientific discoveries. There is at least one other kind of replication that also plays a role, which I call rhetorical replication. The first reports about the opportunistic infections established a classification according to which PCP and KS could be seen as either usual or unusual. Accordingly, the underlying immune deficiency was presented as either known or a newly discovered one. The claim of having discovered something genuinely new depended on this frame. Replicating the claim of discovery implied replicating not only laboratory results, but also the classificatory frame in which these results indicated a new immune deficiency. Without this frame, one could not decide if laboratory results signaled a known or an unknown immune dysfunction.

Without exception, the classificatory system for PCP and KS was reproduced in subsequent scientific articles published by various authors in various journals. They replicated not only the laboratory results confirming opportunistic infections, but also the frame in which these infections were presented as signs of a scientific discovery.

The significance of this classificatory frame should not be underestimated. It was stated from the beginning that the opportunistic infections were accompanied by an immune deficiency. More generally, it was known that immune deficiencies cause opportunistic infections. Yet, the newly signaled deficiency was not presented against a classification of immune impairments (e.g., acquired vs. induced vs. congenital, viral vs. non-viral), but against one of social categories. This rhetorical move was fundamental to further developments. Without risk categories as a key initial element of the scientific discovery, we would have a different social and cultural history of AIDS, different prevention policies, and a different path to the discovery of HIV.

Experimental replication was, however, accompanied by rhetorical replication, which became an intrinsic part of the justification of discovery. Risk categories became a fixture of scientific articles about a new immune dysfunction. Very soon, new categories were added to the initial ones. As I show in Chapter 2, they grew and formed a system, which took on an existence of its own.

In a similar way, Severe Acute Respiratory Syndrome (SARS) was represented in the spring of 2003 in medical journals in a classificatory frame that allowed scientific claims that this was a newly discovered syndrome. SARS was signaled as a very severe, even lethal form of pneumonia in late February and early March 2003 in Hong Kong and Guangzhou. Afterward, cases from other Asian countries, North America, and Europe were signaled, too. But was it just an old form of pneumonia that had become especially virulent in winter, or was it a new syndrome? This time, to show that the syndrome could affect anybody, patients were presented in medical articles as unremarkable, without previous respiratory illnesses, and without a history of cigarette smoking (*NEJM*, May 15, 2003, 348/20, p. 1979). Several articles stressed that only a small proportion of the patients diagnosed with the new disease smoked or had health problems in the past. Patients were classified along travel habits, contacts, profession, and family relationships to show that despite their diversity, they had been infected by the same agent. In the classification of SARS, the risk categories were travelers and healthcare workers (*EID*, September 2003, 9/9, pp. 1064–9; *MMWR*, March 21, 2003, 52/11, pp. 226–8). This time, social stigmatization accompanied the handling of the epidemic: travelers coming from Asia were screened with particular care in airport lounges, and social contacts with them were avoided. This shows that risk categories are not a thing of the past but are still used in framing diseases as new and previously unseen. It also shows that the use of social categories of risk for framing the interpretation of biological phenomena usually entails social stigmatization. As I show in the following chapters, social classifications of risk have important consequences for how prevention and health policies are conceived.

2

The Economy of Risk Categories

In the early 1980s, all at once "new" and "unusual" diseases began to generate an immune deficiency unseen before. As we very well know, this deficiency was not restricted to a single risk category. When reading the clinical reports dating from the 1980s, we can see that the cases were quite diverse with respect to gender, ethnic origin, age, geographic area, and habits. Yet this diversity was channeled and systematized into risk categories. The recognition of the new immune deficiency relied precisely on a classificatory system that would tie it to certain social categories. What was the economy of this system? Which resources did it use and how? What were the relationships between risk categories? How were they constituted with respect to one another? How did they shape knowledge of the causal agent and its transmission?

The Classification of Risks

The first risk categories with which the medical AIDS discourse operated were hardly new or unusual. The term "homosexuals" was established as a medical category at the end of the nineteenth century, occupying an important role in medical models of human sexuality (Conrad 1986; Conrad and Schneider 1985, pp. 181–5; Poirier 1988; Pressman 1990). It was presented both as a disease and as a medical condition liable to attract other diseases. In the 1970s, homosexuality was associated with (and held responsible for) the reemergence of sexually transmitted diseases, especially hepatitis B (Epstein 1988); it was

thus seen more as a general condition favoring the appearance of infectious diseases than as a disease per se. The 1970s also witnessed the
emergence of "homosexual lifestyle" as a medical category. The background of this process was the medicalization of "lifestyle," a larger
and complex process related to the growing interpretation of everyday
life in medical terms (Brandt 1990; Nelkin 1985; Hilgartner 1985).
In turn, this interpretation was a central feature of biomedicalization
(Clarke et al. 2003), understood as a larger socioeconomic process
starting at about the same time. Biomedicalization represents everyday
life in terms of medical risks and relies on standardized instruments for
monitoring health at the collective and individual level.

From this perspective, "homosexual lifestyle" emerged at the inter-
section of two distinct developments. One was the reinterpretation of
everyday life in the gay cultures of big cities in medical terms (Conrad
and Schneider 1985, pp. 199–204). The other was the association with
infectious (and mainly sexually transmitted) diseases. The category of
drug users, although a much newer medical construct, was constituted
essentially along the same lines (Kane and Mason 1992). (Intravenous)
drug use was transformed into a medical category both as a disease
(addiction) and as a bodily and psychological condition favoring other
diseases. In this case, the catalytic factors were the construction of "addiction" and "lifestyle" as medical concepts, in a context larger than
that of drug use.

Because the Acquired Immunodeficiency Syndrome is perceived in
terms of being a sexually transmitted disease (STD), categories already
associated with STDs may have appeared as the "natural" candidates
for (exclusive) AIDS risk[1] (Grmek 1990; Epstein 1988). There are,
however, other categories which do not appear to be "natural" but
played an important role nevertheless: Haitians, women, and infants
were not previously subject to medicalization in the same way "homosexuals" and "drug abusers" were. At the same time, they are seen as
problematic, in the sense that they do not seem to fit a pattern of rationality: "Haitians," for example, were maintained as a risk category
without any apparent reason, whereas "infants" and "women" were
neglected for a long time.

---

[1] The rhetorical construction of AIDS as various diseases is detailed in Chapters 3
and 5.

Therefore, the questions are (1) how were "homosexuals" and "drug users" transformed into risk categories for something that was old and new at the same time? (2) How were the reported infections, along with the underlying immune deficiency, presented as entities with a completely new meaning (i.e., as related to the Acquired Immunodeficiency Syndrome)? (3) How did they form a self-sustaining classification system in 1982–3, which functioned by virtue of its own economy and allowed for apparently paradoxical risk categories? (4) What role did these risk categories play with respect to scientific knowledge?

These questions can help us better understand how classification practices work. Scientific knowledge relies on classifications, those within scientific disciplines, among these disciplines, and between science and non-science. Classifications appear to be a basic operation in every scientific domain. We are confronted here with a relevant case because AIDS risk categories, the outcome of a classificatory system, take such an important place in etiologic and epidemiologic models. By examining their production as a system, their relationship to each other, and their exchanges (that is, their economy), we can gain insights into how classifications work and with what consequences.

I do not detail here the "homosexual" risk category, which has been the object of many studies (Clatts and Mutchler 1989; Treichler 1988a,b; Epstein 1996). Instead, I first examine how the production of a new entity – the Acquired Immunodeficiency Syndrome – was dependent on the newly introduced risk categories; then, how a specific classification system was produced; and finally, the role played by categories such as Haitians, Africans, hemophiliacs, women, and infants.

The distinction between the old and the new *Pneumocystis carinii* (PCP) and Kaposi's sarcoma (KS), respectively, was achieved in part by calling them (and the underlying immune deficiency) "acquired" or "community-acquired" (*NEJM*, December 10, 1981, 305/24, pp. 1425, 1431, 1437). Also, "severe acquired immunodeficiency" was present in the title of clinical reports dating from late 1981 (*NEJM*, December 10, 1981, 305/24, p. 1439). Usually, "acquired" receives its meaning from the contrast with "congenital." It designates a disease or immune deficiency that is not innate or genetically determined but appears at a later moment in one's life, due to non-genetic factors. Both old and new immune deficiencies associated with PCP and KS were acquired; however, the new were "more acquired" than the old ones.

"Acquired immunodeficiency" got its meaning not from any wholly new symptoms associated with it, but from being presented as seen only in certain categories. This circularity is due to the "old" immune deficiencies now being presented as having genetic grounds (p. 1443) – which, ironically, amounts to redefining "acquired" as "congenital" – or as being due to the "lifestyle" of risk categories.

Other expressions were "Kaposi's sarcoma and opportunistic infections in previously healthy persons" (*MMWR*, September 24, 1982, 31/37, p. 507), "KSOI syndrome" (Kaposi's sarcoma/opportunistic infections syndrome) (*MMWR*, June 4, 1982, 31/21, p. 277 and June 11, 1982, 31/22, p. 300), and "gay compromise syndrome" (*The Lancet*, December 12, 1981, II/8259, p. 1338). In these cases too, the syndrome was category-specific, whereas categories were syndrome-specific. A clinical report on the "gay compromise syndrome" justified this name as follows:

This case is a paradigm of the newly recognized syndrome of opportunistic infections and/or Kaposi's sarcoma in homosexual males. Because these patients seem to be severely immunocompromised, we have called it the "gay compromise syndrome." *P. carinii* infection is rare and, before its appearance in homosexuals, was found almost exclusively in malnourished or immunodeficient patients. *C. neoformans* is likewise an infrequent pathogen; it may infect immunodeficient or apparently healthy individuals. (*The Lancet*, December 12, 1981, II/8259, p. 1338)

This was one of the very rare cases where the terms "gay" and "gay syndrome" appeared in the medical articles. Usually, the term "acquired immunodeficiency" was used; when writing about risk categories, the term "homosexuality" was used. The fact that *P. carinii* ("rare," "in homosexuals," "almost exclusively in malnourished or immunodeficient patients") was previously seen in immunodeficient patients did not prevent the name "gay compromise" being given *because* of the category-specific immune deficiency. With the risk category defining the specificity of the syndrome, and the latter defining the specificity of the risk category, they become mutually reinforcing.

In September 1982, the *Morbidity and Mortality Weekly Report* (31/37, p. 507) introduced the expression Acquired Immunodeficiency Syndrome (AIDS), which replaced previous names. Cultural critics (Treichler 1988a,b) and journalists (Shilts 1987) have each offered their versions of how the name was coined in a meeting at the Centers for Disease Control and Prevention. Relevant here is that expressions such as "acquired immunodeficiency" or "community-acquired immune deficiency" were present in the medical discourse from the beginning, helping to distinguish between different categories of immune deficiency.

With the Acquired Immunodeficiency Syndrome as characteristic for some categories, which in turn were *the risk* of a specific immune deficiency, the classification system produced both its criterion and its categories. Within this self-referential frame, the distinction between old and new immune deficiency lost its meaning.

Patterns of Differences: How "Haitians" Were Made Into a Risk Category

The construction of Haitians as an additional "risk group" illustrates the case in point. "Haitians" has been maintained for more than two years as an official epidemiological category by the Centers for Disease Control and Prevention,[2] in spite of strong protests about the absurdity of classifying a whole nation as a risk category. The standard explanations refer either to a circumstantial error or to a bias in the biomedical discourse: in 1982–3, AIDS was perceived as being (among other things) a tropical disease brought to North America by tourists (Treichler 1999). But if we look more closely at the way this risk category was introduced we can see that neither a circumstantial error nor a simple racist bias was behind it. Although certain racist biases in the biomedical AIDS discourse have been documented and analyzed (Treichler 1999, 1993; Seidel 1992), I argue here that explanations based solely on these biases are not satisfactory when we get down to understanding the paradoxes of the biomedical AIDS discourse, such as the long-term maintenance of apparently absurd categories, or the long-term ignoring of relevant ones. Besides, we still have to answer the question of how AIDS was transformed in such a short time from an STD into a tropical disease. How could these contradictory representations be concomitantly maintained? Were they without any consequences for representations of the infectious agent?

---

[2] Medical reports on the "Haitian" risk factors appeared until 1987.

The first report on "Opportunistic Infections and Kaposi's Sarcoma among Haitians in the United States" appeared in the July 9, 1982 issue of *MMWR* (31/26, pp. 353–61). It stated that 19 Haitian patients from a hospital in Miami and 10 Haitian residents of Brooklyn had been diagnosed with opportunistic infections and Kaposi's sarcoma. The enumeration of opportunistic infections for each group of patients was followed by a description of laboratory findings, including those showing "severe T-cell dysfunction." Three additional cases were reported from California, Georgia, and New Jersey. The editorial note stated that:

> The occurrence of severe opportunistic infections among 32 Haitians recently entering the United States is a new phenomenon. The in vitro immunologic findings and the high mortality rate (nearly 50%) for these patients are similar to the pattern recently described among homosexual males and IV drug abusers. None of the 23 Haitian males questioned reported homosexual activity, and only 1 of 26 gave a history of IV drug abuse – substantially lower than the prevalence reported for heterosexual patients of other racial/ethnic groups who had Kaposi's sarcoma or opportunistic infections. (*MMWR*, July 9, 1982, 31/26, p. 360)

Haitians, as a "new phenomenon," have to thus enter a classification system in which mutually exclusive categories reinforce each other. Another clinical report ("Acquired Immune Deficiency in Haitians. Opportunistic Infections in Previously Healthy Haitian Immigrants") stressed the differences between risk categories as relevant for the meaning of the syndrome. "Haitians" were not "homosexuals," nor did they have a history of drug abuse or illness. Moreover, they were recent immigrants and, as such, a clearly defined ethnic group (*NEJM*, January 20, 1983, 308/3, p. 125).

Risk categories were seen as characteristic for the immunodeficiency syndrome. In Haitian men, AIDS was accompanied by a variety of opportunistic infections. These infections (*M. tuberculosis, Pneomocystis carinii, C. neoformans*, and *Candida albicans*) were indicative of a cell-mediated immune deficiency. At the same time, unlike other patients with AIDS, Haitians were "neither homosexuals nor addicted to drugs" (*NEJM*, January 20, 1983, 308/3, p. 127). After discussing CD4+ cell counts in the same section, the report concluded that: "These immunologic findings are characteristic of AIDS among drug addicts, homosexuals, and now Haitians" (p. 127). Other articles, in an attempt to exculpate "Haitians" from homosexuality, argued that "solarium exposure can produce immunological disorders in otherwise normal (and presumably heterosexual) subjects" (*Nature*, June 2, 1983, 303, p. 371). AIDS in "black Africans" and in "Haitians" should be considered against this background.

It is interesting to note that reported cases of AIDS in women and heterosexual men did not affect the risk categories; neither did the case of a Haitian using drugs, reported a few months later (*NEJM*, April 7, 1983, 308/14, p. 842). Cases of infants were reported in this context as "infants born of Haitian mothers" and "Haitian infants," thus classifying them as "Haitians." The fact that some of the opportunistic infections (such as tuberculosis) were considered to be endemic among Haitian immigrants did not prevent the authors of clinical reports from considering them AIDS-related, by virtue of the fact that "Haitians" had already been introduced as a new risk category.

The basic differences that transform "Haitians" into a new risk group are traced with respect to sexual orientation, drug consumption, health, citizenship, and racial status. These classification criteria, when put side by side, may seem completely heterogeneous, even absurd: after all, what is the connection between sexual orientation, citizenship, and race? And how can such a connection sustain the thesis of a new, formerly unseen immune deficiency? Yet it is exactly this heterogeneity that makes the classification system flexible and expandable in several directions at once.

An *MMWR* article distinguished between "Haitians in the United States" and "Haitians in Haiti"; Haitian patients from two hospitals located in Miami and New York became "Haitians in the United States," a general category related to "Haitians in Haiti." Diseases were problematic and new for "Haitians in Haiti" and hence for "Haitians in the United States." Both groups were previously healthy and had no history of immunosuppressive therapy. However, over a period of two and a half years, KS had been diagnosed in eleven cases in Port-au-Prince. In turn, recent Haitian immigrants in the US had had a high prevalence of tuberculosis, associated with immune deficiencies (*MMWR*, July 2, 1982, 31/25, p. 360). Thus, both KS and tuberculosis were new and problematic in Haiti (a country generally known for its extreme poverty). Both were associated with immunosuppression. As a conclusion, "Haitians" were associated with immunosuppression.

In later articles, this syllogism was reversed: diseases and opportunistic infections that are problematic and new for "Haitians in the United States" become problematic for "Haitians in Haiti" (*NEJM*, Oct. 20, 1983, 309/16, p. 949). We encounter here two different arguments, according to different epidemiological theses: to argue that the syndrome was already present in Haiti and then brought by Haitian immigrants to the United States, diseases endemic in Haiti, such as tuberculosis, are called new and problematic for "Haitians in the United States" because they are actually new and problematic for "Haitians in Haiti" (*The Lancet*, October 15, 1983, II/8354, p. 877). Tuberculosis, although systematically presented as endemic in Haiti, was counted in clinical reports among the AIDS-related opportunistic infections by virtue of its association with the "Haitian" risk group and was considered relevant for the immune deficiency.

Conversely, to argue that the syndrome was brought to Haiti from the United States, these opportunistic infections must become new and problematic for "Haitians in Haiti." They were characteristic for "Haitians in the United States":

The recognition of Kaposi's sarcoma and opportunistic infections in Haiti is temporally related to the appearance of AIDS in the United States. The earliest possible case of opportunistic infections in Haiti that is known to our group occurred in July 1978, and the first case of fulminant Kaposi's sarcoma was diagnosed in June 1979. The first cases of Kaposi's sarcoma and opportunistic infections in homosexual men in the United States were documented in early 1978. We do not believe that AIDS was present in Haiti before 1978. This contention is supported by the clinical experience of practicing pathologists and dermatologists in Haiti and by our inability to identify earlier cases through examination of autopsy and biopsy records. It also seems likely that Haitians would have presented to U.S. hospitals sooner if AIDS have been occurring (sic) in Haiti before 1978. (*NEJM*, Oct. 20, 1983, 309/16, p. 949)

Apparently, what we have here are several arguments for the proposed epidemiologic model: (1) a historical one (pushing back the initial moment of the disease), (2) one based on clinical experience, and (3) a commonsensical one. But all of them depend on distinguishing between the risk categories "of Haiti" and those "of the United States," and on arranging them in different temporal and clinical orders. Arguing for one epidemiologic model or another (with completely different consequences) thus depends less on the intrinsic characteristics of the reported diseases and infections than on rearranging the categories of the classification system to change the pattern of differences between them.

In the economy of risk classification, "Haitians" made very good sense: they were integrated by exclusion from other categories, thus both helping to define and being defined by this exclusion. Clinical cases gained their meaning from ascription to one of these categories: there was no room left for ambiguities. In this sense, having "Haitians" be an ethnic and not a medical category did not affect the classificatory system. The representation of infections and diseases (such as tuberculosis or Kaposi's sarcoma) in "Haitians" as AIDS-related helped integrate the new risk category in the given classification. "Haitians" are part of the same risk system, it is argued, because their opportunistic infections (and KS) are common to all risk categories. At the same time, they are different, because in "Haitians" these infections have an "endemic" and "old" form, as well as a "new" and "problematic" one.

Clinical reports written by Haitian physicians argued for integrating Haitian patients into other risk categories. During the 1983 hearings on AIDS in the Subcommittee on Intergovernmental Relations and Human Resources of the U.S. House of Representatives, medical experts argued for the removal of "Haitians" from the epidemiologic classification of the Centers for Disease Control and Prevention; the category was removed from the New York reports in July 1983. Its presence was called "arbitrary," the result of a lack of conclusive scientific data, and of the oral (hence: implicitly biased) denial by Haitian AIDS patients of "any history of homosexuality, drug abuse or hemophilia" (Compas 1983a, p. 41). What was contested was not the classificatory system as such, but (1) that Haitians could be translated into other categories, and (2) the presence of Haitians as an ethnic and not as a socio-medical category. A clinical report ("Characteristics of the Acquired Immunodeficiency Syndrome [AIDS] in Haiti") argued that homosexuality was not as unknown in Haiti as was asserted by other reports:

Some of the risk factors for AIDS in the United States were present in our patients with opportunistic infections and Kaposi's sarcoma in Haiti. Bisexual activity was reported by 15 percent of the men with Kaposi's sarcoma or opportunistic infections for whom such information was available and by 24 percent of the men prospectively questioned by a clinician in the Haitian Study Group. The identification of bisexual Haitian patients who had had sexual relations with American homosexuals in New York and Miami also provides a link between the two populations. There is a very strong bias against homosexuality in Haiti, and our data may underestimate this risk factor. (*NEJM*, Oct. 20, 1983, 309/16, p. 949)

Another clinical report ("Acquired Immunodeficiency Syndrome with Severe Gastrointestinal Manifestations in Haiti") argued that many Haitians will not admit homosexual contacts because they violate Haitian social taboos. Although they denied it, a good proportion of Haitian men (and hence of Haitian immigrants) were homosexuals. Moreover, homosexual prostitution in Haiti was a well known phenomenon. As a consequence, in spite of different clinical symptoms (among which diarrhea and tuberculosis were prominent), the reported patients should be reclassified as homosexuals (*The Lancet*, October 15, 1983, II/8354, p. 877).

In his medical statement before the Subcommittee on Intergovernmental Relations and Human Services of the U.S. Congress, Dr. Jean-Claude Compas argued that "Haitians" were not a proper medical category, but an ethnic one:

Three social/medical groups, homosexuals, intravenous drug abusers and hemophiliacs, and one ethno-national community, Haitian immigrants, were labeled as being responsible for the eruption and the spread of the AIDS outbreak. For the first time in history, a disease was being attributed to a nationality without clear epidemiologic or scientific justification. (Compas 1983b, p. 44)

Haitians should, Compas argued, therefore be integrated into the "homosexual" risk group. The rationale for the reclassification, he continued, was that more than 30% of the "Haitian AIDS population" had actually admitted to homosexual experience. This percentage was reason enough for a redefinition, and it made any questions (such as those about AIDS and heterosexuality) about the other 70% superfluous. This brought "Haitians" from one extreme to the other: from a nation without homosexuals to one with widespread homosexual experience. What it argued for was actually not the abolition of the risk category as such, but its integration into that of homosexuals: a "separate high-risk classification" would lead to the scapegoating of Haitians by the "other high-risk groups."

In all these arguments, the classification system imposes speaking or writing of risk in its own terms; by force of this requirement, the argumentation strategies have to operate continuously with the categories they claim to contest, and reproduce them as such. They speak of two populations ("Haitian patients" and "American homosexuals"), distinguish them from "previously described high-risk groups," and identify a distinct "Haitian AIDS population." This made possible the construction of causal and epidemiological models in the mid-1980s in which Haiti played a central role. The key thesis – namely, that the infectious agent might have passed the barrier between animals and humans – relied heavily on a Haitian setting. This thesis was formulated first in a letter to *The Lancet* (April 23, 1983, I/8330, p. 983) by a Harvard virologist; its main statements were that the infectious agent concerned might have been the swine fever virus (which, like the human immunodeficiency virus, is a retrovirus) and that it might have been passed from animals to humans via the consumption of raw meat, after which it was further transmitted by sexual contact.

Seen from this perspective (which I detail in the Chapters 3 and 4), "Haitians" appears less as a discursive accident than as an important strand in this classificatory network. This category supported a central thesis about the nature of the infectious agent and played an important part in narratives of its origins.

"Hemophiliacs" and Blood Transfusions

Although the relationship between "Haitians" and "homosexuals" was a special one, other categories seemed to be irreconcilable with this classificatory system. How could "hemophiliacs" be brought into such a classification? An explanatory model associating them with STDs or tropical diseases was not available. Their character as a group was not clear at all; they were not identified by a common ethnic origin or by a distinct urban lifestyle.

The first reports about persons with hemophilia A diagnosed with *Pneumocystis carinii* pneumonia were published by the CDC weekly bulletin in mid-1982. Against the background of a classification provided by the risk categories already in operation, hemophiliacs were first presented as clearly distinct, then as similar in diagnosis, and afterwards as part of the same classification. One report stated that hemophilia A patients diagnosed with *Pneumocystis carinii* pneumonia were "all three heterosexual males; none had a history of intravenous drug abuse" (*MMWR*, July 16, 1982, 31/27, p. 365); they were presented as "a 62-year-old resident of Westchester County, New York ... a 59-year-old lifelong resident of Denver, Colorado, and a previously healthy 27-year-old lifelong resident of northeastern Ohio" (pp. 365–6).

They were spatially distinct from the existent "risk groups," which included cases located in New York City, Los Angeles, and Miami. The editorial note concluded that the three patients had clinical and immunological features similar to those of "homosexuals," "heterosexuals who abuse IV drugs," and recent Haitian immigrants. Therefore, it was the same immune deficiency, which in turn suggested transmission of an agent through blood products (*MMWR*, July, 16, 1982, 31/27, p. 366). The representation of risk as spatially distributed played an important role in the construction of etiologic and epidemiologic models of the infectious agent and took the form of risk maps showing which cases were to be found in what cities and boroughs, ordered according to zip codes. This was a combination of epidemiologic models of an infectious agent transmitted through the environment and models of a sexually transmitted disease (more about this topic in Chapter 5). In this context, it was relevant to construct hemophiliacs as a distinct risk category by taking into account spatial location.

The stress placed on spatial distance and dispersion was meant to support the thesis of "transmission of an agent through blood products" (without direct sexual contact), among others. Because one of the main epidemiological models of the time stressed social environmental factors, located in cities such as New York, San Francisco, and Los Angeles, the spatial isolation of persons with hemophilia A was an argument for a different etiology. Six months later, another CDC report emphasized again the spatial distance and dispersion of persons with hemophilia A diagnosed with opportunistic infections and cellular immune deficiency. It was stated that data about the patients did not suggest infection through personal contact with homosexuals, drug users, or Haitian immigrants. Their only common feature was transfusion with factor VIII concentrate (*MMWR*, December 10, 1982, 31/48, p. 644).

The cases discussed here were "a 55-year-old severe hemophiliac from Alabama ... a 10-year-old severe hemophiliac from Pennsylvania ... a 49-year-old patient from Ohio, and a 52-year-old severe hemophiliac from Missouri" (pp. 644–5), respectively. Thus, the new risk group matched neither (1) previously known means of transmission nor (2) the direct contact model. Two classifications are actually in operation here: one lies along a "sexual activities, drug usage, travel, and residence" axis, and the second lies along a "contact with each other, with homosexuals, with illicit drug abusers, or with Haitian immigrants" axis. Each classification matches a risk group with a transmission path. The new risk category had not only special spatial attributes, but also a lack of direct contacts. Although blood components are not explicitly declared a means of transmission, all other known possible ways were excluded. Spatial dispersion, lack of direct contact, and diversity, in their turn, support blood components as a means of transmission: "in most instances, these patients have been the first AIDS cases in their cities, states, or regions. They have had no known common medications, occupations, habits, types of pets, or any uniform antecedent history of personal or family illnesses with immunological relevance" (*MMWR*, December 10, 1982, 31/48, p. 652).

At the beginning of 1983, a different way of presenting the "hemophiliac risk group" appeared. It introduced a distinction between hemophiliacs diagnosed before and after the Acquired Immunodeficiency Syndrome was discovered. The hemophiliacs from "before" were active and mobile, due to medical advances. Danièle Carricaburu and Janine Pierret (1995, 1992, pp. 9–25) confirm, for the case of France, that the medical discourse has constantly presented hemophiliacs as the result of medical technology. This had allowed "risk" to be defined as a technical feature of "product damaging." It is interesting to note that "hemophiliacs" sustained not only the thesis of transmission-at-a-distance, but also of the transmission of the infectious agent through ordinary, occasional transfusions. A clinical report about transfusion-associated immunodeficiency in an infant asserted that the widespread occurrence of AIDS (i.e., in several risk groups) suggested accidental transmission through blood products (*The Lancet*, April 30, 1983, I/8331, p. 956).

Presenting the "lifestyle" of persons living with hemophilia as a product of medical advances and transfusion technology was not a new turn in the medical discourse. New in this context is the shift from the initial undifferentiated construction of "hemophiliacs" as spatially isolated, immobile, and dispersed (all elements which contrasted it to

the other risk categories and sustained the thesis of transmission-at-
a-distance) to a new distinction. This shift, along with reports about
transfusion-related immunodeficiency cases,[3] led to a redefinition of the
group risk, as leading to loss of lifestyle, on the one hand, and on the
other hand as a technical risk, actually associated more with the transfusion technology than with the group as such. The "hemophiliac"
group was consequently given a double status. It was still considered
a risk group and retained its place in the risk classifications, but because risk was also understood as technology-related, this group was
presented as a victim of technology.

This double status led to a double moral status, based on the distinction between self-induced risks (as in the case of the other established "risk groups") and externally induced risks, such as those faced
by hemophiliacs (Miller 1992; Patton 1989; Carricaburu and Pierret
1992). The individual is responsible for self-induced risks, but not for
externally induced ones. In the first case, it is his/her duty to know
about the consequences of his/her actions; in the second case, the individual has to rely on the knowledge of other social actors. This double
status reverses Niklas Luhmann's distinction between risk and danger,
discussed in the introduction: blame is placed upon persons at risk,
whereas persons in danger are exempted from blame.

Another effect was the distinction between technological (transfusion-related) and group risks. From 1983 on, clinical reports and
articles on hemophiliacs with opportunistic infections and/or AIDS
did not discuss transfusion technology. One exception[4] was seen in a
short-lived argument in the medical literature about whether US blood
products imported to Europe were safe or not. It did not concern transfusion technologies, focusing instead on US blood products contaminated by risk donors. This argument was that the infectious agent
was transmissible through blood products. "Risk donors"[5] had to be
identified making use of the existent risk classification.

A closer examination of how this was achieved shows the role of
rhetorical devices in building up a double status for risk. The first

[3] See for example *MMWR*, Dec. 10, 1982, 31, pp. 652–4 and *The Lancet*, April 30,
1983, I/8331, pp. 956–8.
[4] *The Lancet*, June 30, 1984, I/8391, p. 1455.
[5] *The Lancet*, June 30, 1984, I/8391, p. 1453 and January 29, 1983, I/8318, p. 213;
NEJM, February 21, 1985, 312/8, p. 484.

reports on persons with hemophilia A stressed their spatial dispersion, immobility, and lack of contact – all arguments for transmission
through blood products: "the lives of hemophiliacs have been transformed by advances in treatment during the past decade" as a consequence of "techniques of concentrating and storing [factor VIII]."

Remarkable changes have occurred during the past decade with this program
of self-administration of a factor VIII preparation. It has provided a means of
early and preventive treatment and has minimized hospital admissions among
hemophiliacs. The program has given patients a new degree of freedom and in-
dependence in managing their disease. Besides decreasing the need for hospital
admissions, it has diminished the number and severity of complications. The
availability of concentrates of factor VIII has also allowed safe surgical treatment of acute problems and repair of severe joint deformities. Thus, lifestyle
and life itself have changed for many hemophiliacs. (*NEJM*, January 13, 1983,
308/2, p. 94)

The article presented hemophiliacs as a compact group, whose
"lifestyle" was the product of a medical technology. It stated that "the
risk associated with exposure to plasma from multiple donors" is not
new and has "long been a concern in the care of these patients" because of "hepatitis, a common event in the histories of many of these
patients." The etiology of the syndrome was declared to be completely
unclear: "Whether it is secondary to multiple antigenic exposures, to
a specific transmitted agent or to some other mechanism is not yet
known" (*NEJM*, January 13, 1983, 308/2, p. 94). The paper's conclusions about hemophiliacs' risks were that the home-infusion program needed revision and that more cryoprecipitates would be used
and risk thus minimized. This meant that physicians should become
more aware of the problems related to blood-parts concentrates. The
choice was between preventing AIDS and preventing the complications
of hemophilia, and AIDS prevention had priority (*NEJM*, January 13,
1983, 308/2, p. 95).

The study argues for the costlier cryoprecipitate technology, which
excluded self-administration and related single donors to single recipients. But before it came to this argument, the study proposed a
redefinition of risk: it was a "clear fact" that hemophiliacs were at
risk of contracting AIDS. Then it introduced a conditional clause: alternative technologies (i.e., cryoprecipitates) could in the future minimize the risks of this category. Although in vitro abnormalities of

immunoregulation have been shown, case numbers are not statistically significant "for definitive comparison of the risks of different modes of treatment." This actually reverses the initial assertion; it refers now not to abnormalities of immunoregulation in persons, but to those in blood samples, without relating the two. Their statistical insignificance does not allow a definitive comparison of technological risks. In this context, transfusion technology is seen as being conducive to or as favoring risk, and not as risk itself. The assertion about the statistical insignificance of in vitro studies, however, reverses this view in discussing "risks of different modes of treatment." The reversal of perspective allows debate about whether transfusion technologies are risky, irrespective of risk categories.

After the retroviral agent was described as HTLV-III (human T-lymphotropic virus III) in American and British-authored papers, and as LAV (lymphadenopathy-associated virus) in French-authored ones, identifying risk donors decreased in significance and was replaced by direct identification of the retroviral agent in blood products.[6] Because the retroviral agent was not immediately accepted (two different candidates were competing for this role), the debate over transmission through blood products was prolonged until 1985. In later media debates on contaminated transfusions (the "blood scandals" from France, the United Kingdom, and Germany), 1985 was presented as a turning point.[7] Because there was no medical knowledge about transmission through blood products before 1985, nobody could be held responsible for early transfusions. But this knowledge depended, as shown in the preceding discussion, on a double risk status. The disjunction of technological, transfusion-related risk from "hemophiliacs" played a relevant role in this process, until it became possible to identify the retroviral agent directly in blood products. Along with "hemophiliacs," "transfusion recipients" supported the theory of transmission-at-a-distance, reinforcing the viral agent model. At the time of the first reports,[8] this theory was not the only one claiming legitimacy.

---

[6] *The Lancet*, April 7, 1984, I/8380, p. 730 and August 18, 1984, II/8399, p. 397; *NEJM*, February 21, 1985, 312/8, p. 483.

[7] See, for example, the features in the German weekly *Der Spiegel* (10/1991, 47/1991, 25/1992, 48/1992) and in the French weekly *Le Nouvel Observateur* (June 13, 1991).

[8] The first report on a transfusion-associated infection in a non-hemophiliac person was reported in *MMWR*, Dec. 10, 1982, 31/48, pp. 652–4. On pp. 644–52 the same issue reported on hemophiliac cases.

The heterogeneity and complexity of "transfusion recipients" brought about additional problems: e.g., for infants acquiring immunodeficiency as a consequence of blood transfusions, it had to be explained why such cases were not ascribed to the risk category of infants, and why the immunodeficiency was an acquired and not a congenital one. Several types of immunodeficiency syndromes in infants (Nezeloff's, Di George's, and others) were known. Their symptoms were more or less similar to those in cases claimed to be Acquired Immunodeficiency Syndrome. Similarly, in the case of adults classified as transfusion recipients, it had to be argued that transfusion was the only event that could have induced the reported immunodeficiency. Therefore, classifying reported cases as transfusion recipients had to begin with declassifying them as other possible cases; also, the donor had to be classified as a risk too. Thus, a report about an infant with immunodeficiency ("Acquired Immunodeficiency in an Infant: Possible Transmission by Means of Blood Products") declassified the case with respect to other risk categories and simultaneously asserted a causal link to them. Because the patient's parents were heterosexuals, non-Haitians, and did not use IV drugs, there was no risk group with which to directly match the infant's AIDS diagnosis. However, the diagnosis could be matched with a gay man as a blood donor. This was not a one-to-one but rather a list-to-list match. The list of blood donors was compared with that of AIDS patients in the San Francisco area, and a single match was found (*The Lancet*, April 30, 1983, I/8331, p. 957).

There were two possibilities: this was a congenital immunodeficiency or an acquired one. The first was excluded on the grounds of this match. A clinical report of eighteen cases ("Acquired Immunodeficiency Syndrome (AIDS) Associated with Transfusions"), published eight months later, presented the modes of transmission according to the risk classification: between homosexual men, between drug addicts through needle sharing, and from heterosexual men to their female partners (*NEJM*, January 12, 1984, 310/2, p. 69). Its selection of eighteen cases (out of 2157) was legitimated as follows:

Patients with AIDS who did not fit into one of the groups known to have an increased incidence of AIDS were investigated. The medical and social histories obtained included information on receipt of blood or blood products during the five years preceding the diagnosis of AIDS. If no other potential risk factors were identified and the patient had previously received transfusions, he or she was classified as having transfusion-associated AIDS. [. . .] Donors may or may not experience symptoms or have signs associated with AIDS, but most donors transmitting the disease would be expected to come from populations previously recognized as having an increased incidence of AIDS (i.e., homosexual men with multiple partners, abusers of intravenous drugs, persons born in Haiti, or patients with hemophilia). Using the definition of a high-risk donor (a person belonging to a group at increased risk for AIDS or having a reversed ratio [<1.00] of T-helper to T-suppressor lymphocytes), we identified a single high-risk donor during each of the initial investigations, regardless of the number of donors. (*NEJM*, January 12, 1984, 310/2, p. 70)

The classification of donors reproduces exactly that of the risk categories (although a hemophiliac as a blood donor may seem problematic), and the newly created category of "high-risk donor" actually matches the whole classification. The chain is constructed both through one-to-one correspondence (there is one "high-risk donor" corresponding to every recipient) and through category-related correspondence (other categories correspond to one distinct risk category).

In the articles analyzed here, the selection of cases (from large samples) was legitimated by risk categories and, at the same time, reinforced them. Besides the circular character of this procedure, it is striking that the heterogeneity of the classification hinders neither its continuous enlargement, nor its use in apparently contradictory situations. Rather, it is precisely this heterogeneity that makes the classificatory system so plastic. Cases that may seem irrelevant with respect to sexual orientation are classified with respect to ethnic origin, or drug use, and vice versa.

Declassifying transfusion recipients (as "homosexuals," "Haitians," and so forth) in order to reclassify them became common; the construction of causal links illustrating the thesis of transmission-at-a-distance of the infectious agent was common as well.[9] "Transfusion recipients" were thus constituted through a complex set of rhetorical operations, similar to those that served for the construction of other categories – analogies with hemophiliacs, declassification, and causal chains based on indexical and category-related correspondences.

The criterion of mutual exclusivity (i.e., hemophiliacs being non-homosexuals, non-Haitians, and vice versa) played a central role as

---

[9] See also *NEJM*, January 12, 1984, 310/2, p. 115; *The Lancet*, January 14, 1984, I/8368, p. 102.

a device for building up risk groups here. However, it must be seen for what it is, namely as a device for classifying that does not reflect the complex reality of social groups. That this criterion cannot have empirical relevance is convincingly proven by the empirical study of Carricaburu and Pierret (1992, pp. 97–155), who have shown that real people actually do not accurately mirror "risk classifications." Their research was conducted with French hemophiliacs who were also HIV carriers. Although some of them were heterosexuals, others had same-sex or bisexual relationships. In these cases, it was impossible to give a clear-cut account of the relationship between HIV infection and a single transmission path (sexual or transfusion-related). Nevertheless, these persons chose a unique identity as a way of accounting for how they had become HIV carriers: some identified themselves as hemophiliacs, whereas others stressed their sexual orientation. Persons diagnosed with HIV tried thus to recompose their identities around these classifications, so that they could "pass" for members of a clearly defined "risk group." These recompositions of identity (Carricaburu and Pierret, 1992, pp. 201–11) not only were conducted with respect to the present and future, but also implied a reconstruction of the past, so that a person retrospectively ascribed herself to a "risk group." On the other hand, physicians used these classification devices continually to manage clinical diagnoses: in this way, classifications appear as a tool for managing disease used by patients and physicians alike. These classifications have concrete consequences for the ways in which people consulting a physician perceive (or shape) their identities, as well as for how physicians evaluate and diagnose their patients.

Out of Africa: "Africans" and Kaposi's Sarcoma

Another "ethnic" group playing a similar role, but with far larger consequences, is the "African risk group." "Africans" as a medical category was related to rare, tropical infectious diseases (Prims 1986; Patton 1989; Seidel 1992). In the late 1960s and in the 1970s, the term "Africans"[10] was frequently used in reporting and describing a number of virally induced diseases (Marburg disease, Ebola fever, African

---

[10] They were understood in this context as the populations from sub-Saharan Africa.

yellow fever); sub-Saharan Africa was generally presented as a (potentially unlimited) reservoir of disease (an image reinforced by the media reports on the outbreak of the Ebola virus in the late 1990s).

In contemporary epidemiological models, the "African pattern" means the transmission of HIV at accelerated speed through sexual contact from male to female and from female to male, as well as the transmission from mother to child.[11] Like "Haitians," the category "Africans" has been a matter of heated controversies, attracting accusations of racism (Treichler 1992; Chirimuuta and Chirimuuta 1989; Kitzinger and Miller 1992). Several studies have highlighted ethnic biases and racial prejudices in the media treatment of "Africans" (e.g., Patton 1993). In his ethnographic study of AIDS in Tanzania, Philip Setel (1999, p. 21) has characterized the epidemiologic knowledge base of AIDS in Africa as "a hodgepodge of figures from different kinds of studies among numerous population subgroups in scattered locations."

As in the case of "Haitian AIDS," media accounts have tried to identify a geographic origin of the syndrome and to explain it on the grounds of local "socio-medical" factors. These accounts have been criticized because the blame was laid (directly or indirectly) on a number of ill-conceived risk categories, suggesting biased health policies. On the other hand, media narratives of the origins of AIDS have generated counter-models: these claimed, among other things, that homosexual American tourists brought the virus to Africa from North America and not the other way around (Chirimuuta and Chirimuuta 1989).

In the present context, the relevance of "Africans" lies not primarily in the study of media-generated biases (however important these may be for the public perception of AIDS), but in this category's key role with respect to the causal models of the acquired immune deficiency. This category supported a series of narratives which framed the thesis of a viral agent; it also supported narratives of the origins of AIDS, which left an indelible print on today's epidemiological models. Contemporary attempts at providing alternative explanations of how the

---

[11] See Brown et al. 1993; Stine 1993; Barnett and Whiteside 2002, pp. 55–7; Stevenson 2001, p. 319. See also the features from popular magazines such as the German *Der Spiegel* (4/1990, 9/1991, 25/1991) or the French *Le Nouvel Observateur* (June 28, 1990 and November 30, 1989).

HI-viruses appeared (e.g., Hooper 2000a, p. 19; 2000b, p. 73) still stick with this framework, even when giving it a different twist.

The first clinical reports on "Africans" or "Black Africans" with an acquired immune deficiency were published in the spring of 1983, almost two years after those on the first risk groups. "Africans" had already played a role in the presentation of Kaposi's sarcoma as new and problematic, when it was asserted that KS was usually seen in Equatorial Africa, in an aggressive form similar to the one reported from New York and Los Angeles. From March 1983 onward, a series of articles described cases of opportunistic infections in Europe-based Africans as fulfilling the CDC criteria of AIDS.[12] A month later, cases of African patients examined years before in Zaire were retrospectively diagnosed as AIDS cases. A Danish surgeon who had worked in Zaire until the mid-1970s and died in Europe in 1977 got the same retrospective diagnosis.[13] A year later, cases of Kaposi's sarcoma among natives in Zaire, Zambia, and Uganda were reported as indicative of AIDS.[14] In these reports, "Africans" as a category was introduced as new, distinct, and formerly unseen. This category was related to some important new developments: (1) the re-presentation of past cases as having actually been AIDS cases and (2) the reworking of the initial classification. The first development, although not exclusively related to "Africans," made it possible to push the origin of the disease further into the past, asserting that AIDS had been present in Africa for a long time and had ancestral origins. The second, not less interesting, development shows that Kaposi's sarcoma was differently presented and negotiated at different moments in the discourse: in the beginning it played a decisive role in constructing risk categories (the KS seen in North American patients looked like, but was not, the old KS seen in African patients). Later, the old KS, which looked like, but was not, the new Kaposi's sarcoma, became the new "new" KS. Different medical entities were constituted out of fairly similar symptoms and clinical signs.

More generally, the retrospective description of clinical cases as AIDS cases, which identifies the origins of infection in a more or less

---

[12] *The Lancet*, March 19, 1983, I/8325, p. 642 and March 26, 1983, I/8326, p. 701.

[13] *The Lancet*, April 23, 1983, I/8330, pp. 925–6.

[14] *The Lancet*, June 16, 1984, I/8320, pp. 1318–20; March 17, 1984, I/8377, pp. 631–2, and March 3, 1984, I/8375, pp. 478–80.

remote past, was used for negotiating the definition of disease and various transmission models. A paper published by *The Lancet* in 1986 (May 31, I/8492, p. 1279) pushed back evidence for HTLV-III/LAV as far as 1959. In the case of a Frenchman who was diagnosed with AIDS in Paris in 1983, the moment of infection was presented as a blood transfusion received four years earlier in Haiti – that is, in 1979 (*The Lancet*, October 15, 1983, II/8354, p. 883). The thesis of transmission by blood transfusion was supported by the reconstruction of a past event as the original moment of infection, and by connecting it to a risk category. The absolute origin of AIDS, as the place where the infectious agent was born a long time ago is unequivocally related to "Africans" (see, for example, *Science*, March 20, 1992, 255, p. 1505).

At first glance, the construction of "Africans" seems not to differ very much from that of other categories: it is introduced by presenting a classification in which they are not homosexuals, hemophiliacs, or transfusion recipients. They have been healthy and have a new form of immunodeficiency:

Acquired immune deficiency syndrome (AIDS) has been described in homosexual or bisexual men, in drug addicts, in hemophiliacs, and in Haitian immigrants. To our knowledge there is no report of AIDS and opportunistic infections in previously healthy Black Africans with no history of homosexuality or drug abuse. (*The Lancet*, March 19, 1983, I/8325, p. 642)

After data on the patients' residence and their "good socioeconomic status," the opportunistic and viral infections, and the laboratory results, the paper asserted that "these patients fulfilled all the criteria of AIDS." But the criteria, which are supposed to be grounded in the description of opportunistic and viral infections, gain their relevance only as correlates of the risk classification. It is precisely risk categories, their mutual exclusiveness, and the incompatibility of the new category with other disease definitions that allow for "criteria of AIDS" and for opportunistic infections as being AIDS-related. Conversely, these criteria make "Black Africans, immigrants or not . . . another group predisposed to AIDS." Relevant in this respect are the transformations in the regime of representation. "Africans" begins with "previously healthy Black Africans with no history of homosexuality or drug abuse"; then, it becomes "Black patients seen in Brussels and who were from Central Africa." Toward the end, it becomes "Black Africans, immigrants or not," defined as a "group predisposed to AIDS." This is the new risk category to be added to the classification. In arguing for unusual immunosuppression in Africa, medical papers reinforced categories already in use: they argued that, because homosexuality, promiscuity, drug use, or transfusion were unknown in the reported cases, the whole of Central Africa "might be an endemic zone for the AIDS agent."[15] Moreover, because AIDS had been reported in a "Black Malian who had never been to Central Africa," the epidemiological frontiers of AIDS were open.[16]

In other instances, "Africans" were used to argue for a certain infectious agent: Robert Gallo used them for his human T-lymphotropic virus III (HTLV-III), and Luc Montagnier used them for the lymphadenopathy-associated virus (LAV). A paper authored by Luc Montagnier and his team opened with a direct invocation of the special position of "Africans" in the classification:

Evidence of a role for retroviruses in acquired immunodeficiency syndrome (AIDS) has been supported by the isolation of a new human T-lymphotropic retrovirus (lymphadenopathy-associated virus; LAV) from high-risk populations such as homosexual men with lymphadenopathy syndrome and from AIDS patients such as a young hemophiliac. [. . .] Many cases of this disorder reported in Europe since 1983 have been in Black patients from Central and Equatorial Africa or Whites who have traveled in this area. They have none of the usual risk factors. Clearly, the isolation of LAV in AIDS patients from the African group, which has geographical, ethnic and epidemiological characteristics distinct from those of the other AIDS risk categories, would be strong support for its role in the disease. (*The Lancet*, June 23, 1984, I/8391, p. 1383)

The competition (in the form of a paper by Robert Gallo and his team, published a year later) answered in a similar way; the special character of the "African" risk category legitimates HTLV-III. Usually, AIDS occurred in homosexuals, bisexuals, IV drug users, their infants, female sexual partners of men with the syndrome, Haitians, and patients with hemophilia. But it had been recently reported in Africa, where there was a high prevalence of KS. KS in African children was similar to KS in homosexual men with AIDS. HTLV-I (the first human retrovirus identified by Robert Gallo) was highly frequent in Central

---

[15] *The Lancet*, April 23, 1983, I/8330, pp. 925–6.
[16] *The Lancet*, October 29, 1983, II/8356, p. 1023 and March 17, 1984, I/8377, p. 631.

Africa too (*Science*, March 1, 1985, 227, p. 1036). Hence, HTLV-III is the causal agent of AIDS. The components of this argument were: (1) dissociation between "Africans" and other risk categories, which reinforces again the special character of the former; (2) association between AIDS-related KS and African KS, which reinforces the special character of "Africans"; (3) HTLV-I is present in Central Africa; and (4) HTLV-I and HTLV-III belong to the same family. Conclusion: the distinctiveness of "Africans" and the copresence between them and a human retrovirus support another retrovirus as the causal agent.

A particular role in making "Africans" an older, special category was played (and not only here) by the "African" Kaposi's sarcoma as the new, AIDS-related KS; this reconfiguration supported the idea that KS (and AIDS too) were much older, endemic phenomena in Equatorial Africa. The identity of the viral agent is supported by the special position of "Africans;" conversely, the African origin of the viral agent reinforces this position. Under these circumstances, "Africans" was a much more stable category than "Haitians." The logic of classification did not require homogeneity; in other words, categories were not included by virtue of certain intrinsic properties, but were defined ad hoc. According to this logic, cases of women and infants of African origin were also classified as "Africans," whereas other similar cases were classified as "Haitians," "women," or "infants." Similarly, cases of homosexual patients of Haitian origin were classified as "Haitians" and not as "homosexuals."

Why Women Were "Discovered" So Late

In January 1983, cases of women with opportunistic infections were clinically described under the heading "Female Sexual Partners of Males with Acquired Immune Deficiency Syndrome" (*MMWR*, January 1983, 31/52). In December 1982, cases of infants with opportunistic infections and immune deficiencies were reported under the heading "infants" (*MMWR* 31/49). Previous reports about opportunistic infections and immune deficiencies in women and children ascribed them to risk categories such as "Haitians" or "transfusion recipients." In spite of early identification, such cases were classified as "risk groups" only in the mid-1980s. This time sequence, among those for other categories, is in contrast to that for "Haitians," which was introduced early and remained a category for two and a half years. Sociologists and cultural critics have tried to explain this paradox either as the effect of moralization (Perrow and Guillen 1990), or of a gender bias (Treichler 1999; Patton 1990). The first explanation essentially claims that the stigma associated with "homosexuals" led to the peripheralization of other risk groups. Women and infants were simply ignored because the strong stigmatization of homosexuals monopolized the attention. The second explanation is that biomedical representations of AIDS were actually gender biased, leaving little or no place for women as a "risk group": AIDS was seen as an essentially male sexual disease with lethal effects, whereas cases of women were a kind of secondary effect.[17] Consequently, they were affixed to the category to which their male partners belonged – i.e., as drug users, Haitians, or sexual partners of bisexual males. According to this logic, cases of infants were classified according to the mothers' status.

The problem with this account is that it is not clear whether AIDS was represented exclusively as a male sexual disease. The empirical evidence seems to inform this thesis: intravenous drug users and hemophiliacs were not represented as gendered, being part of the classification system all the time. Moreover, the syndrome acquired different meanings with respect to "Haitians," "Africans," and "homosexuals": AIDS was presented as a tropical disease, as an endemic state, as related to tribal practices, and much more. Consequently, the place women occupied in the economy of discourse seems to be more complex; although for a long time they were represented as "secondary effects," this does not completely account for them being first ignored and then made into a risk category.

Looking more closely at the first reports and articles on cases of women with opportunistic infections and immune deficiency, we can see that they relate to other risk categories in a specific way. Consider for example the first clinical descriptions. They established a classification for "opportunistic infections or Kaposi's sarcoma (or both) associated with the acquired immune deficiency syndrome (AIDS) in

---

[17] Authors such as Paula Treichler have convincingly shown that the biomedical discourse included a gender bias, AIDS being represented as a male sexual disease related to the "homosexual lifestyle." The question is whether this bias is characteristic of all medical representations of AIDS. Treichler, like other authors, seems to adopt this view, but she restricts her analysis mostly to the "homosexual risk group."

previously healthy persons," which included "white male homosexuals living in urban areas," "heterosexual intravenous drug abusers, a disproportionate number of Haitian immigrants, and a small number of hemophiliacs" (*NEJM*, May 19, 1983, 308/20, p. 1181). Accordingly, the possible causes were defined as "environmental and host factors, including viral or other transmissible agents, illicit drug use, and genetic factors." The main claims were that:

The distribution of the syndrome best fits the hypothesis that AIDS is caused by a biologic agent transmissible by a variety of routes, including sexual contact and intravenous injection. To define further the populations affected with this syndrome and explore the possible role and routes of transmission of a biologic agent, we studied the regular female sexual partners of our male patients with the syndrome. (*NEJM*, May 19, 1983, 308/20, p. 1181)

We encounter several rhetorical strategies here: first, the paper introduces the classification as a framework for representing (1) AIDS and (2) the possible causes, which are of an environmental and/or genetic nature. Two contradictory statements are joined: that the exact cause is unknown and that there are environmental and/or genetic causes. Further, (3) the risk classification ("actual distribution") sustains the thesis of a biologic agent transmissible by different routes. Thus, (3) actually denies (2) and states that a unique agent is the cause of AIDS, on the basis of (1), so that when it comes to formulating the explicit aim of the paper, this already requires taking the unique agent hypothesis for granted.

(1) The construction of a new risk category is announced before it actually begins ("define further the populations affected"); (2) then the thesis of the biological agent is taken for granted; (3) it is defined with respect to the transmission routes; and (4) after this definition, the new risk category is given a name – i.e., "female sexual partners." These four steps can be grouped in the construction of (1) a new risk category and (2) the biologic agent, supported by the representation of transmission routes. At the same time, "female sexual partners" are the grounds for representing transmission routes (it is affirmed that they were studied to define the latter). At a time when the viral model (sexual transmission) clashed with the environmental one (contagious transmission), "female sexual partners" was a strong argument for the former.

Further on, the article stated that the women were exclusively heterosexual, did not use IV drugs, and did not inhale drugs; they did not manipulate drug paraphernalia, were monogamous, and practiced (with the exception of a minority) only vaginal intercourse. By contrast, their male partners used IV drugs, and one of them had had homosexual encounters (*NEJM*, May 19, 1983, 308/20, p. 1182).

The category of "women" was coextensive with "female sexual partners," as the negation of "male partners." The discussion section stated that risk factors like promiscuous male homosexuality and illicit drug use were absent in the women reported by the study: "None were Haitian and none had hemophilia. The only common risk factor we could identify in all the subjects was prolonged monogamous contact with a male patient who had documented AIDS" (*NEJM*, May 19, 1983, 308/20, p. 1183). If one resists the temptation of ruminating about women who were neither male homosexuals nor hemophiliacs, one can see that "women" (or "female sexual partners") as a risk are part of a system which defines them by exclusion from any of the other categories. At the same time, they serve to represent (and confirm) a transmission route. The article states that "subjects who are sexual partners of heterosexual men with AIDS are at risk of acquiring the syndrome." This is repeated twice: "this syndrome is transmissible from men to their female sexual contacts" and the "study suggests that AIDS may be sexually transmitted between heterosexual men and women" (*NEJM*, May 19, 1983, 308/20, p. 1184).

This reveals a more complex situation than that of simply ignoring cases of women with opportunistic infections and immune deficiencies. "Women" is coextensive only with "female sexual partners" here, and the latter is meant as an instrumental representation of a means of transmission. This can work only if female "sexual partners" are at the same time a link in transmitting the disease, a way of transmitting the infectious agent per se, and a "risk" integrated in the given classification.

Other reports proceeded in a similar way: they first presented the cases as "steady sexual partners of males with the acquired immune deficiency syndrome" and of risk groups (*MMWR*, January 7, 1983, 31/52, p. 695), as "heterosexual patients who could not be included in any of these known risk groups" (*JAMA*, September 9, 1983, 250/10, p. 1310), "wives of patients with ARC and AIDS," and "female sexual

partners of male members of high-risk groups" (*JAMA*, October 18,
1985, 254/15, p. 2094). Women were "steady sexual partners" or had
"only one sexual partner," "only had sexual relations with [her] husband" "limited to genital intercourse" (*JAMA*, September 9, 1983,
250/10, p. 1310) or "vaginal–penile intercourse" (*JAMA*, October 18,
1985, 254/15, p. 2095). The infectious agent was "transmitted sexually
or through other intimate contact" (*MMWR*, January 7, 1983, 31/52,
p. 698); a "new transmissible agent . . . spread parenterally and through
sexual contact in a fashion similar to hepatitis B" (*JAMA*, September 9,
1983, 250/10, p. 1312). This allowed AIDS to be identified first in
risk groups like the "bisexual, homosexual, and drug-abusing population." From them, the immune deficiency would spread via heterosexual contacts, but at a diminishing rate, in the "general population."
Because risk factors are characteristic to risk groups, the general population does not know risk factors (*JAMA*, September 9, 1983, 250/10,
p. 1312).

"Female sexual partners of males with AIDS" stood for one-way
transmission. Other models relied on completely different categories,
such as "prostitutes," "Haitians" or "African" women. These were
gender categories and subdivisions of "Haitians" or "Africans" at the
same time (*The Lancet*, March 17, 1984, I/8377, p. 631). Whereas
"female sexual partners" supported male-to-female transmission,
"Haitian" and "African" women supported two-way transmission,
albeit in a complex way, depending on whether they were presented as
prostitutes or not (*JAMA*, March 15, 1985, 253/11, p. 1571). Moreover, the latter two categories supported the argument that the immune
deficiency was expanding in several directions. In turn, "prostitutes"
stood as an intermediary link in a heterosexual male-to-male transmission model. "Mothers with known risk factors" upheld the model
of vertical transmission.[18] These categories relied on different ways of
presenting male and female sexual organs with respect to the infectious
agent and its action.

Because "normal sexual intercourse" was constantly associated with
spouses (who were the only women having "normal intercourse"), it
was an argument against female-to-male transmission. Transmission

---

[18] *JAMA*, May 6, 1983, 249/17, p. 2350 and August 3, 1984, 252/5, p. 643; *NEJM*,
January 12, 1984, 310/2, p. 76.

of the infectious agent from female to male is possible only if the male partner's penis is bruised (as a consequence of past or present STDs).[19] Another argument was that anal intercourse is more infectious than vaginal intercourse: this infectiousness increases when one is having sex with an unknown person. But because anal sexual intercourse is not a great risk factor for heterosexuals, the choice of sexual partner is more important. This, again, marginalized "spouses" with respect to female-to-male transmission (*JAMA*, April 22/29, 1988, 259/16, pp. 2430–31). Besides, female-to-male transmission reported from Africa simply did not match "western culture":

Evidence cited in support of female-to-male transmission is unsubstantiated. Maternal-to-infant transmission of HTLV-III is not analogous to a sexual route of transmission [. . .] Moreover, data from Zaire, where a 1:1 sex ratio of AIDS cases (there is a 9:1 male–female ratio in New York City) may be consistent with female-to-male transmission, do not necessarily apply to Western culture. In central Africa, the role of unsterile needles in the spread of HTLV-III remains unclear. Furthermore, citing the presence of HTLV-III infection in prostitutes does suggest male-to-female spread or IV acquisition of infection; it does not substantiate female-to-male spread. (*JAMA*, April 4, 1986, 255/13, p. 1704)

Prostitutes were then the main argument in favor of female-to-male transmission. They were a "reservoir" of the infectious agent, from which men got infected. The term "reservoir" was used in reports in a double sense: on the one hand, metaphorically, designating an accumulation of infection in this particular "risk group." Thus, "prostitutes constitute a reservoir of HIV, particularly in Central Africa" (*The Lancet*, July 16, 1988, II/8603, p. 164) and "female prostitutes could be an important human reservoir of HTLV-III among the heterosexual population" (*JAMA*, June 21, 1985, 253/23, p. 3378). "African prostitutes" had (unspecified) "abnormal sexual practices" (*The Lancet*, July 16, 1988, II/8603, p. 164), which could facilitate female-to-male transmission. On the other hand, prostitutes were a "reservoir" in the literal sense of the word, with the sperm of customers being deposited in their vagina and directly infecting further clients. They were reservoirs of STDs, facilitating the infection of their clients (*JAMA*, 1986, April 4, 255/13, p. 1704), susceptible to "loss of epithelial integrity"

[19] See *JAMA*, Dec. 13, 1985, 254/22, p. 3177; also, *NEJM*, Feb. 13, 1986, 314/7, p. 417 and Oct. 30, 1986, 315/18, p. 1167.

(that is, bruises of the vagina) which could ease transmission of the virus:

The associations between certain sexually transmitted diseases and HTLV-III antibody in the prostitutes are of interest. These results are consistent with those of a case-control study, which identified a significant correlation between AIDS in homosexual men and a history of syphilis or a reactive microhemag-glutination assay for *T. palladium*. It may be that epithelial integrity is an important barrier to viral transmission and that diseases such as gonorrhea, chancroid or syphilis, which cause mucosal or squamous epithelial discontinu-ity or bleeding, are risk factors for AIDS virus infection. (*NEJM*, February 13, 1986, 314/7, p. 417)

Because female sexual organs were little more than a reservoir of toxic sperm, it was only logical that the latter was the immunosup-pressive agent. Female sexual organs (and hence the female body) were much more suited for dealing with sperm than the male body, which produced it but had no natural mechanisms to filter the sperm's tox-icity, as does the female body. Therefore, women received, deposited, and passed on infectious sperm (which could not penetrate the double barriers of the vagina). The female body was presented not so much as being affected by the infectious agent, but as a kind of store where the latter is deposited over fairly long periods of time and then passed over to male bodies through sexual contact. Women as stores and carriers of sexually transmitted infectious agents was hardly a new concept in the medical discourse on sexually transmitted diseases (Treichler 1988a); medical representations of female sexuality have been entangled with moral judgments and stigmatization of prostitution at least since the nineteenth century (see, e.g., Bernheimer 1989). Cultural representa-tions of female prostitution, and of the prostitutes' bodies, were thus adapted and embedded in the economy of the risk categories.

Women's "natural resistance" to sperm was challenged twice: once in the mid-1980s, by the concurrent two-way transmission model, according to which the infectious agent was transmitted both ways, although at different speeds (*JAMA*, October 18, 1985, 254/15, pp. 2094, 2096). The thesis of two-way transmission at different speeds was also reinforced by the theory that sexual contact might not be the only form of "intimate contact" that could lead to transmission. Other contacts, such as kissing, could lead to infection with the virus. At the beginning of the 1990s, this thesis was challenged a second time, when women were presented as naturally vulnerable to sperm. This theory operated on reversed premises – i.e., that under certain circumstances the female sexual organs might actually be badly equipped for handling sperm and the infectious agents it carried.[20] This "natural vulnerability" was illustrated by "African women"; they were vulnerable to sperm because of the sexual techniques through which they increased sexual satisfaction (techniques of tightening the vagina), their "amoral" or "promiscuous" sexual life with many partners, and rituals such as female circumcision.[21] The thesis of "immunosuppressive sperm" was challenged by the viral agent in the mid-1980s and was reconfigured in the context of "homosexual" risk practices (or factors) at the beginning of the 1990s (see Meyer-Bahlburg et al. 1991). As Philip Setel (1999, p. 184) has convincingly shown, stigmatizing notions such as "promiscuity" or "prostitution" do not adequately apply to the situations of many young African women, who have been dislocated from their traditional village contexts and had to find new means of subsistence in the precarious context of menial trades and services.

We can thus see that there was no unique and coherent etiologic model based on "women." This fact, among others, can explain the paradox of reporting cases without making them into a risk category. And with several subcategories sustaining different, contradictory models, there could hardly be a single, consistent "women" category. "Female sexual partners" supported only male-to-female transmission because they were supposed to have only one steady, already infected sexual partner. "Female sexual partners," "spouses," and "mothers with known risk factors" supported "infants" as a distinct category, but they were a strong counterargument to transmission through "household contact" (*JAMA*, March 15, 1985, 253/11, p. 1573), a thesis sustained by the first reports on "infants." "Prostitutes" sustained the idea of a "reservoir for HTLV-III infection for heterosexually active individuals" (*JAMA*, Oct. 18, 1985, 254/15, p. 2096). "African" women, in turn, meant that the infectious agent circulates by both of these

---

[20] See, for example, *NEJM*, August 20, 1992, 327/8, p. 572; also, *JSTD*, 1992, 20, pp. 96–9.
[21] *NEJM*, July 18, 1985, 313/3, p. 182; *Science*, Nov. 21, 1986, 234, p. 955 and March 14, 1986, 231, p. 1236.

means – a theory upheld by reports of Kaposi's sarcoma in women patients of African origin (the new, immunosuppression-related KS was considered to be male-specific).

"Infants at Risk"

Cases of infants with opportunistic infections and immune deficiencies (unrelated to transfusions) were signaled only very shortly before "female sexual partners" of men with AIDS. In the beginning, these categories were sometimes represented as separate, sometimes as related. It looked as if in some cases infants and newborns could acquire the immune deficiency on their own, independently of their mothers' immune deficiency or of transfusions. Infants of Haitian origin were presented as "Haitian"; being affected by the Acquired Immunodeficiency Syndrome as a newborn did not automatically mean that the mothers were presented as a related category – that is, as "mothers-with-AIDS" (*NEJM*, April 7, 1983, 308/14, p. 842). In the mid-1980s, newborns and infants with the acquired immune deficiency were presented as "infants" and related systematically to "mothers with known risk factors." They supported the vertical transmission of the infectious agent, and a horizontal one (male sexual partner to mother). Thus, infants were sometimes treated as "infants" and sometimes as something completely different; sometimes they supported a specific transmission model, and sometimes they were an additional argument for a given category.

Immune deficiencies in newborns and infants have been known for a long time; several syndromes of congenital immune deficiencies, such as Di George's, Nezelof's, Wiscott-Aldrich's, and SCID (severe combined immunodeficiency disease) were known and described at the time when the first cases of infants were reported. Acquired immune deficiencies in infants and newborns were considered to be, among other things, a consequence of poor diet and living.[22] Both congenital and acquired immune deficiency syndromes in infants lead to the appearance of various opportunistic infections and the depletion of blood cell populations. At the beginning of the 1980s, papers describing

---

[22] See, for example, *AIM*, 1973, 79, pp. 545–50; *JP*, 1974, 85, pp. 717–23.

"cell-mediated immune defects" (*AJDC*, 1980, 134, p. 824), "immunologically compromised children" (*AJDC*, 1980, 134, p. 1149) or "antibody deficiency" (*AJDC*, 1981, 135, p. 618) were frequent in pediatric journals. These syndromes were characterized (in the context
of *AIDS*) as "well-defined," "rare, poorly characterized" (*MMWR*,
December 17, 1982, 31/49, p. 667), "recognized laboratory patterns
for known congenital immune defects" (*JAMA*, May 6, 1983, 249/17,
p. 2347), "readily diagnosable," and "sporadic and of uncertain etiology" (*The Lancet*, April 30, 1983, I/8331, pp. 957–8). The problem
was to present opportunistic infections and laboratory findings indicative of immunodeficiency in infants as AIDS-related, and not as related
to other syndromes of pediatric immune deficiency. One could suppose
that "infants" appeared in this context as a consequence of laboratory
evidence and arguments made about the specific characteristics of the
opportunistic infections – in other words, that it was derived from
and enforced by "facts." But let us examine how the first report from
MMWR presented "Unexplained Immunodeficiency and Opportunistic Infections in Infants – New York, New Jersey, California."

The case descriptions stated the ethnic status of infants (Black/
Hispanic, Haitian, and White), followed by short descriptions of *Pneumocystis, Mycobacterium avium-intracellulare*, and *Candida* infections
(*MMWR*, December 17, 1982, 31/49, pp. 665–6). The mothers of the
infants were described according to residence and to the "sociodemo-
graphic profile" – that is, according to ethnic status, drug abuse history,
and prostitution history. The editorial note stated that the nature of the
immune dysfunction is "unclear" and compared it with other congenital immunodeficiency syndromes described in children (Di George's
and Nezelof's). It also asserted that "they [the immunologic features
of high-normal or elevated immunoglobulin levels and T-lymphocyte
depletion] have, however been described in a few children with variants
of Nezelof's syndrome." The conclusion was that:

It is possible that these infants had the acquired immune deficiency syndrome
(AIDS). Although the mother of the infant in case 1 was not studied immunologically, her death from PCP was probably secondary to AIDS. The mothers
of the other three infants were Haitian or intravenous drug abusers, groups
at increased risk for AIDS. The immunologic features described in the case
reports resemble those seen both in adults with AIDS and in a child reported
to have developed immunodeficiency following receipt of blood products from

a patient with AIDS. [. . .] Although the etiology of AIDS remains unknown, a series of epidemiologic observations suggest it is caused by an infectious agent. If the infants described in the four case reports had AIDS, exposure to the putative "AIDS agent" must have occurred very early. [. . .] Transmission of an "AIDS agent" from mother to child, either in utero or shortly after birth, could account for the early onset of immunodeficiency in these infants. (*MMWR*, December 17, 1982, 31/49, p. 667)

The whole structure of the argument is (1) to make an assertion (that a patient has AIDS), (2) to then state it as a possibility, (3) to then deny it as a mere possibility on the grounds of the given classification, and (4) to state similarities with immunologic features in the classification. Simultaneously, it is stated that: (1) the cases belong to this classification, (2) therefore, it is the same disease. The first line of argument negates the opening assertions of the "editorial note" and excludes the immune deficiency from being a congenital syndrome. The second line of argument concerns the etiology of AIDS. It is made possible by the classification of the immune deficiency as AIDS. It first states that the etiology is unknown, and then negates this statement by asserting that (1) there is a causally acting infectious agent (2) supported by epidemiologic observations. Afterward, it states that early exposure to the infectious agent depends on whether the described infants had AIDS. This is already taken for granted, and the argument takes the form of a syllogism. The transmission (i.e., the "early exposure") is "either in utero or shortly after birth" and accounts for the early onset of immunodeficiency. Simultaneously, this is used as a counterargument to the possibility of a congenital syndrome. Thus, the thesis of a new (intra- or extrauterine) means of transmission is the result of a complex string of arguments which, paradoxically enough, identify the reported cases as instantiations of given risk classifications.

"Facts" such as opportunistic infections or laboratory evidence for depletion of blood cells are presented here in a classificatory frame that actually made them possible as "facts" and as evidence for AIDS. In turn, they enforce the classification, along with "infants" as empirical evidence. The possibility that laboratory findings and clinical symptoms are related to other congenital or acquired immune deficiencies appears as incompatible with the frame and is rejected. Journal articles argued that the association between malnutrition, poor living, and immune deficiencies was known for many years, whereas that between AIDS and the reported symptoms in the "children's communities" was new (*JAMA*, May 6, 1983, 249/17, pp. 2348–9). This news was a strong argument for AIDS in infants. Others argued that the observed immune deficiency was not congenital; it was like the one reported in homosexuals and drug addicts (*JAMA*, May 6, 1983, 249/17, pp. 2353–4). Several cases had been initially diagnosed with Nezelof's syndrome, a diagnosis which had to be revised. The means of contesting such diagnoses was to assert that syndromes such as Nezelof's were unknown and contested in the medical community (*JAMA*, August 3, 1984, 252/5, pp. 642–3). Because the report of such symptoms in children coincided with the appearance of AIDS, the coincidence itself was a powerful argument in favor of an AIDS diagnosis (*NEJM*, January 12, 1984, 310/2, p. 80).

This reversed the characterization of pediatric immune deficiencies as well known or well defined and put them on a par with AIDS. Both were unknown; consequently, they could not be distinguished from each other. This reversal transformed AIDS – one might say with a single stroke – into a pediatric immune defect. Relevant here is the fact that the classification of the reported cases is paralleled by a reclassification of AIDS as another form of immune deficiency. When children and infants are no longer "Haitians" or "offspring of drug abusers," it becomes important to redefine AIDS too, so that it can fit the new category. The two – "children" and "pediatric AIDS" – become now mutually reinforcing, without affecting the meaning of "adult AIDS."

The result of these transformations in the line of argument – i.e., a new category in the risk classification based on the empirical evidence – is the premise allowing the argument to unfold from empirical evidence to its conclusion (Pêcheux 1975).

"Infants" as a distinct category was confronted with pediatric immunodeficiency syndromes that have similar opportunistic infections and symptoms; therefore, "infants" could not have the syndromes they can have as infants. The possibility of congenital immune defects (Nezelof's and Di George's syndromes) was mentioned in articles. Lab results were compared both to known pediatric immune syndromes and to the risk group of "homosexuals and drug addicts with AIDS." The classificatory frame, however, made it possible to present the syndrome as a distinct pediatric disease and as a variety of AIDS at the same time. Later reports used the expression "pediatric AIDS" to designate this double status, which was usual throughout the 1980s. A clinical report stated that "the hypothesis that these children (i.e., the cases described) have a pediatric form of AIDS is most strongly supported by associations with adults with AIDS" (*JAMA*, August 3, 1984, 252/5, pp. 642–3), thus using risk classification as the strongest argument. Writing in the comment section about the fact that some children were initially diagnosed with Nezelof's syndrome, the report concluded:

A few of the children included in our survey had a provisional diagnosis of Nezelof's syndrome, a variant of severe combined immunodeficiency (SCID). This syndrome, when originally put forth, was described as a condition of cell-mediated immunodeficiency in a child with embryonic thymus. There is disagreement in the literature as to the diagnostic criteria for Nezelof's syndrome, and rather than being considered a distinct entity, it is characterized as a variant of SCID. [...] Nothing is known of the etiology of Nezelof's syndrome. Until a specific diagnostic test for either Nezelof's syndrome or pediatric AIDS becomes available, a clear distinction between these two entities may not be possible. (*JAMA*, August 3, 1984, 252/5, p. 643)

The report pleads here directly for "pediatric AIDS" as a variety of Nezelof's syndrome, and therefore as a pediatric disease; at the same time, it invokes risk classification as the strongest argument for the described condition being a form of AIDS. (The paper refers throughout to the difficulties of diagnosing congenital infection and congenital immune deficiency.)

The paradox is that to show that infants do have the acquired immunodeficiency syndrome, they have to be presented as non-infants, and if they are presented as infants, then it cannot be shown that they have AIDS. Conversely, AIDS in "infants" has to be the Acquired Immunodeficiency Syndrome of the adult risk categories and, at the same time, a pediatric syndrome distinct from other pediatric syndromes. Thus, "infants" are similar to "women," where the central risk figure is supported by different representations that are parallel and at times contradict each other.

This explains why AIDS historians had the impression that "infants" and "women" were latecomers, neglected or inconsistent, although they were in fact central categories enforcing theses such as the universal or the vertical transmission of the infectious agent. They were actually a multiplicity of discourses running in different directions, intersecting, and retaining traces of each other. Their manifold and contradictory character made possible central claims about AIDS as having universal, two-way, or vertical transmission.

Classification Practices and the Meaning of AIDS

Did these classification practices produce different meanings for AIDS? If one takes into account only the official definitions provided by the Centers for Disease Control and Prevention and by the World Health Organization (which have also changed several times over the past two decades), the answer is no. According to these definitions, there are precise criteria (periodically updated) for diagnosing AIDS (McGovern and Smith 2001, p. 33). The official definition of the syndrome seems to provide a precise meaning for the Acquired Immunodeficiency Syndrome. It is grounded in empirical evidence (provided by lab results) for the presence of antibodies to the HI-viruses and/or the presence of opportunistic infections. The definitions of AIDS have also been differentiated according to the laboratory technology available in different countries. We now have an advanced definition of AIDS, appropriate for technologically developed countries, and a less advanced one, for the less developed countries. This sometimes gives occasion for open controversies about the interpretation of opportunistic diseases, or about whether there is actually any opportunistic disease at all (Crystal and Jackson 1992; Miller 1992). Nevertheless, the definitions (and hence the meaning) of the syndrome do not seem to be shattered by such incidents, assuming that the advanced definition always works in advanced countries, and the less advanced one works in less advanced countries. Upon closer examination, this very definition appears to be not only a matter of negotiation, but also rhetorically constituted.

I briefly discuss here an empirical example that shows how the meaning of the retroviral agent and the definition of the syndrome are constituted. The reported case is one of a patient whose death has been diagnosed as due to renal failure. The report simultaneously negotiates two different, contradictory aspects of the case: it contests the diagnosis of renal failure and argues that the official definition of AIDS should be enlarged to cover apparent cases of renal failure:

It is recognized that renal failure leads to impairment of host defenses, including cell-mediated immunity. Therefore, the occurrence of *Pneumocystis carinii* pneumonia or other opportunistic infections in a patient with preexisting renal failure would not meet the case definition for AIDS. A patient seen recently at our clinic illustrates this problem. [. . .] This patient was a member of a group (intravenous drug abusers) clearly at risk for AIDS and had one of the characteristic opportunistic infections, the characteristic immunodeficiency and a positive ELISA for antibodies to the causative virus. It was assumed that he had infection caused by HTLV-III/LAV, and he was treated accordingly. However, because of renal failure he did not meet the case definition for AIDS. (*NEJM*, May 22, 1986, 314/21, p. 1386)

We encounter here a strong argument: antibodies to HTLV-III/LAV were identified through a test. But the problem is whether these antibodies were produced as a reaction to the retrovirus entering the body after an immune impairment caused by renal failure, or whether renal failure was a consequence of the presence of HTLV-III/LAV in the body. The first possibility means rejecting the causal role of the retrovirus, which appears only as a consequence of an already existing immunodeficiency. The dilemma cannot be decided on the grounds of a laboratory test for antibodies to HIV. The two claims of the paper are mutually exclusive: if the patient did not die of renal failure, an extension of the definition would not be necessary, and if the definition has to be extended, then it would not be necessary to contest it anymore. Nevertheless, the article actually succeeds in supporting both claims. First, it contrasts renal failure to AIDS and stresses similarities with other cases (impairment of host defenses); then, it defines the patient in a way that denies a relationship between renal failure and IV drug consumption. The latter, as a risk factor, is associated with AIDS. Thus, renal failure is conducive to immunosuppression, which in turn leads to *Pneumocystis* pneumonia. This excludes the case from being AIDS. This argument is contradicted by a second: belonging to a risk group, taken along with the presence of PCP, immunosuppression, and the positive result of the ELISA test, makes the case for AIDS. The conjunction is at the same time an implication: belonging to a risk group means that *Pneumocystis*, immunosuppression, and a positive ELISA test mean AIDS.

Thus, (1) renal failure as a diagnosis is denied and (2) an inconsistency of the AIDS definition is emphasized. The definition does not succeed in covering consistently the risk group to which it refers. The device of risk manages in this case to (1) enforce a classification,

(2) successfully challenge a possible causal model, (3) argue for an alternative model, and (4) demand a revision of the definition. The identity of the retrovirus, its role in the immune deficiency, and the significance of the test are enforced by an apparently paradoxical rhetorical move: contesting and reconstructing the definition of AIDS with the help of "risk." This shows that risk groups are not derived from the definition of the disease; the latter is dependent on how one operates with risk groups. Although the definition as such does not explicitly refer to risk, but rather to opportunistic infections and to test results, what counts as relevant is negotiated and decided by using the device of risk.

The construction of categories such as "homosexuals," "Haitians," "hemophiliacs," or "Africans" did not necessarily imply presenting the syndrome in one and the same way everywhere (Brandt 1988; Gilman 1993). "Haitians" and the first accounts of a virus passing the barrier between animals and humans relied on a tropical setting. In "homosexuals," the infectious agent was tied to histories of sexually transmitted diseases, sexual acts, and frequencies of sexual contacts. These are only two examples of how the meanings of the syndrome vary depending on risk classifications.

With respect to "homosexuals," AIDS took the meaning of a sexually transmitted disease supported by the history of other sexually transmitted diseases, the environment of sexual contacts, the "sexual lifestyle," and the spatial organization of sexual acts. Even the retroviral agent was presented as the agent of a sexually transmitted disease and, simultaneously, of an immune deficiency. It could induce immune deficiency only if it induced STDs. On the one hand, AIDS was presented as a syndrome and therefore as a general condition that led to the further development of various diseases and infections. On the other hand, it was ascribed the status of a sexually transmitted disease. Opportunistic infections such as *Pneumocystis* pneumonia or Kaposi's sarcoma were represented as sexually transmitted diseases, related either to sexual orientation or to a known sexually transmitted agent.[23] The first reports on opportunistic infections and Kaposi's sarcoma, while presenting them as new and problematic phenomena, stressed the significance of the sexually transmitted cytomegalovirus and sexual

[23] *JAMA*, March 26, 1982, 247/12, p. 1741 and April 2, 1982, 247/13, p. 1861.

orientation. Several epidemiologic studies took hepatitis B (as a sexually transmitted disease) as a pattern for AIDS in the "homosexual" group; this similarity supported the idea of a viral agent. Interestingly enough, the possibility of multiple, simultaneous means of transmission (present in the hepatitis B model) was ignored, although it meant that a virus can be transmitted through sexual contact and blood transfusions at the same time. Reports argued instead for sequential transmission, first through homosexual contact and then through transfusions. Hepatitis B–modeled AIDS remained essentially a sexually transmitted disease.

The virus was transmitted first through homosexual, as well as heterosexual, contacts and afterward through IV drug consumption (shared needles) and blood transfusion. Frequency of sexual contacts among homosexuals played a key role as a trigger of this chain reaction (*NEJM*, January 12, 1984, 310/2, p. 69). However, risk-specific gender differences made it very difficult for the infectious agent to be transmitted through heterosexual sex.[24] Hence, the syndrome had a double, paradoxical status: it was a particular condition of the immune system, leading to various diseases and infections, and a group-specific sexually transmitted disease, explained through special risk factors. One might believe that such theses have long since been abandoned and constitute nothing more than a kind of historical curiosity now. This is in fact not the case. I show in Chapter 3 how the "resistant vagina" thesis was replaced by that of the "fragile vagina" in the late 1980s and early 1990s. The contraposition of the former (i.e., the "fragile anus" thesis) was still used in the 1990s in prevention research, with results that sometimes seem absurd. Thus, a study on "risk behaviors" published in 1991 (Meyer-Bahlburg et al. 1991, pp. 18–9) correlated different types of sexual acts in HIV-positive and HIV-negative "homosexuals" with blood cell counts. The results were that $CD4+$ lymphocytes correlated positively with unprotected anal sex and that the $CD4/CD8$ ratio was positively correlated with the variables "troubles with climax" and "troubles with ejaculation."

My argument here is that the view of AIDS as an STD has led to specific approaches in prevention research and policies that do not always

---

[24] *JAMA*, May 6, 1983, 249/17, p. 2372 and January 13, 1984, 251/2, pp. 240–1.

seem to be very effective. As recently noted,[25] this approach does not work at all well with gay people in their early and mid-twenties. The STD-based prevention policies represent condoms as a means of protection against STD *and* AIDS. Condoms help prevent the unwelcome, scary consequences of infection. Although this scare-based strategy worked well with earlier generations (which had direct, concrete experience of what it means to live with HIV and AIDS), it remains abstract and ineffective in younger generations, which may not perceive condoms as protection against AIDS anymore.

Classifications as Boundary Objects

Another effect of this classification system was that at least in certain instances it brought together scientists from various disciplines. It created a frame in which heterogeneous research interests and perspectives could talk to each other. The property of scientific objects of accommodating heterogeneous interests, time horizons, and perspectives is expressed by the notion of boundary object (Star 1989, p. 47). Boundary objects can be engineering blueprints, software codes, maps, or classifications (but not only these). They are heterogeneous, expandable, and recombinable. They are not given once and for all, but are continuously modified in the process of their use. Due to their plasticity, they can be used by scientific practitioners from different disciplines, thus enabling scientific cooperation and the production of knowledge. At least in the case of "pediatric AIDS," the classification of AIDS risk displays the properties of a boundary object.

Even if the association STD/AIDS has been noticed and discussed by sociologists, the significance of AIDS for the risk group of infants and children has remained relatively obscure and neglected. Children were a paradoxical group: they were presented as belonging to a known category (such as "Haitians," "Africans," or "drug users") and as a special category at the same time. Apparently, the description of opportunistic diseases, infections, and symptoms was uniform. For many cases of children and infants, the diagnostic of Acquired Immunodeficiency Syndrome was accompanied by the description of opportunistic

---

[25] See Erica Goode: "With Fears Fading, More Gays Spurn Old Preventive Message." *The New York Times,* August 19, 2001. Section 1, p. 1.

infections and other diseases. The blood cell count was a ubiquitous argument. Laboratory results of antibody tests for HTLV-III, LAV, or HIV appeared later (and were discussed at various times in various journals), so that until 1988–9 arguments relied mainly on cell counts and laboratory evidence for opportunistic diseases. Another important factor was the evolution of the diagnosed opportunistic infections and their response to treatment. This is a widely established canon in clinical reports; its significance here was augmented by the necessity of showing the problematic or different character of the respective infections, or their resistance to therapy. Against this background, reported cases were classified according to the parents' ethnic status, addiction, social situation, weight, and developmental milestones, all mixed together (*JAMA*, May 6, 1983, 249/17, pp. 2351–2). Openings also contained short descriptions of the mothers' risk status ("drug addict," "promiscuous," "alcoholic," "heroin addict"), which reclassifies the cases as belonging to different risk categories.

The classifications were followed by detailed descriptions of the opportunistic infections, the infants' actual condition and, occasionally, the therapy. At first sight, there is nothing unusual about the case descriptions; but such mixed-up classifications in the case openings project the opportunistic infections and diseases against the background of typical infant diseases. Data about birth weight and pregnancy term, along with "normal developmental milestones," created a pediatric frame for the descriptions of infections (*JAMA*, May 6, 1983, 249/17, p. 2356). At the same time, case descriptions opened up the possibility of reordering cases according to the mother's risk status. They created thus two representational tracks, one pediatric and one AIDS-related, so it became easy to shift "infants" back and forth between them. This also allowed shifting the description of clinical symptoms back and forth between the two tracks (*JAMA*, May 6, 1983, 249/17, p. 2354).

"Acquired Immunodeficiency Syndrome in infants," equated with "pediatric AIDS," became a condition with a double status: an infant-specific disease and at the same time one characteristic of the risk group background. It was made possible by the abandonment of "household risk" in favor of integrating households or families in risk areas (that is, in risk categories). The "household risk" thesis did not compare the described immune deficiency symptoms in infants with known congenital immunodeficiencies, but rather considered only the possibility of the said symptoms being due to neglect and malnutrition. This possibility was rejected because poverty, neglect, and malnutrition in children had been present for a long time, while the Acquired Immunodeficiency Syndrome was recent (*JAMA*, May 6, 1983, 249/17, p. 2348). The double status of infants was maintained until the end of the 1980s, well after serologic evidence for antibodies to the retrovirus became possible. Cases of children with opportunistic infections were continuously presented against the background of adult risk groups.[26] The expressions "infants at-risk" and "mothers at-risk," or "at-risk population," were used simultaneously in medical articles at the end of the 1980s, meaning one and the same thing: the ascription to established risk categories. Infants were designated as being at risk (which made them a somewhat autonomous category) and at the same time as "at-risk infants," which ascribed them to pre-existing categories. Individual case presentations retained the form discussed previously: the openings created a pediatric frame (developmental milestones, birth weight, pregnancy term, infant-specific diseases),[27] against which the syndrome was to be evaluated. Nevertheless, the ambiguity of the distinctions between the diagnosis of "pediatric AIDS" and that of congenital immunodeficiency syndromes, between adult and pediatric AIDS, was clear in later clinical reports and articles:

The major difficulty in diagnosis of HIV infection in infants results from placental transfer of maternal IgG to the fetal circulation, thereby preventing accurate diagnosis by routine enzyme-linked immunosorbent assay or Western blot. (*AJDC*, 1989, 143, p. 1147)

The paper acknowledged the difficulty of a "conclusive diagnosis of congenital infection": a clear-cut identification of the immune deficiency as acquired or congenital was difficult for practitioners. At the same time the presence of antibodies to HIV was regarded as a mere confirmation of the mother's status (*AJDC*, 1989, 143, p. 1151). The double status of acquired immune deficiency in infants also made it possible to argue for perinatal (or vertical) transmission of the infectious agent as an additional means of transmission, complementing

---

[26] See for example *AJDC*, 1988, 142, p. 29 and 143, pp. 775, 1147.
[27] See *AJDC*, 1988, 142, pp. 32–3.

the model of horizontal transmission (sexual and through blood/blood products). In turn, vertical transmission reinforced this double status, providing a satisfactory explanation for how an adult disease could be transformed into an infant one.

This rhetorical strategy made it possible to bring researchers with quite different interests into the same cognitive frame: it connected AIDS researchers, mainly oriented toward male adults, with pediatricians, who were interested in children's and infants' diseases and immune deficiencies. A common frame for discussion and debate was created for specialists who otherwise would not have had any contact and continued to work separately. Moreover, in introducing a problem (Is there a pediatric AIDS?), it legitimated the collaboration between different fields of expertise.

From this perspective, it can be argued that this strategy (distributed over several articles), with its double representational track, indecisiveness, openness, and multiple and continuous reclassifications, acted as a boundary object in the sense described by Star and Griesemer (1989): it brought together specialists from different medical fields, created a common pool of problems and expectations, legitimated a research area, and contributed to the coordination of knowledge production.

How Classifications Work

How do these classifications work? How do they produce knowledge? A classical argument about classifications is that the categories with which people make sense of the natural world mirror their social organization (Durkheim 1965 [1915]). In other words, social actors represent natural phenomena according to the categories in which they structure their lives. These categories are stable and orderly; therefore, they allow social actors to produce stable, reliable knowledge about the natural world.

The medical representations of the Acquired Immunodeficiency Syndrome, of its accompanying symptoms, and of its character as a new disease were certainly framed by classificatory operations which produced risk categories. The historically determined cultural background of these categories played a significant role here. At the same time, their plasticity is surprising: classifications were not made according to a strict definition or scheme, but rather according to the ad hoc requirements of concrete contexts of argumentation. The completely heterogeneous character of the risk categories was not a hindrance, but rather a significant element in advancing the thesis of a new immune deficiency. Categories were not monolithic; they were made up of various, and not seldom contradictory subcategories. As previously shown, "women" comprised several subcategories, supporting contradictory representations of how the causal agent worked.

Therefore, we cannot conceive of classifications as consisting of given, immutable categories, in the way Émile Durkheim and Marcel Mauss (1963) saw them operating in "primitive societies." In the Durkheimian tradition, Mary Douglas (1992b, p. 263) sees the categories according to which the natural world is classified as an unambiguous, "perfect notation system" on which theories are built. The classifications examined here, however, are neither clear-cut nor immutable. Rather, classifications are hybrids, in the sense that they mix up formal and informal, clear-cut and fuzzy criteria (Bowker and Star 1999, p. 54).

The view I propose here is a practice-ground one: we should not see classifications as sets of categories, but rather as networks of classificatory operations. These operations stabilize and expand the classificatory system by making it plastic and adaptable. In the course of these transformations, categories may change locally, while the stability of the system as such is increased. In the economy of AIDS risk categories, definitions and characterizations of particular groups changed all the time; this, however, did not affect the stability of the system. Risk categories continued to be used in medical articles well into the 1990s.

A helpful analogy may perhaps be provided here by thinking of the ways in which viruses survive and adapt by changing small portions of their protein structure. Classifications may be said to possess the same property of effecting local, context-bound changes. This allows them to remain stable, reproduce, expand, and absorb various, even contradictory explanatory models. It is not so much logical coherence, underlying general principles, and immutability that make classifications work. Rather, it is adaptability, local changeability, expandability, and absorption of contradicting categories. As I show in Chapter 3, classifications played an active role in the hybridization and transformation of causal and epidemiologic explanations, as well as in controversies about the AIDS infectious agent. A key criterion for their epistemic success and relevance was the ability to support heterogeneous representations of the agent. Without this ability, little additional knowledge could be gained. As it turned out, the classificatory system was able to support not one, but several (contradictory) representations. How, then, did this happen?

3

The Etiologic Agent and the Rhetoric of Scientific Debate

The Sociology of Scientific Debates

In this chapter, I show how the system of risk categories generated and supported a number of contradictory theses about the etiologic agent. One of the first questions arising here is: how were these theses debated in medical articles? Did they unleash a controversy? How was it resolved, and what factors played a role in this process?

Scientific controversies have been studied intensively in the sociology of science (e.g., Collins 1988; Latour 1988; Barnes, Bloor, and Henry 1996). A scientific controversy is usually understood as "a publicly and persistently maintained dispute... concerned with a matter of belief" (McMullin 1987, p. 51). It implies an ongoing disagreement, with continuing argument and counterargument, usually on two sides. These sides have public exchanges, so that the scientific community can judge the case. In many cases, scientific controversies involve the replication of a key experiment (Gieryn 1999); the mobilization of material, social, and cultural resources; or changes in group competencies and social relations as major factors influencing the controversies' outcomes.

Some controversies are decided in a couple of months or even weeks; others may take several years or even decades. Controversies may be resolved or closed: in the first case, the scientific community agrees on the merits of the case. In the second case, there is no community agreement, yet the topic at stake becomes less important, slips quietly out of the limelight, or does not receive the material and time resources it needs to be resolved. A scientific disagreement or debate is different from a controversy: although they are public, scientific debates do not involve a direct challenge to one thesis by its opposite (McMullin 1987, p. 53). Several positions may be involved in scientific debates: these positions are not necessarily clear-cut, and resolution may not always take the shape of an unequivocal decision. Generally speaking, debates may involve beliefs, attitudes, or both. Scientific debates, however, are mostly concerned with beliefs about the nature, way of working, or properties of an entity.

Because debates, as well as controversies, imply the public expression of beliefs, they are intrinsically tied to the use of argument and persuasion. They require the public presentation of data and facts, the formulation of hypotheses, and the construction of ties from these hypotheses to the conclusion. Students of scientific controversies (e.g., Latour 1988; Clarke 1990; Pickering 1995) have stressed the role played by (1) the mobilization of various resources, including rhetorical ones, and (2) the negotiation of problem boundaries. These elements are relevant with respect to how a scientific explanatory model becomes dominant while others are rejected.

The first element essentially means that capacity of scientific persuasion depends on the weight of the assets a scientist can accumulate: these include journal articles, but also laboratory probes, instruments, research money, social relations, and her position at a prestigious research center. The more persuasive means a scientist has, the better she will disseminate her results in the community. In the case of a debate or controversy, she will be able to tip the balance in her favor by using these resources. The second position claims that the definition of scientific problems and the distinctions between different kinds of problems and between problems and non-problems are not given but rather subject to negotiations in the scientific community. In fact, scientists spend a great deal of time tracing these boundaries (Galison 1996a). Deciding what is a scientific problem and what is not plays a decisive role in many scientific controversies; therefore, scientists will seek to persuade the community of their definition of the problem. In this respect, again, rhetorical resources are used to define problems and to trace boundaries between science and non-science and between the relevant and the irrelevant, in order to win debates and controversies.

Therefore, an important feature of the sociology of scientific debates is examining the rhetorical resources and strategies, as well as the broader cultural representations, that intervene in debates in the scientific community. In this chapter, I analyze the debates about the nature of the etiologic agent of AIDS. In Chapter 4, I focus on the full-fledged scientific controversy about the discovery of the HI-virus.

The common wisdom is that it took a long time to identify the etiologic agent of AIDS as a human (retro)virus because of the extraordinary complexity of the syndrome; that at first there were several hypotheses about the nature of the agent, mere errors in the development of medical knowledge. In time, the empirical (that is, laboratory) evidence led to the correct identification of the retrovirus. Some notions about "risk factors" (such as those concerning the role of amyl nitrites) may have initially led medical researchers up a dead-end street, but in the end the human retrovirus was almost unanimously accepted as the causal agent. There was of course some messy controversy between Dr. Robert Gallo and Dr. Luc Montagnier, but this is secondary with respect to the unanimous acceptance of the retrovirus idea.

AIDS historians consider that, in the mid-1980s (when the retroviral agent was identified), the notion of "risk factors" replaced that of "risk groups" (Oppenheimer 1992). This replacement played an important role in the identification of the HI-virus because it allowed more accurate representations of how it entered the body and how it acted upon the immune system. Therefore, the shift from a focus on collective to individual behavior stimulated the advance of medical knowledge. Most of the time, "risk factors" have been interpreted as forms of (sexual) behavior (Wermuth, Ham, and Robbins 1992; Meyer-Bahlburg 1991; Estep, Waldorf, and Marotta 1992; Connors 1992): the sexual behavior of men who have sex with men (equated by most empirical studies with "homosexuals"), the sexual behavior of African women, that of sex workers, and that of intravenous drug users. But it is not at all clear whether "risk factors" ever actually did surplant "risk groups": both have continued to be used to date.

Between mid-1981 and mid-1983, two clusters of etiologic models were dominant: (1) viral and (2) environmental models. After mid-1983, a hybrid emerged, combining elements of the two. The result is known today as the explanatory model of a family of human retroviruses (human immunodeficiency viruses), whose effects on the immune system are favored (and accelerated) by a series of factors. The first reports of Kaposi's sarcoma stipulated a viral cause for this skin cancer form; opportunistic infections such as PCP, in turn, were clearly associated with an immune deficiency. Bringing together KS and opportunistic infections contributed to a model in which a viral agent, favored by sexually transmitted diseases, led to an immune deficiency. This infectious agent affected certain categories, according to their specific "risk factors"; these provided the facilitating environment in which the agent could affect the immune system and pass from individual to individual.

Viruses and Lifestyles

The environmental model asserted that the agent responsible had to be sought in the social environment of "risk groups." This environment consisted of category-specific "risk factors," which were sufficient and necessary conditions for the immune deficiency. The viral agent was related to the "history of sexually transmitted diseases" of risk groups, which was either directly associated with the infectious agent (as in the cytomegalovirus thesis) or constituted the antecedents of the viral infection. A "history" of STDs was also considered proof of multiple sexual partners. The "disease history" of the body was understood as being the social history of the patients and as providing a profile of their risk. Environmental discourses stressed risky "lifestyles," circumscribed by certain social spaces. The use of inhalant drugs and sexual practices in baths or in clubs were seen as being intrinsic to the definition of risk groups, as constituting their social environment, and as being the cause of the immunodeficiency.

After mid-1983, environmental risk factors were seen as related to a viral agent, irrespective of whether there was a history of sexually transmitted diseases. The result was that the viral agent thesis was reinforced by behavior- and lifestyle-determined, group-specific "risk factors." These were seen as forms of (sexual and non-sexual) behavior produced in and by a social environment favorable to the transmission of the human retrovirus. An example: throughout most of the 1980s, female sexual organs were considered a biological environment much more resistant to HIV than the male sexual organs of "homosexuals."

Because of this natural resistance, it was very improbable that the virus could pass into blood through the vaginal walls. At the beginning of the 1990s, when the rates of infection among women rose, it was argued that the female sexual organs are much more sensitive and vulnerable to infection than the male sexual organs (Brown, Ayowa, and Brown 1993). But this made it difficult to explain how the virus could be passed from women to men. "Women" were overwhelmingly represented as receivers or "reservoirs" of the retrovirus; an account was needed for how they managed to pass it to men, if penises are more resistant. The "history of sexually transmitted diseases" made it possible to explain how the virus could get through the cuts and sores of the penile skin and enter the bloodstream. The differences in the "natural vulnerability" of heterosexual men and women were thus constituted as translations of the differences in the nature and character of risk factors. On the one hand, there was the "female vulnerability," provoked by environmental factors (circumcision rituals, sexual practices of "African" women, and so forth); on the other hand, there was the "male vulnerability," determined by the history of STDs.

Another significant aspect of this model was the spatialization of risk factors. These were initially conceived as given by the history of sexually transmitted diseases. The environmental model saw them as spatially arranged factors – that is, as forms of behavior that in certain social spaces are specific to each "risk group." Thus, the risk behavior of the "homosexual" risk group was produced in clubs, bars, and saunas. That of IV drug users was given by the shooting galleries. For Africans, it was remote rural places. Spatial models of contagious agents were not a novelty: they have been used since the nineteenth century in order to make sense of contagious diseases such as diphtheria, typhus, or tuberculosis (Hardy 1993). The environmental model was to a large extent similar to these action-at-distance models: all asserted that the social environment propagated the immune deficiency. It is no coincidence that theses such as "household transmission" or "transmission through casual contact"[1] were formulated in this model. Relevant in this context is that the STD model was combined with a contagious one – a hybridization with important consequences for the idea of a retroviral agent.

---

[1] See *JAMA*, May 6, 1983, 249/17, pp. 2345–49 and Sept. 20, 1985, 254/11, p. 1429.

Against this background, a series of puzzles arises: how was it possible that two such contradictory models should appear and coexist (for a while at any rate) in the same system of categories? The differences between the "viral agent" and the "lifestyle" theses have long been noted by commentators; however, the fundamentally different assumptions on which they rely have not been discussed in detail. Their hybridization appears then even more puzzling. How was it possible to combine them? In the case examined here, however, the "lifestyle" model was not completely rejected; rather, some of its key elements became incorporated in explanations of how the viral agent worked.

Scientific Knowledge, Debates, and the Financing of AIDS Research

In many cases, the debates between proponents of the viral and the environmental thesis, respectively, did not take the form of open controversies, with each party explicitly attacking the opponents' arguments. Rather, these debates were conducted as oblique attacks on the fundamental assumptions of the opponents. In mid-1983, the debates gained in significance, due to the decision of the U.S. Public Health Service to spend an extra $14.5 million on AIDS research. Critics pointed out that, actually, these were not additional research funds but money taken from other research programs and redirected to AIDS research (*Nature*, August 11, 1983, 304, p. 478). The problem was determining on which AIDS research topics this money should be spent. At about the same time, in August 1983, the Subcommittee on Intergovernmental Relations and Human Resources of the U.S. House of Representatives held a series of hearings on AIDS research, where passionate arguments were made for research funding.[2]

The decision to redirect the research money came at a time when (1) the AIDS research community still debated the viral vs. the environment

---

[2] The Reagan administration had been strongly criticized for its lack of interest in funding AIDS research and for ignoring the social dimensions of the epidemic. The hearings before the Subcommittee on Intergovernmental Relations and Human Resources of the U.S. House of Representatives assembled prominent AIDS researchers and activists; moreover, they revealed the amounts spent between 1981 and 1983 by the Centers for Disease Control and Prevention and the National Institutes of Health on AIDS research.

thesis and (2) the first papers by Dr. Robert Gallo and Dr. Luc Montagnier, respectively, were published in *Science* (see Chapter 4 for a detailed analysis). Dr. Robert Gallo claimed that he had discovered a retrovirus, HTLV-III, that caused AIDS. In turn, Dr. Luc Montagnier claimed that he had discovered a retrovirus, called LAV, that caused AIDS. Journal articles on AIDS research funding, as well as the statements before the subcommittee of the U.S. House of Representatives made reference to Dr. Robert Gallo's discovery of HTLV-III.

Should then the new research money be directed to research on retroviruses? Or should it be directed to research on the immune system and on immune cell functions, or maybe even better, to research on lifestyle factors? The U.S. Public Health Service's decision to redirect money to AIDS research came after sustained criticism of the federal government for its lack of interest in AIDS research. Although $14.5 million was a modest sum, it was nevertheless welcome, additional research money. This decision did not go unnoticed in scientific journals, which debated the kind of research on which the money should be spent. Because the participants in these debates include both authors and reviewers of research grant proposals, the debate's outcome and the terms in which the arguments are formulated are not without consequences for the financing of future research.

Relevant in this context are the arguments for and against channeling money into research on lifestyle factors, or retroviruses. Scientific debates usually center upon a topic that is made into an object of contestation. Generally speaking, this is true of other debates too, such as political ones. Starting with political debates as models, classical rhetoric has defined the object of contestation as stasis (Gross 1999; Prelli 1989) and considered its treatment crucial for the outcome of debates. The way in which this object is defined and the way the definition is used to support each position considerably influence the course and outcome of debates.

In the case examined here, Robert Gallo and Luc Montagnier published their respective articles in *Science* only a month before the funding decision was announced. Therefore, the general question was whether to fund research on retroviruses; the particular question was whether to fund research on the HTLV family of retroviruses, believed at the time to include the causal agent of AIDS. The object of contestation, however, was not whether to fund research on retroviruses or on the HTLV family. The object of contestation was whether there was enough scientific knowledge about retroviruses and their effects on the immune system to justify channeling research money in this direction.

Proponents of the environmental model argued that very little was known about immune cell functions and that the proven presence of antibodies to a (retro)virus did not necessarily mean that this was the cause of the immune dysfunction. After all, the virus could have entered the body in the presence of an already existing immune deficiency (*Nature*, April 28, 1983, 302, p. 749). Besides, very little was known about cell immune functions "in real life." These arguments simply stated that there was no proof of a retrovirus as a causal agent and that the state of knowledge at that time did not justify this as a preferred direction of research. Areas of investigation such as immune cell functions were considered equally important. Other position articles made an analogy with the drive to conquer cancer in the 1970s, which had generated "a lot of poor research and, on the whole, poor returns" (*Nature*, August 25, 1983, 304, p. 672 and September 29, 1983, 305, p. 349). It was argued that funding of AIDS research should not abandon the peer-review process and that money should not be given to a few prominent researchers without due review of grant proposals. These arguments pleaded for funding several research tracks in an open manner.

Proponents of the viral model acknowledged lack of knowledge about immune cell functions and that the existence of antibodies was no proof of the causal role of the retrovirus, whether it was HTLV or not. Nevertheless, it was argued that money should be channeled into research on this topic. Lack of knowledge was no proof that a retrovirus did not cause AIDS. "Sheer ignorance of the cause" justified the hypothesis of a retrovirus: "The search for antibodies among representative samples of the groups which are apparently susceptible to AIDS is plainly an urgent matter" (*Nature*, June 2, 1983, 302, p. 364). This search alone is not sufficient; it has to be accompanied by a "fuller understanding of the consequences of retroviruses capable of causing malignancy for the biology of the infected cell" and by research on the biology of immune cells. The latter, however, was already being researched by many people.

During the hearings before the Subcommittee on Intergovernmental Relations and Human Resources, Dr. Edward Brandt, the U.S. Assistant Secretary for Health stated that research and funding efforts were concentrated at the National Cancer Institute (NCI) and at the National Institute of Allergy and Infectious Diseases (NIAID), because "this is an infectious disease, and a sexually transmitted disease" (Brandt 1983, p. 384). At the fundamental level, research funds were directed at identifying the etiologic agent, for which three candidates stood up: cytomegalovirus, the Epstein–Barr virus, and HTLV (Brandt 1983, p. 385). The Epstein–Barr virus was never a serious candidate; of the remaining candidates, HTLV was the strongest. As Brandt stressed,[3] two meetings had already taken place at the NCI on the topic of retroviruses and AIDS, involving intramural research staff and university scientists (1983, p. 295).

Relevant here is that where AIDS research is done depends on the definition of the disease: it is an infectious disease, but also a sexually transmitted one. Therefore, research money and programs are divided between two institutes: the NCI and the NIAID. This is relevant for the funding of fundamental AIDS research: a certain institute is defined not only through the specific competencies of its research staff and specific technologies, but also through very specific research interests, all of which influence the further direction of research. In our case, retroviral research was being done at the NCI. At the time of the hearings and the funding debates, HTLV-III was emerging as the etiologic agent of AIDS. At the same time, it was at the center of a bitter discovery dispute along with LAV, its French counterpart (more about this in Chapter 4). Although the decision to divide funds for research between the NCI and the NIAID (with all the consequences entailed by this) cannot be attributed to rhetoric alone, it was clearly legitimated by the definition of the syndrome.

The object of contestation (there is not enough scientific knowledge) was made into an argument for supporting research on retroviruses and their effects upon cell biology. This is, actually, the course taken by AIDS researchers in the 1980s: research efforts (and money) were mostly directed at the structure of retroviruses (HIV, SIV) and their effects upon the immune system at the cellular level. In the late 1980s, the standard view, supported by Dr. Robert Gallo and other prominent researchers, was that AIDS fundamental research should focus

---

[3] In his statement, the Secretary of Health had ruled out amyl nitrites as a serious candidate for the role of etiologic agent (Brandt 1983, p. 382).

on the HIV retrovirus and on the development of a vaccine against it
(see, e.g., Gallo et al. 1987, p. 27; Curran and Morgan 1987; Letvin
et al. 1987; Levy et al. 1987). Research on cell immunity was not
mentioned as a priority anymore, although some French researchers
stated that the cell protection mechanism is not known (Klatzmann and
Gluckman 1987). Twelve years after the 1983 debates, a book written
by a former member of the staff of the President's Commission on the
HIV Epidemic complained that the immune system was still poorly
understood and that researchers had just started to work on immunity at the cellular level (Grady 1995, pp. 93–4). Reviewing the efforts
to develop a vaccine against AIDS, Christine Grady considered them
futile in the absence of an understanding of how the immune system
works (p. 95). The idea of a preventive HIV vaccine, characteristic for
AIDS research in the late 1980s, relied exactly on the assumption that
research should focus on the structure of the retrovirus and on how
it works. This meant that the structure of the retrovirus is the main
thing worth knowing to prevent and heal the immunodeficiency syndrome. Other topics, such as immune functions at the cellular level,
were not relevant. This assumption, however, has its roots at least in
the scientific debates of 1983, when the retroviral thesis, boosted by the
articles of Dr. Robert Gallo, was combined with the argument that lack
of knowledge about retroviruses justifies focusing all research efforts
on them.

AIDS, Sexually Transmitted Diseases, and Viruses

A major problem for the viral model of AIDS was to bring together
viruses, STDs, and immune deficiency in a (more or less) coherent
causal account. This was no easy task, because an immune deficiency
can be presented as the background against which a virus enters the
body *or* as the effect of a virus. If the second was the case, what role
did STDs play? And how could a virus be tied to STDs? What was the
order of the pieces in the puzzle?

The first reports on "Kaposi's sarcoma in homosexual men" dating
from September 1981 – a period when KS was presented as a problematic, new disease – associated KS with ethnic origin, sexual orientation,
and number of sexual partners, thus establishing a link between the
viral cause of KS, STDs, and homosexuality (*The Lancet*, September
19, 1981, II/8247, p. 598).

The ethnic as well as the age determinants served to enforce the new and problematic character of KS; the sexually transmitted diseases and number of sexual partners seemed to have little place in the description of a skin cancer form not usually associated with sexually transmitted diseases. Without any explicit association, the report referred to them twice, then stated that the etiology and pathogenesis of KS were unknown; it then formulated the thesis of a viral etiology, supported by evidence for cytomegalovirus (CMV) in the tumor cells. It continued by asserting that the increased risk of KS and the immune function of homosexuals had not been studied in sufficient depth. Because they, homosexuals (explicitly defined as a "population" – that is, as a distinct group), had a high prevalence of STDs and there was the hypothesis that CMV might be venereally transmitted, the "homosexual population" might be at an increased risk of contracting KS (*The Lancet*, September 19, 1981, II/8247, p. 600). CMV antibodies in the reported patients were presented as an argument for the "viral cause of KS" (which at the time of the report was a matter of scientific controversy). Because KS is tied to AIDS, the argument went, the viral cause of KS must be tied to AIDS too.

"Homosexuals" were now a group at risk for Kaposi's sarcoma, a risk that was defined through a high prevalence of sexually transmitted diseases. Because all the patients had "histories of a variety of sexually transmitted diseases," the thesis of a viral origin of KS was supported by putting together disparate entities: the cancer was associated with the cytomegalovirus, and CMV in turn was associated with sexually transmitted diseases. Henceforth, Kaposi's sarcoma was discussed as though it could have a viral origin, and it was believed that the virus "might be venereally transmitted," in a population which had both the respective skin cancer form and the risk factors.

The association of cytomegalovirus with KS had already been discussed in medical journals before 1981.[4] In that debate, however, CMV was seen as only one factor in the triggering of KS, with additional factors such as malaria needed to induce "persistent infection"; factors such as "genetic background" and "immunodisbalance with persistent heterogenic stimulation" were needed to provoke "persistent heavy infection." It was this combination of several factors, over a long period

---

4 See, for example, the journal *Cancer*, 1980, 45/6, pp. 1472–7.

of time, which would finally lead to "multiple primary malignancies in
KS patients." The novelty of this article was that it associated a skin
cancer form *both* with a viral cause and with sexual transmission. It
relied for its argument on bringing together apparently disparate definitions of a risk category. The causal model, in turn, relied on "risk
factors" and "groups" forming a mutually reinforcing, self-sustaining
construction. Various rhetorical devices converge to construct risk factors: there are successive substitutions of categories, simultaneously
creating different classifications (of KS and of sexually transmitted diseases) and extrapolating causal chains from them.

By the end of 1981, opportunistic infections associated with Kaposi's
sarcoma supported the thesis that the unusual or problematic disease
was actually a syndrome, defined as a "new acquired cellular immunodeficiency," "a potentially transmissible immune deficiency," "cellular immune dysfunction," or a "severe acquired immunodeficiency"
(*NEJM*, December 10, 1981, 305/24, pp. 1425, 1431, 1439). These
names coexisted with those of "opportunistic infections and Kaposi's
sarcoma" in the same issue of the journal (p. 1465).[5] Contrary to what
has been stated by other authors, I did not find designations such as
GRID (gay-related immune deficiency) or "gay cancer" in the medical press. The only time that I encountered a similar designation was
in a letter published by *The Lancet* on December 12, 1981 (II/8259,
p. 1338), which used the syntagm "gay compromise syndrome." With
this exception, from the end of 1981 medical reports and articles alternately used names such as "immune deficiency" (with variations) or
"Kaposi's sarcoma and opportunistic infections." An examination of
medical articles shows how the rhetoric of risk factors promoted these
theses. A report on "evidence of a new acquired cellular immunodeficiency" presented the immunodeficiency–cytomegalovirus connection[6]
as follows:

The fact that this illness was first observed in homosexual men is probably
not due to coincidence. It suggests that a sexually transmitted infectious agent
or exposure to a common environment has a critical role in the pathogenesis

[5] See also *NEJM*, January 28, 1982, 306/4, p. 250.
[6] The connection was already signaled in the summary as: "A high-level exposure of male
  homosexuals to cytomegalovirus-infected secretions may account for the occurrence
  of this immune deficiency."

of the immunodeficiency state. Sexually transmitted infections, including cytomegalovirus, are highly prevalent in the male homosexual community. In a recent study, 94 per cent of exclusively homosexual men had serologic evidence of cytomegalovirus infection, as compared with 54 per cent of heterosexual men attending the same venereal disease clinic. (*NEJM*, December 10, 1981, 305/24, p. 1429)

The paper ties cytomegalovirus and immune suppression in "homosexuals" to sexually transmitted diseases, which in turn are a risk factor because they belong to the history of this group. Although two etiologic factors are stated ("sexually transmitted infectious agent or exposure to common environment"), only the former is detailed in the "discussion" section. The only factor with respect to which the patients did not differ from one another is the "history of sexually transmitted disease."

The immunodeficiency–cytomegalovirus connection emerged as the only coherent model: the virus enters the body with the sexually transmitted diseases, after which it remains in "the semen of asymptomatic subjects for more than a year," being activated later. Repeated sexual contact would lead to "overdoses" of the viral agent and therefore to "overwhelming chronic infection and immunodeficiency or Kaposi's sarcoma." Alternatively, there is a specific strain of cytomegalovirus "transmitted initially in the male population" (*NEJM*, December 10, 1981, 305/24, p. 1430). The real alternative, which was acknowledged but not taken seriously, was that "cytomegalovirus infection was a result rather than a cause of the T-cell defect, and that some other exposure to an undetected microorganism, drug or toxin made these patients susceptible to infection with opportunistic organisms, including cytomegalovirus." This would mean that the supposed viral agent becomes just another opportunistic infection and that risk factors are conceived as collectively shared environments. The grounds for rejecting this thesis are that "cytomegalovirus is highly suspect, in view of its prevalence among male homosexuals and its previously documented potential for immunosuppression." Interestingly enough, the transmission of the infectious agent through sexual contact and its inactivity in asymptomatic subjects, which are not pursued further, later become part of the HIV etiology.

This article was cited in other clinical reports (*NEJM*, December 10, 1981, 305/24, p. 1443), which regularly presented cases as (former) patients at clinics for sexually transmitted diseases. As some articles acknowledged, many epidemiological studies selected STD patients as AIDS-relevant simply because (inner city) clinicians had addresses of venereal medical practices, where patients were more easily reached.[7] Until the second half of 1982, reports linked immunosuppression to a viral agent on the grounds that it entered the body together with sexually transmitted diseases; at the same time, the cytomegalovirus was seen as an oncogenic agent, causing both the immune deficiency and KS. CMV's role as an oncogenic agent, but not an agent for STDs, had been debated in the medical press through the 1970s and at the beginning of the 1980s. CMV had a double, completely paradoxical role: it caused KS in an already immunocompromised host and was a major cause of immune deficiency in the same KS patients. Thus, CMV produced cancer and immune deficiency, together with STDs, all at the same time (*The Lancet*, July 17, 1982, II/8290, p. 126). In this strange constellation, the cytomegalovirus was ascribed almost magical powers, in a process not dissimilar to the patterns of shamanistic thinking discussed by Bertrand Hell (1999). Hell argues that evil phenomena (such as a virus) cause disorder, which is not only an ontological but also a cognitive disorder. The task of the shaman is to master cognitive disorder by providing an account (however illogical) of the origins of the evil.

Another medical paper asserted that the cytomegalovirus was widespread among homosexual men. The majority of these men already had antibodies to CMV when they were in their twenties. Promiscuity, combined with CMV infection, led to the spread of immune suppression: "There is convincing evidence that active CMV infection suppresses cell-mediated immunity. Thus, frequent sexually transmitted exchange of multiple strains of CMV among promiscuous homosexual men is likely" (*The Lancet*, September 18, 1982, II/8298, p. 632). Because the cytomegalovirus had been identified in tumor cells, it acted in combination with cancer viruses, and was itself such

---

[7] A "special report" on the epidemiology of the "current outbreak of Kaposi's sarcoma and opportunistic infections" described the selection methods it used as follows, in its "surveillance and reporting methods" section: "In several of the metropolitan areas, physicians who serve large numbers of homosexual men were known by the staff of clinics for sexually transmitted diseases or by other health-care personnel" (*NEJM*, January 28, 1982, 306/4, p. 249).

a virus (*The Lancet*, September 18, 1982, II/8298, p. 633). Others stated that the "homosexual" risk group was exposed to more varieties of cytomegalovirus than the general population, because it also had a higher rate of infection and exposure to sexually transmitted diseases. Therefore, this "risk group" experienced a "more profound" immunodeficiency:

> It [CMV] may be transmitted sexually, and homosexuals may have high rates of infection by CMV, up to 95% in some studies. Moreover, CMV is immuno-suppressive, although the milder immunosuppression it causes has not been associated with Kaposi's sarcoma or opportunistic infections. [...] Another possibility is that the homosexual population at risk for AIDS experiences a more profound immunosuppression than members of the general population who might contract a viral infection, because they are exposed to many variants of CMV and other viruses. (*Science*, August 13, 1982, 217, p. 619)

Multiple, repeated STDs also induced a state of immune deficiency which, in turn, led to KS (*The Lancet*, May 15, 1982, p. 1086). According to this pattern, sexually transmitted diseases played a causal role, whereas the action of a KS-related virus was only the consequence of a weakened immune system. The cytomegalovirus, it was argued, was effectively inducing immunosuppression in the context of a genetic predisposition of the "homosexual" risk group to immune deficiencies. In discussing the possibility of the body overproducing antigens, because of repeated infections with the Herpes simplex virus and the cytomegalovirus, and speculating about whether this overproduction led to immunodeficiency, one paper concluded that such cases were "rare even among homosexuals" and that additional factors, such as genetic background, have to be taken into consideration. This background would consist in hyporesponsiveness to the action of viruses. As a consequence, persistent viral infection would lead to immune deficiency, which would open the gate for other infections. Alternatively, the paper proposed, a "latent, broad-based cellular immunodeficiency" may exist among homosexuals (*NEJM*, December 10, 1981, 305/24, p. 1443).

Sander Gilman (1998, p. 21) has argued that anxieties about STDs have a long tradition in literary representations of the male body and of "natural" (i.e., heterosexual) sexual relationships. We are confronted here not with the domain of literature and poetry, but with the more restricted (though no less important) one of medical representations. A whole group, one which does not have "natural" sexual relationships, is assigned a genetically determined immune deficiency, associated with a collective history of STDs. The cultural "otherness" is translated into a biological one, supporting (and justifying at the same time) the thesis of a viral agent.

The "certain factors" making the immune deficiency clinically active were sexually transmitted diseases in the past 20 years, which were a sign for this "predisposition." Still another variety of the viral model emphasized the significance of hepatitis B for identifying the agent responsible for the acquired immunosuppression: hepatitis B was seen in the 1970s as a sexual disease, transmissible through repeated sexual contact (Epstein 1988). Moreover, it was considered that hepatitis B and immunosuppression had a similar transmission pattern and that in some of the reported cases antibodies to the hepatitis B virus (HBV) had been identified. The claim that the AIDS agent and the hepatitis B virus had a similar genetic structure was advanced with the argument of risk categories too:

In the USA and in most developed countries transmission of HBV is mainly horizontal, with high-risk groups comprising intravenous drug abusers, homosexual males, intimate heterosexual contacts of HBsAg carriers, people living in institutions for the mentally retarded, patients on haemodialysis, and patients who require large numbers of blood transfusions, such as those with haemophilia and thalassaemia. The common factor in all of these groups is contact with potentially infected blood, blood products or body fluids. Vertical transmission occurs less frequently. However, in developing countries vertical transmission is more important; the virus is most likely to be acquired by neonates at parturition. In many parts of the world, including Southeast Asia, parts of Africa, and the Caribbean basin, detectable HBV markers may be found in half or more of the population. In homosexual men the virus is probably transmitted when mucosal surfaces are breached during intercourse. In homosexual men the risk of acquiring hepatitis B is statistically related to the number of different sexual partners. The groups at highest risk of acquiring AIDS are male homosexuals, intravenous drug users, Haitians and haemophiliacs. There is evidence that blood transfusion is an additional risk factor and that AIDS can be acquired through heterosexual contact. Vertical transmission may also occur. In homosexual men the risk of acquiring AIDS is also related to the number of different sexual partners. Thus, the epidemiology of AIDS is remarkably similar to that of HBV infection. It is possible that AIDS and hepatitis B are unrelated blood-borne viral infections, since these same groups are also at risk of acquiring other potential blood-borne infections such as cytomegalovirus (CMV). However, for reasons discussed below, we favour an association with HBV. (*The Lancet*, October 15, 1983, II/8354, p. 883)[8]

The infectious agent, identified as cytomegalovirus, as an oncogenic virus, as both, or as HBV-related, simultaneously plays the roles of an agent that

1. is sexually transmitted,
2. induces sexually transmitted diseases,
3. induces cancer forms,
4. induces immunosuppression, and
5. is triggered by a genetically determined immune deficiency.

All these are variations on the history of sexually transmitted diseases, characteristic for "homosexuals." Their presence here is to be explained in relationship to representations of homosexuality as genetically determined that have been current since the 1970s. As Steven Epstein and Sander Gilman (Epstein 1988; Gilman 1988, p. 247) have shown, the 1970s witnessed a series of debates about the relationship between sexually transmitted diseases, psychic dysfunctions, genes, and homosexuality. The medical history of the risk group – a "history of sexually transmitted diseases" – acts as the frame in which the etiologic agent, opportunistic infections, and immune deficiency can be meaningfully differentiated from other, apparently similar infections and deficiencies.

The multifaceted viral agent – sometimes similar to the HB-virus, sometimes identical with CMV, and sometimes a mere STD agent – was adaptable to various situations and characteristics of the risk groups. In this sense, contradictions and paradoxes were an advantage rather than an obstacle: they allowed the thesis of the viral agent to persist and incorporate whatever laboratory evidence was available. And here "homosexuals" played a key role: the "otherness" of their genetic constitution was paired with STDs to explain why all of a sudden a virus was inducing immune deficiencies. In her exploration of the cultural repertoire of genetic determinism, Elizabeth Shea (2001, p. 526) has stressed the metonymic character of "genes": that is, the capacity of this

---

[8] See also p. 885; *NEJM*, Sept. 8, 1983, 309/10, p. 609 and January 12, 1984, 310/2, p. 69; *JAMA*, Oct. 18, 1985, 254/15, p. 2095.

rhetorical figure to synthesize and condense the representation of radical differences. In this sense, it can be argued that the thesis of a special genetic constitution was a metaphor for disease-stricken otherness – and a significant one with respect to etiologic models.

What this account lacked, however, was an explanation of how the infection could be passed on to persons with no history of STDs who were not necessarily "genetically different." The solution came from the competition: the environmental account of AIDS provided exactly the explanation sought, subsequently being incorporated into viral explanations and becoming standard wisdom.

AIDS as a Contagious Disease

Let us now turn to the "social environment" as the competitor of the viral agent. A crucial element in the viral model was the history of sexually transmitted diseases; the environmental model did not put great emphasis on this history. Present risk factors were at the same time present causes of the immunodeficiency. A reliable device was contrasting "homosexuality in the past" with "homosexuality in the present." This, along with a redefinition of homosexuals, produced the aggregate designated as "lifestyle." "Lifestyle" as a risk factor was introduced in the 1970s too (Conrad and Schneider 1985), when it competed with psychiatric diseases as an explanation of homosexuality. The same decade also witnessed several medical discourses on "lifestyle risks," which created a general frame of speaking about risk: dietary risks, smoking risks, environmental risks, and so forth (Brandt 1990; Hilgartner 1985). In this framework, individual actions and decisions had positive or negative health outcomes; as a consequence, health became a matter of individual responsibility, requiring informed decisions.

The first articles about an environmental agent and "lifestyle risks" still referred to "opportunistic infections and Kaposi's sarcoma in homosexual men" and rejected the cytomegalovirus thesis with the following arguments, which I reproduce here in their entirety:

The cytomegalovirus hypothesis suffers from an obvious problem: It does not explain why this syndrome [Kaposi's sarcoma] is apparently new. Homosexuality is at least as old as history, and cytomegalovirus is presumably not a new pathogen. Were the homosexual contemporaries of Plato, Michelangelo, and Oscar Wilde subject to the risk of dying from opportunistic infections? Certainly, a few cases caused by unusual microbes would have passed unnoticed among the welter of other deaths caused by common infections before the advent of modern microbiology, but what of recent times? *Pneumocystis* has been known for almost 30 years, and, given the right specimens and correct stains, it is fairly easy to identify. Present indications are that we are seeing a truly new syndrome, not explainable simply by failure to diagnose earlier cases. Therefore, we must suspect that some new factor may have distorted the host-parasite relation. So-called recreational drugs are one possibility. They are widely used in large cities where most of these cases have occurred, and the only patients in the series reported in this issue who were not homosexuals were drug users. Fashions in drugs change frequently, and experimentation with new agents is common. Perhaps one or more of these recreational drugs is an immunosuppressive agent. The leading candidates are the nitrites, which are now commonly inhaled to intensify orgasm. Users of amyl nitrite are more likely than nonusers to have hundreds of sexual partners and to contract venereal diseases. Preliminary data indicate that this "liberated" subgroup may be at highest risk for immunosuppression. (*NEJM*, December 10, 1981, 305/24, p. 1466)

We encounter several contrasts: one of them, amply developed, is homosexuality "in the present" vs. "in the past." This line of argument was used later in a *Science* article ("Disease that Baffles Medical Community," August 13, 1982, 217, pp. 618–21) in calling the role of cytomegalovirus into question. Other contrasts concern numbers ("maybe a few cases in the past" vs. those of the present) and qualitative differences between the opportunistic infections (i.e., *Pneumocystis*) and Kaposi's sarcoma of the past, on the one hand, and those of the present, on the other. Whereas the infections of the past have been known for a long time and are easy to identify ("given the right specimens and correct stains"), those of the present are problematic. This strategy of contrasting the known/the usual with the unknown/the unusual was consistently used. In introducing "recreational drugs," "homosexuals" are redefined. This group consists of "users" and "nonusers" of amyl nitrite; it is even asserted that the only non-homosexual cases reported in the same issue were drug users (actually intravenous drug users, which makes a radical difference with respect to the means of transmission). With respect to the opportunistic diseases, KS, and immunosuppression, this is a "homosexual" group; with respect to environmental risk factors and immunosuppression, it is a "drug users" group. This double status, validated solely by the place it occupies in the rhetorical economy, supports drug use (1) as a risk factor and (2) as the cause of immunosuppression. As a risk factor of an environmental nature, drug use is accompanied by residence ("large cities"), number of sexual partners ("hundreds of sexual partners"), and sexually transmitted ("venereal") diseases. Together, they constitute the social profile of a "liberated subgroup," not far removed from "lifestyle."

Soon enough, "cortisone creams" (used by "homosexuals" for treating the results of traumatic sexual acts) appeared on stage as a possible causal agent (*NEJM*, April 15, 1982, 306/15, p. 935). But the path was not further pursued; in the meantime, researchers were busy showing how the use of amyl nitrites can (entirely or partially) affect the immune system.[9] Starting from the same premises as the viral model, these studies offered a completely different view of the nature of Kaposi's sarcoma, opportunistic infections, and immunosuppression. The first examined (1) "hyperinfection with cytomegalovirus and other sexually transmitted agents" and (2) "the long-term use of amyl nitrite (AN), currently in vogue as a sexual stimulant," as possible causes of immune deficiency (*The Lancet*, February 20, 1982, I/8269, p. 412). Nevertheless, only amyl nitrites were discussed at large, because they had been widely used since the late 1960s and were readily available in bars and baths. A study reported fifteen cases, of which only eight involved the use of amyl nitrites. However, the eight persons concerned had more sexual partners than the other seven, a fact which justified the association between amyl nitrites, homosexuality, and a "promiscuous lifestyle" (*The Lancet*, February 20, 1982, I/8269, p. 413).

Factors such as the history of sexually transmitted diseases, length of sexual activity, and age were dropped as irrelevant. Sexually transmitted diseases were derived from drug use. Interestingly enough, the viral agent model, which also discussed the possible role of nitrites, operated in the reverse mode: the use of nitrites appeared as depending on the history of sexually transmitted diseases and the number of sexual partners. In the environmental model, STDs depended on the amounts of nitrites used. After discussing the role of the cytomegalovirus at length, another paper examined the possible role of nitrites in the

[9] *The Lancet*, February 20, 1983, pp. 412–15; *NEJM*, September 30, 1982, 307/14, p. 893.

larger context of general use of drugs: using surveys of STD clinics in three major U.S. cities, it found that, compared with heterosexual men (14.9%), a far larger proportion of homosexual and bisexual men (86.4%) used nitrites. The fact that the survey included only patients who had visited STD clinics, or used generalizations such as "homosexual," "bisexual," or "heterosexual" men, was not regarded as problematic. Because the frequency of nitrite use was correlated with the number of sexual partners over one month, it had to be correlated with STDs, as well as with "types of sexual behavior" and the places where this behavior happened:

> The interest in a causal role for inhalants containing amyl nitrite or isobutyl nitrite or both ("poppers," as they are commonly called) stems from the hypothesis that they are used as sexual stimulants or recreational drugs by some homosexual men. In a recent survey of 420 men attending clinics for sexually transmitted diseases in New York, San Francisco and Atlanta, we found that 86.4 per cent of homosexual and bisexual men (242 of 279) as compared with 14.9 per cent of heterosexual men (21 of 141), reported the use of nitrite inhalants within five years. However, the frequency of nitrite use was closely correlated with the number of sexual partners reported during the previous month. This suggests that the use of nitrites may be associated with other hypothetical etiologic factors, such as sexually transmitted infections, antimicrobial agents for treatment or prevention of these infections, types of sexual behavior, attendance at places where partners are encountered, and perhaps the use of other drugs. (*NEJM*, January 28, 1982, 306/4, p. 252)

Nitrites are defined as being used in "homosexual" spaces, and the role of a viral agent (cytomegalovirus) is downplayed. This is explained in terms of a "hyperimmunisation of homosexual men to CMV" (*The Lancet*, February 20, 1982, I/8269, p. 414). In the viral model, there was no "hyperimmunisation," but "persistent heavy infection." Whereas in the viral model there was a genetic predisposition to becoming infected with CMV, the "lifestyle" account saw things exactly the other way around. Paradoxically, to acquire an immune deficiency, "homosexuals" had to have a well-functioning immune system. The argument opened the way for the environmental agent to produce immune "abnormalities" and explained why a viral agent cannot cause immunosuppression:

> The time and space clustering of this syndrome has not yet been explained. Although a CMV mutant is clearly a possible cause, no point source has been

identified and no genetic relations among CMV strains from patients with KS or *P. carinii* pneumonia have been established. Other viruses have not been epidemiologically linked with KS. There are no data on recent changes in homosexual lifestyle apart from the casual observation of case-clustering in the more openly homosexual U.S. coastal cities. AN (amyl nitrites), on the other hand, has come into widespread use during the past 10–15 years. Half of our healthy AN users and patient B never used the drug before 1975; this suggests that AN use is becoming more widespread. If AN causes immunosuppression, then the latency period between the start of AN use and development of KS might be about 5 years. Similar latency periods have been reported between use of immunosuppressive drugs such as corticosteroids and development of KS. (*The Lancet*, February 20, 1982, I/8269, p. 414)

Concentration in "homosexual U.S. coastal cities" and the widespread use of nitrites "in the past 10–15 years" define the "time and space clustering." Therefore, nitrites cause immunosuppression, with a latency period similar to that of a viral agent. Later papers used a similar line of argument when sustaining the causal role of amyl nitrite (*The Lancet*, May 15, 1982, I/8281, p. 1083).

Frequency of sexual contacts was depicted as depending on drug use (*The Lancet*, May 15, 1982, I/8281, pp. 1084–5). Nitrites were seen as (1) a direct cause of immunosuppression, with an oncogenic agent entering the already immunodeficient body; (2) allowing a "carcinogenic agent, otherwise controlled by the immune system, to operate"; or (3) a "surrogate for...overall drug use or exposure to an oncogenic virus at present confined to the homosexual community" (*The Lancet*, May 15, 1982, I/8281, p. 1085). Social spaces, risk groups, and the causal agent mutually define each other: in "homosexual discotheques," there is active as well as passive exposure to amyl nitrites. These were used far more intensively by homosexuals than by heterosexuals anyway and were clearly associated with promiscuity. On these grounds, it was argued, "chronic exposure" to amyl nitrites leads to immune suppression, which in turn allows the induction of cancer (*The Lancet*, May 15, 1982, I/8281, p. 1086). Nitrites are characteristic for certain social spaces, which are characteristic for a certain risk category, which characterizes the use of nitrites.

Papers supporting the immunosuppressive role of amyl nitrites and other "lifestyle factors" argued that the presence of antibodies against a virus (such as HTLV-I) is no proof of its causal role in the immune deficiency (*Nature*, April 28, 1983, 302, p. 749). The presence of a virus could be the consequence of an already impaired immune system; besides, very little is known about the various functions of different types of blood cells, or about their genetic origins. "Male homosexuals" carry antibodies against other viruses anyway. By contrast, much is known about the "lifestyle" of this group (which has a "pathetic promiscuity") and about amyl nitrites as immunosuppressants.

Thus, the environmental agent acts through direct use and exposure in social environments. The use of amyl nitrites defines the risk group ("much more common among homosexual men") and is at the same time an etiologic agent. It explains why immunosuppression appears with predilection among homosexual men and how it is caused. Although the number of sexual partners may be relevant in the short term, the use of amyl nitrites is significant in the long run. Chronic, longtime exposure to amyl nitrites induces immunosuppression, whereas a sexually transmitted agent induces cancer against this background.

This circular explanation separates the cause of cancer (KS) from the cause of immunosuppression and orders the two hierarchically: whereas they were mixed up in the viral model, here they become quite distinct. This explains how the "lifestyle" model, which could not (and did not) ignore CMV or STDs, arranged them in such a way as to obtain completely different results. In the late 1980s, the association between KS and amyl nitrites was integrated into the larger viral model: the use of amyl nitrites was a "lifestyle factor" that favored the action of the HI-virus and the occurrence of KS as an opportunistic infection (Jaffe et al. 1987, pp. 139–40).

AIDS and "Immunosuppressive Sperm"

Let us now turn to the thesis of the "alloantigenic sperm." This thesis, along with the amyl nitrites one, is described today as a curiosity in the development of medical knowledge on AIDS; it may have affected this knowledge in the beginning, but it played no further role. Such curiosities are sociologically relevant in a double sense: first, they are embedded in the economy of the medical discourse; second, they are not without consequences, but they exercise considerable influence on subsequent developments. Indeed, "alloantigeneic sperm" was still being referred to in epidemiological papers at the beginning of the 1990s

(Meyer-Bahlburg et al. 1991, p. 5). Moreover, it has become a component of the Duesberg (1996) theses which, however marginal with respect to the medical establishment, continue to attract attention. In the late 1980s Peter Duesberg, a respected biochemist at the University of California at Berkeley, published several articles (followed by a book in 1996) arguing that retroviruses could not cause immune deficiencies. AIDS was caused instead by lifestyle factors. The immunosuppressive character of sperm played here a prominent role. Duesberg's theses attracted considerable criticism from mainstream AIDS researchers, but he became a sort of hero in the gay community and got wide media exposure (Epstein 1996, pp. 117–18). His theses were not abandoned in the 1990s but continued to be disseminated outside the main scientific journals.

"Alloantigeneic sperm" is also at the core of the "multifactorial theses" developed in the late 1980s (Oppenheimer 1992). Moreover, "African dry sex" as a risk factor (Brown, Ayowa, and Brown 1993; McGrath et al. 1992) is directly influenced by the idea of a weakening of the "natural" resistance of the sexual organs. The main claim regarding "alloantigeneic sperm" was that human sperm had different effects on the male and the female body, respectively; it induced immune deficiency in men and was responsible for the Acquired Immunodeficiency Syndrome. "Homosexual behavior, specifically the passive role in anal intercourse" was connected to immune deficiencies (*Nature*, June 2, 1983, 303, p. 371). In a complementary fashion, it was claimed that sperm had "immunopotentiating effects" on the female body, preventing, among other things, the development of breast cancer. Alternatively, the female reproductive tract had evolved "mechanisms to minimize the entry of spermatozoa or sperm antigens into the blood stream, to guard against induced infertility and also perhaps AIDS" (*Nature*, August 25, 1983, 304, p. 678). Because both "homosexual lifestyle" and "cultural environment" implied the exchange of large quantities of sperm, this led ultimately to the appearance and large-scale spread of immune deficiency. Other infectious agents, such as the cytomegalovirus, could enter the body with the sperm but were not the main factors responsible for immunosuppression. Sperm was the main culprit:

We have, therefore, postulated that under the special circumstances of anal intercourse, the chronic, repeated exposure of some young homosexual males to sperm alloantigens may be equivalent to the effect of allogeneic kidney grafts. The frequent laceration of the sperm's recipient rectal mucosa, coupled with the presence of colonic bacteria, may not only create a better contact between the sperm and the immune apparatus present in lymph and blood but also provide an adjuvant effect toward enhanced alloimmunization. (*JAMA*, January 13, 1984, 251/2, p. 237)

AIDS appeared at the beginning of the 1980s and not earlier exactly because "a subset of men" (read: gays) had been subjected to a massive "sperm attack" since the rise of "unprecedented promiscuity" in the late 1960s. In this perspective, AIDS was an immune deficiency similar to those induced by malnutrition, the recreational use of drugs, or organ transplants (*JAMA*, May 6, 1983, 249/17, p. 2373). Readers' letters claimed that animal experiments had provided good evidence about the connection between immune suppression and sperm and about the role of "frequent anal intercourse as a causal factor in the immune deficiency characteristic of AIDS" (*Nature*, June 30, 1983, 303, p. 748).

Alloantigenic sperm was an intrinsic component of the "homosexual lifestyle" that developed in certain urban areas; it was simultaneously a risk factor *and* the agent responsible for immunosuppression. A direct consequence, discussed on television shows (Treichler 1988a; Bersani 1988), was the thesis of the "resistant vagina." It claimed in essence that the female vagina (being multi-layered) was much more resistant to the sperm's immunosuppressive effects than the single-layered male anus; hence, heterosexual intercourse did not lead to immunosuppression. In the late 1980s and early 1990s, this thesis was replaced by that of the "fragile vagina" (Piot and Mann 1987, p. 153; Brown, Ayowa, and Brown 1993), which claimed that the vagina was a fragile organ, easily made vulnerable by sexual practices, sexually transmitted diseases, and sexual activity. This fragility explained how the HI-virus was passed from male to female during sexual intercourse. In the mid-1990s, medical researchers called for systematic research on the mucosal immunity of the sexual organs, considered crucial for developing effective AIDS therapy (Grady 1995, p. 94). The call acknowledged lack of scientific information about mucosal immunity and considered that research had been unilaterally focused on the HI-virus.

Three rhetorical strategies can be seen as fundamental in the development of the "alloantigenic sperm" thesis: (1) presenting the immunosuppressive agent (i.e., sperm) as starting a chain reaction, in which

gender-determined body differences intervened; (2) describing risk as
a geographic concentration that favors such a chain reaction; and (3)
reversing the analogies with immunosuppression in kidney transplant
recipients. I now briefly discuss these strategies.

Both the environmental and viral agent theses operated with one
main etiologic factor assisted by a cluster of cofactors. In the alloantigenic discourse, cofactors ("profound promiscuity") not only favored,
but also amplified the immunosuppressive effects of sperm. One article presented a graphic scheme that showed how "profound promiscuity" starts a chain reaction in which microbes and drug abuse enhance the immunosuppressive effects of sperm (*JAMA*, May 6, 1983,
249/13, p. 2371). In a first phase, great quantities of sperm enter
the body, which in turn builds up antigens. Various infectious agents
(and especially those of sexually transmitted diseases) associated with
"profound promiscuity" act as an additional strain on the immune
system. In a second phase, the immune system has already been weakened; infectious agents from previously acquired sexually transmitted
diseases are reactivated and become virulent; the system, becoming
even more weakened, cannot defend the body against the effects of
sperm, which amplifies the effects of other infectious agents. Gender-
specific body differences intervene in this phase of avalanche-like immune suppression: the lining cells of the anal mucosa are destroyed
more easily than those of the vaginal mucosa. In a feedback loop,
these differences also confirm the role of "profound promiscuity"
in starting the chain reaction. One clinical study on "alloantigenic
sperm" compared 26 male sperm recipients with one female anal
sperm recipient and concluded that their similarity confirmed gender
differences:

The demonstration of similar immune dysregulation concomitant with the
presence of serum antibodies against her husband's sperm in a heterosexual
female who routinely practiced anal-genital intercourse not only lends further
support to the concept of sperm-induced immune dysregulation but also un-
derscores the critical structural difference between the rectum and the vagina.
While the lining of the vaginal mucosa comprises a squamous multilayer epithelium capable of protecting against any abrasive effect during intercourse,
the inner lining of the rectum is made of a single layer of columnar epithelium.
The latter, unlike the vaginal epithelium, is not only incapable of protecting
against any abrasive effect but also promotes the absorption of an array of

sperm antigens, thus enhancing their exposure to the immune apparatus in the lymphatic and blood circulation. The high immunogenicity possessed by spermatozoa, coupled with the microbiological flora of the rectum, can work in synergism to generate a state of chronic antigenic stimulation. (*JAMA*, January 13, 1984, 251/2, pp. 240–1)

The ordering of sexual acts reflects these differences: because the linings of the mouth are different from those of the anus, oral sex is less risky. In this respect, and in contrast to the anus, vaginal and oral linings provide a similar degree of protection.

The comparison with "heterosexual anal intercourse," decisive for the thesis of gender-specific differences, led to the conclusion that immunosuppression is specific to each risk group ("homosexuals, Haitians, hemophiliacs, drug addicts, and certain women") in a unique way (*JAMA*, January 13, 1984, 251/2, p. 241). "Profound promiscuity," the primary risk factor in this model, was spatially ordered; it was presented as areas favoring large numbers of sexual contacts. Risk groups were thus made equivalent with risk areas. This explained how spatially concentrated, repeated exposure to sperm could have taken place, after many years of sexual activity: the epidemic had its epicenter in Greenwich Village, where promiscuity had attained unprecedented levels in the past decades: "In a first phase, repeated exposure to sperm and STD agents impairs the immune system. Continued promiscuity triggers a second phase, when the immune system is weakened even further" (*JAMA*, May 6, 1983, 249/17, pp. 2370–1).

Concentrations of "promiscuity" also explained how the immune suppression process could become self-sustaining, with various agents boosting the effects of one another. A third, not less relevant strategy was the comparison with the immunosuppression effects seen in kidney transplant recipients. Mostly, transplant recipients emphasized the differences between the old and the new immune deficiency. These recipients were associated with the "old" and "well known" immune deficiency, whereas AIDS was a completely new one. The arguments were reversed: in transplant recipients, the foreign body part triggered an immune response leading to organ failure. In "young homosexual males," foreign sperm produced a violent immune reaction which in the end led to the body's failure. This time, analogies were emphasized: in both cases, the immunosuppressive reaction was due to a foreign element (i.e., transplanted kidney or sperm, respectively) stimulating the production of antigens:

A striking resemblance seems to exist between the young homosexual males and the group of kidney transplant recipients in terms of their increased susceptibility to both opportunistic (including cytomegalovirus) infection and the development of Kaposi's sarcoma. In the kidney transplant recipients, a growing body of evidence now suggests that the underlying immune dysregulation is governed by a process of chronic antigenic stimulation mediated through the allogeneic graft rather than exclusively by the immunosuppressive chemotherapy. (*JAMA*, January 13, 1984, 251/2, p. 237)

Kidney transplant recipients and "homosexual males with AIDS" have in common an increased incidence of Kaposi's sarcoma and other opportunistic infections. This common element "definitely raises the possibility" that allogeneic sperm may affect the male immune system. Sperm antigens induce a "chronic immune stimulation" and open the way for KS and opportunistic infections (*JAMA*, January 13, 1984, 251/2, p. 238; see also p. 241). The analogy between transplant recipients and "homosexuals" is superimposed on that between "homosexual" and "heterosexual" anal sex, to the effect that risk is not ascribed to a sexual practice as such, but to the sexual practice which circumscribes a risk group. Anal-genital contact is successively compared to other sexual acts and to kidney transplant recipients, thus legitimating gender-specific differences in sensitivity. The elements of the picture – immunosuppression, Kaposi's sarcoma, opportunistic infections, cytomegalovirus – are arranged in a totally different way than in the viral model. The latter presented immunosuppression as being induced by a viral agent that was favored by previous sexually transmitted diseases. Secondary risk factors (such as number of sexual partners) were derived from STDs (supposing that a history of sexually transmitted diseases weakened the immune system and was associated with higher numbers of sexual partners). These factors only favored the spread of the infectious agent. The immunosuppression and the opportunistic diseases were both provoked by infectious agents of a viral nature. In the environmental model, risk factors are the infectious agent and the circumstances favoring it. The risk factors of the "homosexual lifestyle" favor the use of nitrites; this in turn produces immunosuppression and is one of the risk factors. Viral agents play a subordinate role. Immunosuppression is socio-environmentally induced and opens the way for the action of infectious agents.

The frame of reference with respect to which these arrangements are produced is given by risk categories. The viral model depended on defining "homosexuals" in the first place as a medical group, with respect to its disease history; all other elements are derived from it. The environmental model defined it as a social group and derived risk factors from the social environment or "lifestyle." The nature of the etiologic agent and the relationships between the agent and its effects are different in the two models; these differences do not result from different clinical or laboratory data, but rather from different ways of arranging risk factors.

Against this background, it is relevant to note the representation of sperm as a pollutant, in a way which reminds us of the "primitive" distinctions between the pure and the impure (Douglas and Wildawsky 1982, p. 35). What is at stake is not the fact that sperm carries the (unidentified) causal agent. Sperm itself is the cause of the infection, because anal sex is a transgression. Although harmless (or even fertile) in vaginal intercourse, sperm becomes destructive when the domain of "acceptable" intercourse is transgressed. In this respect scientific knowledge cannot be said to be immune to culturally determined representation of the human body and to the taboos these representations carry with them. The notion that only media debates on AIDS activated such taboos proves to be wrong: they were present in a place purported to be immune to them. This can be seen as another confirmation of Steven Epstein's thesis (1996) that medical AIDS research has been less than "pure" – pure in the sense of not being susceptible to any contamination through cultural representations or prejudices. Instead, we discover "cultural pollution" at the very heart of scientific knowledge.

The New Etiologic Model

After mid-1983, a new model crystallized, in which the causal role of environmental factors was abandoned in favor of a viral agent. Yet environment and lifestyle as factors did not disappear. The new etiology was actually a combination of both models. In this case, immunosuppression was due to a viral agent whose transmission was facilitated by environmental risk factors. The social environment, as a premise for immunosuppression, was combined with an infectious agent as a cause of the immunosuppression. How did such a combination become possible?

The new model, which started from a universal infectious agent, explained how opportunistic infections, Kaposi's sarcoma, and immunosuppression appeared in each risk group, favored by specific environmental risk factors; it also explained how the universal infectious agent was transmitted from one risk group to another. Because risk groups were characterized through spatial clusterings or agglomerations, group-to-group transmission was to be explained by mobility. Travel to risky places was constantly presented as a feature of the "homosexual" risk group, which allowed for the infectious agent to be transmitted from Haiti to North America, and from North America to Western Europe. The same explanation was used in later epidemiologic models, to show how the virus came from Africa to Haiti. On the one hand, "Haitians" were presented as immobile and living in a traditional social environment; on the other hand, they were presented as immigrating to North America, or as circulating between Central Africa and Haiti. The category of "hemophiliacs" was presented as rather immobile and dispersed, in contrast to the other groups. It was a receiver rather than a carrier of the infectious agent, and it was an argument for transmission through blood products. Thus, the new model managed to be general and specific at the same time, overcoming some of the previous difficulties.

"Haitians" played a key role in the transmission chain: they were (1) the *link* through which the virus could pass between categories otherwise unrelated, (2) the *setting* in which this took place, and (3) the *necessary condition* for the future transmission of the virus. Besides, they supported the theory of a virus transmitted from animals to humans. In other words, "Haitians" (and later "Africans") became the necessary past for explaining the present and foreseeing the future. Let us first examine how the virus passed the barrier between animals and humans. In 1983, a letter to *The Lancet* stated that an animal virus (the African swine fever virus, ASFV) was the infectious agent for AIDS. It was followed by several extensive papers which debated the subject. The echo in the medical press was large and, although its core thesis (that the AIDS virus was the African swine fever virus) was quickly rejected, its significance was much broader. This thesis (1) was the first thesis of a viral agent passing the barrier between animals and humans (seen as valid until today); (2) provided an explanatory model for how this happened, a narrative structure later adopted by "African AIDS"; and (3) provided an epidemiologic model, consistent with the etiologic one, which explained how the virus was transmitted among risk groups. The letter stated a parallel course between the first cases of AIDS in Haiti (pushed back to 1978) and the introduction of the African swine fever virus to Haiti (from Cuba) in 1979. The clinical description of ASFV in Haitian pigs mentioned a mortality rate of 80–100%; the pigs did not produce neutralizing antibodies to the virus; the special character of the Haitian ASFV isolate was singled out. The etiologic model was formulated as follows:

> A possible cycle for the accidental introduction of ASFV into the human population might relate specifically to the Haitian isolate. Perhaps an infected pig was killed and eaten either as uncooked or undercooked meat. One of the people eating the meat, who was both immunocompromised and homosexual would be the pivotal point, allowing for the disease to spread to the vacationing "gay" tourists in Haiti. As the virus is stable in blood, urine and faeces, it might be then transmitted via traumatic sexual practices. Among pigs, ASFV is most easily transmitted in stressed populations. Humans with concurrent viral infections or who are in other ways physiologically stressed appear to be most vulnerable to AIDS. Certainly blood transfusions would be an ideal mode of transmission. (*The Lancet*, April 23, 1983, I/8330, p. 923)

Here again, etiology and epidemiology rely on redefining the "Haitian" risk category. At least one "Haitian" may have eaten the raw or undercooked meat of an infected pig; this suggests a "traditional" lifestyle, which explains how the virus passed the barrier between animals and humans. Afterwards, a homosexual and immunocompromised Haitian who also ate the meat spread it through sexual contact to the "vacationing gay tourists." This explains how the virus was transmitted to the "homosexual" risk group. Thus, ad hoc redefinitions produce risk factors according to every segment of the explanatory model.

The biological account (the virus passing from pigs to humans) is embedded in an anthropological one, which combines poverty-related elements with sexual ones and with ritual practices. In the fashion described long ago by Émile Durkheim and Marcel Mauss (1963) for the aboriginal societies of Australia, cultural categories are applied to the natural world to make sense of how transgression happens – that is, in such a fashion that the cognitive order is restored.

If "transfusion recipients" accounted for how the agent passed from risk to non-risk categories, "Haitians" accounted for a more complicated, intercontinental transmission route. Consider with respect to this an "extraordinary case." The patient, a "heterosexual Frenchman" and "French geologist" who had been working in Haiti, was diagnosed with opportunistic infections four years after returning to Paris. The presentation of his case formulated a strong argument in favor of blood transfusion as a causal agent; the new case was excluded from the classification and then added as a new category, thus showing the role of blood transfusion:

Most individuals with AIDS are homosexual or bisexual young men, and the syndrome particularly affects those who have a great number of sexual partners and a great incidence of sexually transmitted diseases. Other identifiable groups of AIDS patients include users of intravenous drugs, Haitians living in Port-au-Prince or Haitian immigrants to the United States, and haemophiliacs. It is noteworthy that Haiti is a favourite vacation spot for many US homosexual men [...] Our patient, however, does not belong to any of the affected communities, but has spent eight months in Haiti where he was transfused with Haitian blood. The possibility that AIDS may be transmitted by blood has already been suggested by its occurrence in haemophiliacs ... but our case shows in addition the potential danger of ordinary blood transfusions. (*The Lancet*, May 28, 1983, I/8335, pp. 1187, 1190)

The case is first a "heterosexual Frenchman," then a "French geologist," and then a "transfusion recipient." These rhetorical operations present the reader with several chains of transmission. Homosexuals vacationing in Haiti get the virus from the Haitians and, along with Haitian immigrants, bring it to the United States. On the other hand, Haitians pass the virus on to non-risk persons through ordinary transfusions. Looking closer at the rhetorical construction, we can see that there is no explicit statement about how Haitians managed to pass the virus on to homosexuals vacationing there. Rather, the paper performs several, apparently disparate operations: (1) it classifies AIDS risk (which is a canonical operation) and (2) it associates and dissociates the categories it operates with several times, in a way which presents them as related or unrelated to Haiti. Thus, homosexuals are vacationing there; the reported case does not belong to a risk category, *but* (negation) has spent some time in Haiti (as a "French geologist") and has received "Haitian blood." The reported case gains its identity from being declassified several times as non-risk; at the same time, it has to retain all the other identities to support the paper's claims.

Thus we have a complete narrative of how the virus was passed from animals to humans and then from the "primitive" to the "developed" world. In this narrative, each risk category accounts for a future step or link in the transmission chain; at least one means of transmission corresponds to each of these steps. The narrative is not to be found in a single article, but rather is constituted in a network of texts: each of them provides the reader with some elements of the plot, with a partial view of the characters involved. The whole picture, however, emerges from this textual network. Although many authors see narratives as "tales mapped onto tellings of personal experience" (Ochs and Capps 1996, p. 21), the narratives of the origins that unfold here are, rather, tales of culture mapped onto tellings of nature. They enlist knowledge resources about society in the production of knowledge about nature and, as such, engage social actors in continuing them (Myers 1991, p. 45).

The Hunt for the Origins of the Virus

As previously pointed out, "Africans" played a seminal role in (1) building up an origin of AIDS as a geographical, social, and cultural location where the infectious agent has been present (in a more or less dormant form) for a long time, and (2) reconstructing Kaposi's sarcoma in this context as a disease entirely relevant for AIDS. In the first reports, Kaposi's sarcoma was presented as a "usual" and "ubiquitous" skin cancer form with "lesions considered benign"; at the same time, it was "unusual" and "rare." The "African form" of Kaposi's sarcoma was presented in this context as different from (and incompatible with) the newly seen "North American form." In the new context of the "African" risk, a redefinition of "African" Kaposi's sarcoma as AIDS-relevant had to take place. This redefinition maintains a direct relationship to the construction of an origin of the disease. The old KS thus becomes the new, problematic KS (the two having been previously seen as incompatible): "African KS" is no longer opposed to the "AIDS-related KS" (an opposition which actually supported the AIDS-related KS); it is identical with it.

Past cases were unearthed from hospital files and presented as AIDS cases. This enterprise began with the reconstruction of the case of a Danish woman surgeon who had worked for several years in Zaire in the 1970s. Six years after her death in Copenhagen, her medical file was reinterpreted as an AIDS case, being frequently cited in epidemiological journals and in the general press as the proof that AIDS had existed in Africa for a long time already. It is this reconstruction that is examined here first. To make it work, the relationship between AIDS and KS had to be reversed. An initial step in this process had to be the redefinition of AIDS-related KS as similar (and not completely unrelated) to the "hyperendemic focus of KS in Central Africa." This achieved, a questioning of the status of AIDS in Africa is implied. The argument unfolded as follows: because of a lack of technical equipment, AIDS without KS could not be detected in Africa. It could be seen only in those patients who already had KS, because the clinical identification of KS could be done without sophisticated technical equipment. Hence, AIDS and African KS must be related. Moreover, Central Africa was already known as a reservoir of deadly viruses. KS was thought to be caused by a virus. The conclusion: a virus causing KS and AIDS traveled from Africa to Haiti and from there to North America (*The Lancet*, April 23, 1983, I/8330, p. 925).

Although up to that date Kaposi's sarcoma had been described neither in hemophiliacs nor in Haitians, and although it was already seen as indicative of AIDS, the two were now presented as parts of the same epidemic, a fact which changed the relationship of the terms. The cause (of the epidemic, and consequently, of AIDS and/or Kaposi's sarcoma) was now a viral one. The "hyperendemic focus of KS in central Africa" was put side by side with the "epidemic of AIDS and KS"; this made them compatible and comparable. (Remember that the opposite was the case in the first reports on Kaposi's sarcoma.) AIDS in disjunction from KS is hardly identifiable, which, conversely, amounts to the claim that AIDS in conjunction with KS is identifiable.

The structure of the argument was to state a conjunction (AIDS and KS) for given categories, then to assert compatibility with an (until then) unrelated category, and to state that AIDS without KS would not be identifiable. Because it is precisely this conjunction that makes AIDS identifiable, the problem is how to see African KS correctly. Deadly viruses of Central African origin appear as a middle term connecting the viral agent with the importance of Kaposi's sarcoma in Central Africa. The "connection between African and American AIDS/KS," along with the thesis of an "African virus," is specified in a concrete model. Thus, AIDS and Kaposi's sarcoma are brought together; the "African" and "American" KS are then joined with a viral cause, leading to "another deadly, but slow-acting, African virus" being viewed as responsible for AIDS. This account integrated two different explanations, an etiologic and an epidemiologic one, on the basis of a reversal in the understanding and significance of "African KS." With the latter transformed into a sure sign of AIDS, the African origin of the immune deficiency moved to the core of explanatory models.

The only question that remained to be answered was whether the case was a victim of a viral agent in an African setting. She was a "previously healthy Danish woman" who, during most of the 1970s, had worked as a surgeon in a rural hospital, as well as in the capital of Congo (Zaire). During her stay, "she had repeated episodes of diarrhea . . . progressive therapy-resistant diarrhea, fatigue, wasting, and, later, universal lymphadenopathy." At the end of 1977, she died in Copenhagen; the cause of death was diagnosed as *Pneumocystis carinii* pneumonia. This is commented on as follows:

Pneumocystis pneumonia is rare in healthy people. Before her *Pneumocystis* pneumonia this woman had had other symptoms of AIDS (chronic diarrhoea, weight loss, lymphadenopathy). She could recall coming across at least one case of KS while working in northern Zaire, and while working as a surgeon under primitive conditions she must have been heavily exposed to blood and excretions of African patients. She had not been to the USA or to Haiti, and did not abuse drugs. (*The Lancet*, April 23, 1983, I/8330, p. 925)

The entire presentation of clinical and lab results seems to contradict the "African AIDS/KS" thesis, because there is no mention of findings which could point to the presence of Kaposi's sarcoma. What the presentation actually supports is not the conjunction of AIDS and "African Kaposi's sarcoma," but the assertion that "cases of AIDS without KS stand little chance of being detected locally." It confirms an inference and indirectly supports an identifiable conjunction of AIDS and KS. Instead of proof positive of the latter, proof positive of its negation (nonidentifiable disjunction) is constructed (the nonidentifiable disjunction was not noted). Note that the case is not an object of negotiation about whether it is AIDS or not; it is reconstructed as such a case, and the arguments for it are precisely the same as those that sustain the disconnectedness from Kaposi's sarcoma. The final arguments of the "case description" are the diagnosis of *Pneumocystis* pneumonia together with diarrhea, weight loss, and lymphadenopathy. During her work as a surgeon, the patient had come into contact with "at least one case of KS" and with "blood and excretions of African patients"; this explicitly suggests that the infectious agent was transmitted from an "African patient" (with KS, because the patient had not been to the US or Haiti and had not taken drugs). Finally, the report formulates an epidemiological research program, which, although future-oriented in form, serves to enforce the thesis of an "African virus," which has relied, in turn, on re-presenting past events. Accordingly, flying research teams should be sent to Central Africa to search for "killer viruses" and explore the connection between AIDS/KS in Africa and North America. The rationale for doing this was that the "US homosexual community" had a high frequency of tropical infections and that as early as 1968 Manhattan was given the nickname "tropical isle" (*The Lancet*, April 23, 1983, I/8330, p. 925).

The "possible connection" between endemic and epidemic AIDS/KS, which seems to negate the previous argument, actually reinforces it by reversal. What was taken as given when reconstructing the past is supposed possible with respect to the future, and this possibility depends on the given facts of the past, so that stating that a "possible connection" is to be explored by flying teams amounts to stating that the connection exists. This is made clear by the frequency of infections "usually seen only in the tropics" that made Manhattan into a "tropical isle." Originally, the new form of Kaposi's sarcoma relied on distinctions between "seen" and "unseen," "ubiquitous" and "new." In the final argument, there are no more unexplainable varieties of disease, but only the same disease seen in different places, so that we can explain now how it traveled from place to place.

This argument wipes out geographic differences and generates an order in which the "US homosexual community," substitutable with "Manhattan," becomes equivalent to "Central Africa." The thesis of a new, unknown virus originating in Africa is framed and sustained by a social order of the unknown – or, rather, of the "other." The "homosexual community" is as unknown, exotic, and as much a harborer of killer viruses as Central Africa.

Several lines of argument unfold in the article analyzed above:

1. an epidemiological argument, according to which the disease originated in Africa long before it was detected in North American patients; consequently, it was somehow transported from Africa to North America and to Europe. The immune deficiency has an endemic, as well as an epidemic form
2. an etiologic argument, according to which the AIDS agent is a virus, present in Africa for a long time
3. an argument about Kaposi's sarcoma, which in its African form is the same as the AIDS-related one
4. item 3. that is not a simple consequence of the AIDS-related form but rather coexists with it.

Both (1) and (2) rely on (3) and (4); they have been accepted until today as valid and, in a modified form, lay the basis for more sophisticated epidemiological models that distinguish between different patterns of virus transmission (Stine 1993, p. 157). They also have several peculiar features: (1) they rest on the reconstruction of a past case which relies in turn on (2) using the classification not only for redefining AIDS and for (3) generating a new risk category, but also for (4) introducing another classification of Kaposi's sarcoma that contradicts the initial one. By mid-1984, essentially one KS was associated with and indicative of AIDS. One of the first articles that contributed to blurring the distinction between different forms of KS apparently intended to maintain it:

In the United States Kaposi's sarcoma is intimately linked with AIDS, and a common infective aetiology has been postulated. In these cases the tumour is characteristically aggressive and affects the viscera. In central Africa Kaposi's sarcoma is a common tumour, possibly the third-commonest tumour in Uganda. Epidemiological studies have suggested an infective aetiology. Although the tumours occur most commonly in the elderly in a localised cutaneous form, the aggressive disseminated form does occur in younger people. AIDS has been described in Central Africa; previously no association between AIDS and "African" KS has been noted. Our case links AIDS and "African"

KS, thus lending some support to the view that in Africa, as in America, AIDS and aggressive Kaposi's sarcoma might have a common aetiology. If this is true it adds weight to the suggestion that AIDS may be endemic in Central Africa, and must extend the horizons of those investigating the disease. Our patient had no cutaneous tumour, and so may have escaped diagnosis had endoscopy and a full pathology service not been available. The incidence of aggressive KS in Africa may be higher than is generally believed. (*The Lancet*, March 17, 1984, I/8377, p. 632)

There is thus a "United States Kaposi's sarcoma" and a "Central Africa Kaposi's sarcoma": the first is "intimately linked with AIDS" and shares a "common aetiology" with it. It has an "aggressive character," which it shares with the "Central Africa Kaposi's sarcoma." The latter has a very common form, which "occurs in the elderly in a mostly localised cutaneous form," and an "aggressive form," which occurs in the youth. What happens here is that "African KS" is identified with "United States KS" on grounds of "aggressiveness." A single form emerges: aggressive, AIDS-associated KS, induced by the same infectious agent. This is an argument for the long-standing presence of AIDS in Africa in an endemic form. Because "aggressive" KS is difficult to identify without appropriate lab technology, AIDS might have remained unidentified for a long time in Africa. Concerning the question of the identification of KS, the reader will recall that other articles argued that AIDS could be identified in Central Africa exactly because of its association with KS, the diagnosis of which did not need sophisticated lab technology. The thesis of a long-standing presence of AIDS (and hence of the infectious agent) in Africa, formulated in the first reports on the "Danish woman surgeon in Zaire," is thus redeveloped in a context that (1) redefines the relationship between AIDS and Kaposi's sarcoma and (2) provides a model of the origins of the syndrome.

The distinction between the "aggressive" and the "common" African KS was re-presented in later articles as distinguishing between the full-fledged and the endemic, or dormant, form of KS. KS would begin in a dormant state, corresponding to the "common form," which would more or less gradually evolve into an aggressive one. A paper defined Kaposi's sarcoma as "endemic in "equatorial Africa," with a "generally indolent course" (*The Lancet*, June 16, 1984, p. 1318) and then substituted "endemic KS" for "Kaposi's sarcoma in equatorial

Africa." Then, the "endemic disease" is equated with the "classical disease" (a subsection of the "results" section is even titled "Classical (Endemic) Disease"). AIDS-related KS was different from the form reported as endemic in adult African men, but it had "obvious similarities" with KS as reported in African children. The distinction between adults and children equals that between endemic and epidemic and justifies once again the special character of African KS.

We encounter the following categories: (1) KS in young homosexual men; (2) KS in elderly Americans; (3) endemic KS in adult men; (4) KS in African children; (5) KS in North America and elsewhere; and (6) KS in equatorial Africa. Because (5) combines only with (1), and (6) with (3), a double opposition is produced: North America vs. Africa and elderly people/adult men vs. young homosexual men/African children. The only similarity is that between the "KS of young homosexual men" and that of "African children," and it is described as follows: "cutaneous lesions are few in number and occur in unusual sites, generalized lymphadenopathy and visceral lesions are common, and the disease has shown aggressive behavior and a poor response to treatment" (*The Lancet*, June 16, 1984, I/8390, p. 1320). This is the aggressive form of KS, as opposed to the "classical endemic" form found in "African adult men." The aggressive form of KS is accompanied by unusual symptoms and signs which complicate the clinical diagnosis. This KS is as aggressive as the KS characteristic for "immunosuppressed homosexuals." It is encountered in young, well-to-do, educated Africans. The overall conclusion is that AIDS has been identified in Central Africa and that "the transmissible agent responsible may be endemic in Africa" (*The Lancet*, June 16, 1984, I/8390, p. 1320).

Evident here is the association of "aggressive KS" in Africa with "aggressive KS in young (then immunosuppressed) homosexuals," which supports the association of the "aggressive" or "African KS" with AIDS and therefore the thesis of an endemic presence of the infectious agent in Africa. The opposition pairs consist of (1) *classical KS* – longtime presence, endemic – vs. *aggressive KS* – recently recognized, explosive evolution, and (2) *AIDS* – recently recognized in Zambia and Zaire – vs. *infectious agent of AIDS* – long-standing presence in Africa, endemic (see also Figure 2). The conclusion: Africa represents the reservoir of the infectious agent which, favored by risk factors, expanded to Europe and North America. A European reservoir was unlikely,

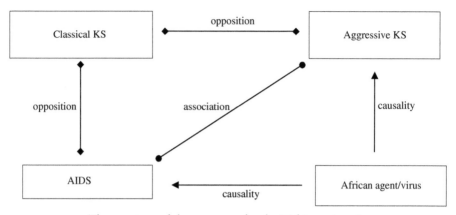

FIGURE 2. The structure of the argument for the "African virus."

because European patients traveled, were homosexuals or hemophiliacs, or had blood transfusions. African patients were none of the above, and Europe-based African patients traveled regularly to their country of origin. At the same time, KS was frequent in equatorial Africa (*NEJM*, February 23, 1984, 310/8, p. 496).

Additional arguments, such as (1) defining hepatitis B as a tropical disease and (2) rejecting malnutrition and parasitic diseases as possible causes of immunosuppression (because patients were "of upper socioeconomic status") supported the case of an "African" infectious agent. The "African" agent left no place for environmental causal factors. It is relevant to note how the need to locate the origins of the virus in Africa requires reversing the distinctions between the usual and the unusual. Travel or same-sex relationships were strong arguments for an "abnormal," unusual, risky lifestyle. Making "Africans" unusual requires regarding same-sex relationships as usual in the given AIDS context. As regards the supposed lack of spatial and social mobility among Africans, Philip Setel (1999, p. 51) has clearly shown that African societies have known a great degree of spatial and social mobility in past decades: displacements, cross-continental trade routes, civil wars, and the search for economic opportunities have forced many Africans into migration across the continent.

From this moment on, environment was assigned the role of a catalyst and shifted from etiologic to epidemiologic models. The identity of the (retro)virus remained to be established, but in a certain sense, it was already known. It could not have been anything else but an identity related to Africa and (skin) cancers, to sexually transmitted diseases, and to the barrier between animals and humans. The debate of the mid-1980s could not have avoided this frame, which pre-established how the AIDS virus can be *the* AIDS virus. Indeed, all the parties in the said debate made plentiful use of all these arguments: at the time of its discovery, the AIDS virus had already been discovered.

How Scientific Debates Work

The debates about the nature of the etiologic agent did not take the form of open clashes between clear-cut positions (environmental vs. viral theses). In many cases, the attacks were oblique: the proponents of the "lifestyle" theses contested the general possibility of a virus playing a causal role in the immune deficiency, or they questioned the state of general knowledge about immune cell functions. Their adversaries claimed that the state of the knowledge about immune cell functions simply required more research money channeled into the topic. Lack of present knowledge about the causal role of a retrovirus is not a proof that this is not the cause. What we encounter in these debates is boundary work in which rhetorical resources are mobilized to define the problem confronting the scientific community: is this an infectious disease, caused by a virus? Is it a contagious disease, caused by non-viral factors?

A key role in deciding these questions was played by three kinds of narratives. (1) The first is about viruses inducing immune deficiencies. This counteracted the view that viruses enter human bodies weakened by already existing immune deficiencies. (2) The second narrative is about environmental factors (lifestyle, sexual activities) weakening the immune system and working to the advantage of immunosuppressive agents (sperm, drugs, or a combination thereof). (3) The third is a narrative of origins: a viral agent already present in a remote (or isolated, or unmonitored) part of the world crosses the barrier between species, mutates, and induces a new immune deficiency.

Each of these narratives has several subordinate plots which confer a concrete shape upon them: these plots involve, in turn, characters such as the Danish woman surgeon who had worked in Zaire, or the nameless Haitian who ate raw pork meat and had homosexual sex. The characters of these plots, however, must not necessarily be human: amyl nitrites, the cytomegalovirus, and the African KS are prominent figures in environmental and viral plots, respectively.

The debate is not decided by one or more of these narratives leaving the stage. In the end, we are not left with a single, triumphant story. What we have in the end is a cognitive frame with a combination of narratives (1) and (3) at its core and narrative (2) playing a subordinate role. Crucial to this frame is the perception that the etiologic agent of AIDS is a virus that originated in a remote part of Africa, crossed the barrier between species, and was carried to other continents, where, in the presence of STDs and intense sexual activity, as well as other lifestyle factors, it induces immune deficiency. This frame provides the necessary elements for the interpretation of clinical data. It is grounded in cultural representations of sexual practices, disease, and otherness.

That scientific debates imply the use of rhetorical resources and devices has been long recognized. My first argument here was that, at least in the AIDS debates, the demarcation of the scientific problem (infectious vs. contagious) played a crucial role. The work of demarcation, of tracing the boundary between problem and non-problem was done, to a very large extent, with rhetorical resources.

My second argument concerns the notion that scientific debates end with the triumph of the right thesis and the demise of the wrong one. The corollary of this position is that the work of demarcation is closed. It implies that some of the actors in the debate use their (rhetorical) resources more successfully than their opponents. In the end, the latter adopt the arguments of the winning party. What happened in the case examined here was not that an unsuccessful line of argumentation was abandoned. Rather, three different narratives were recombined in such a way that one of them took a subordinate position.

In Chapter 2, I used an analogy with a virus to characterize the property of classifications to incorporate local changes, recombine, expand, and absorb contradictory explanatory models. I argue that the same property becomes visible in the debates about the etiologic agent. The successful model made local adaptations, recombined some of its elements, expanded, and absorbed competing models. In other words, at least at the rhetorical level, it displayed the same "viral" properties that characterize classifications.

The outcome of early debates about the etiology of AIDS was the thesis of a retrovirus playing the causal role. In this frame, the discovery of HIV not long after was accompanied by a bitter scientific controversy between two prominent scientists. I turn now to the arguments with which this controversy was carried on.

4

Retrovirus vs. Retrovirus

The Arguments for HTLV-III, LAV, and HIV

The HIV Controversy Revisited

In 1983, *Science* published a paper by Dr. Robert Gallo and his team, which stated that an antigenic reactivity to the human T-cell leukemia virus had been detected in AIDS patients (220, pp. 865–7). This meant that their immune system was producing antigens to a human retrovirus. This was human T-cell leukemia virus, whose existence was detected by the same Dr. Gallo in the mid-1970s. In the same issue, *Science* also published a paper by Dr. Luc Montagnier and his team from the Institut Pasteur in Paris (220, pp. 868–71). They claimed (1) the identification of a human retrovirus in the lymph tissues of an AIDS patient, and (2) that the retrovirus was responsible for the immune deficiency. In 1984, the same journal published another paper by Dr. Gallo and his team, claiming that a human retrovirus had been identified (a different one from that of Dr. Montagnier) and that it was causing the acquired immunodeficiency (*Science*, 224, pp. 497–500). Dr. Montagnier named the virus lymphadenopathy-associated virus (LAV), emphasizing its detection in the lymph tissues. Dr. Gallo in turn named his virus the human T-lymphotropic virus III (HTLV-III), stressing its membership in the family of human T-cell leukemia viruses. The first member of this family (HTLV-I) had also been isolated by Dr. Gallo. What followed has been amply discussed in the sociological and political literature:

1. Robert Gallo and Luc Montagnier each claimed that it was his virus that induced AIDS.

2. Dr. Gallo claimed that his virus was completely different from Dr. Montagnier's, whereas other researchers argued that they had an identical genetic structure: they were not exemplars of the same retrovirus, but practically the same exemplar.
3. It was therefore widely believed that Dr. Gallo had rediscovered Dr. Montagnier's retrovirus in a laboratory probe sent from Paris.
4. A political controversy between France and the United States ensued over which country had first discovered the retrovirus.
5. In 1987, the president of the United States and the prime minister of France settled this matter through a political agreement: both countries were to be regarded henceforth as codiscoverers.
6. Some observers have also stressed the fact that Dr. Montagnier's paper submitted to *Science* (reviewed by Dr. Gallo) had been delayed in publication and had its claims softened in the review process (Connor and Kingman 1988; Grmek 1990).

Up to 1988, medical papers made reference to HTLV-III, LAV, HTLV-III/LAV, or HIV. Afterward, the term HIV (human immunodeficiency virus) gained wide acceptance and replaced the other names. For some time, medical papers and reports argued that either HTLV-III or LAV was the agent responsible for AIDS, thus indirectly arguing against LAV, or HTLV-III, respectively. After 1985, the label HTLV-III/LAV was used much more frequently than the other two designations (Rawling 1994).

The controversy surrounding the discovery of HIV was not the only one in the history of AIDS: another prominent example is the controversy between the scientific mainstream and the biochemist Peter Duesberg about whether retroviruses can cause immune deficiencies or not. Started in the late 1980s, this controversy continued well into the 1990s. Although they received much media exposure, the Duesberg theses actually never had an impact comparable to that of the HIV discovery, which was settled in not only the scientific but also the political sphere. The HIV controversy raises a whole series of questions related not only to the political ramifications of scientific research and to its symbolic status at the national level, but also to research ethics and the peer review process at premier scientific journals.

The following fact needs to be borne in mind in this context: we know now that the parties in this controversy had discovered not varieties of the same virus but practically the same exemplar of the same retrovirus. Regardless of whether they were aware of this at the time of publishing the discovery claims, they were obliged to argue that the same exemplar of the same virus was not identical with itself. Of central significance in the controversy over the discovery of HIV is the claim of each participant that "my virus is not identical with your virus and it is my virus which causes AIDS." How then were distinct identities of the same exemplar of the same retrovirus created? This was not a controversy of fact, not a controversy of theory, and not one of methodological principle (McMullin 1987, pp. 64–73). It was a controversy of identity. In the following, I examine how the controversy about the virus's identity made use of rhetorical strategies and how these were a key element in establishing a retrovirus as the causal agent for AIDS.

Let us recapitulate the elements of the picture: the claim that a human retrovirus was inducing the acquired immune deficiency did not appear against an empty background. In the first place, human retroviruses had been known since the mid-1970s (Grmek 1990). Moreover, various theories about the viral agent's origins had already been put forward, among them those that postulated the exotic "African" and "Haitian" viruses. According to proponents of this view, then, a viral agent induced the immunodeficiency, aided by a constellation of risk factors and cofactors. In the mid-1980s, a kind of osmosis between apparently incompatible elements occurred: (1) a virus was presented as the agent of a sexually transmitted disease and of an immune deficiency at the same time; and (2) the risks of transmission were described in spatial terms, like those of a contagious disease. These elements are incompatible, because regarding the virus as an STD agent implied transmission through direct and intimate contact, rendering space irrelevant. In this case, relevance is ascribed to the temporally arranged string of sexual contacts – that is, to the history of STDs. Seeing the virus as a contagious agent meant that space, instead of time, became relevant: the agent is transmitted through space-determined social clusters. The debates on HTLV-III, LAV, HTLV-III/LAV, and HIV saw the virus as the agent of an STD (or of a tropical disease), but one restricted to certain social spaces. There is an additional aspect of this view, related to Africa. Legitimating the retrovirus (in one of its varieties) as the causal agent of AIDS meant accounting for its appearance in an African setting. The debate about the retrovirus relied to a large extent on a narrative of its origins. This took various forms, from simple stories[1] to more complex ones, combined with genetic analyses of the virus in "African" cell cultures. The identity of the retrovirus had to be established according to three risk dimensions: (1) the risk of sexually transmitted diseases, (2) the social spaces of risk, and (3) the "African" risk. A fourth dimension, related to (3) was added in the mid-1980s, when arguments concentrated on simian models – that is, on the attempt to induce an exact reproduction of the immunodeficiency syndrome in monkeys. The aim of this was to show that the retrovirus was causing the same type of immunodeficiency and that it had crossed the barrier from the animal to the human realm.

The Competition Between HTLV-III and LAV

A central task in establishing the identity of HTLV-III and LAV, respectively, was to show how each of them is related to sexually transmitted diseases. If the retrovirus was like an STD agent, then it was transmitted, among other such agents, through sexual contact between persons who lived in different places on the planet (but who at the same time traveled or frequented the same environments or spaces). Identifying such contacts would then be a strong argument for the retrovirus as the causal agent of the syndrome. Clinical reports and articles stressed the importance of "clusters" in which the virus was transmitted from "person-to-person" through sexual contact (*NEJM*, September 8, 1983, 309/10, p. 609). This required identifying and reporting clusters with HTLV-III or LAV as the common element. Medical reports often included charts of sexual contacts; e.g., patients from the United Kingdom were tied to persons from Australia and the United States, some of whom had been diagnosed with AIDS-related symptoms or had antibodies to HTLV-III (*The Lancet*, September 1, 1984, II/8401, p. 481). Clusters as constellations of (sexual) relationships with a center or a "main carrier" provided an STD-like model of continuous

---

[1] See "Africa and the Origin of AIDS" in *Science*, December 6, 1985, 230, p. 1141.

transmission and supported the thesis that HTLV-III is the sexually transmitted causal agent:

> Several of our findings are consistent with the hypothesis that HTLV-III is the sexually transmitted agent responsible for both AIDS and PGL and that it may be associated in certain cases without symptoms. These include: the observation that 16/19 homosexual men in the two clusters who were tested for HTLV-III had antibodies to the virus and that the PGL carrier (case 11), who seems well, is among them; and the findings that 8/9 (89%) other homosexuals with sexual contact with patients with AIDS or PGL had HTLV-III antibodies and that PGL had since developed in 3 out of these 8. In contrast, only 19 of 86 (22%) promiscuous homosexuals without a known history of sexual contact with AIDS or PGL have detectable HTLV-III antibodies. (*The Lancet*, September 1, 1984, II/8401, p. 483)

HTLV-III is presented here as the causal agent of AIDS not because antibodies to it have been detected in patients, but because they have been detected in clusters of individuals from different parts of the planet who had sexual contact with one another. The "history of sexual contacts," like the one of sexually transmitted diseases, forms the core of the argument for the identity of the retrovirus here. HTLV-III in the semen of patients with AIDS was also a very strong argument for its causal role. Transmitted sexually, the agent had to act like an STD agent and, therefore, be detectable in sexually transmitted fluids (such as sperm). This, in turn, confirmed both the retrovirus as the causal agent of AIDS and the sexual transmission route. Moreover, it showed that risk categories and the causal agent were practically coextensive, with apparently healthy "risk persons" carrying the virus. Risk categories appeared as a proof of the retrovirus's causal role, and the latter confirmed, in turn, their relevance. One paper, bearing the title "HTLV-III in the Semen and Blood of a Healthy Homosexual Man," asserted that AIDS is sexually transmitted through contact with semen (which does not necessarily imply sexual contact). On these grounds, the main culprit must be HTLV-III, to which LAV was closely related (*Science*, October 26, 1984, 226, p. 451). This argument, coming from Dr. Gallo's camp, presented LAV as subordinate and of secondary importance to HTLV-III.

The case on which the argument rested was "a 30-year-old homosexual male," whose "past medical history includes gonorrhea, hepatitis, and sexual contacts in 1982 with a man who subsequently developed

Kaposi's sarcoma." The patient did not present any AIDS-related symptoms, clearly belonged to a risk group, had his sexual contacts traced to a KS patient, and had HTLV-III detected in his semen. These were strong arguments for the causal role of HTLV-III, as well as for a closer monitoring of "urban male homosexuals." The implication was that HTLV-III might be far more widespread than the number of AIDS cases suggested (*Science*, October 26, 1984, 226, p. 453). By suggesting an immediate, unseen danger (larger undetected presence) the article not only called for concrete health policy measures ("asymptomatic carriers should be closely followed") but also, more importantly, implied the ubiquity of HTLV-III. This implication was taken as proof of its causal role. Thus, through metonymy, a whole social category was substituted for one case. The metonymy also moved the detection of HTLV-III in semen from the realm of the accidental into that of the regular and the ubiquitous, entrenching the causal role of the virus. The laboratory evidence (detection in semen) derived its relevance and strength (that is, as an empirical proof of causality) from this rhetorical frame.

If the HTLV-III camp was to win, it had to succeed in promoting two interrelated arguments: one with regard to the HTLV-III/LAV relationship, the other concerning the connection between retrovirus and STD. I begin here with the latter. The tenor of the argument was that the epidemiologic data actually supported the demonstration of HTLV-III in semen; consequently, the syndrome was STD-like, and the presence of the retrovirus in semen was relevant. Not only was it relevant, but it also was inextricably tied to "urban male homosexuals." Because the retrovirus (HTLV-III) was STD-like, it was relatively hard to get; a lot of sexual contacts were needed for infection. In an interview published in the *Journal of the American Medical Association* ("AIDS-associated Virus Yields Data to Intensifying Scientific Study," November 22/29, 1985, 254/20), Dr. Malcolm Martin, chief of the Laboratory of Molecular Microbiology at the National Institute of Allergy and Infectious Diseases, sought to alleviate fears that the virus could be transmitted through casual contact. He declared that "important is the way the virus is spread 99.9% of the time"; this was the sexual (and predominantly homosexual) way. Moreover, the virus "doesn't strip off its jacket and infect a cell in its shirtsleeves" (*JAMA*, November 22/29, 1985, 254/20, p. 2868). Because the genomic structure of the virus is heterogeneous, and because many particles are defective, "multiple contacts are needed to make a hit." One has "to work hard" at getting the virus (p. 2870). Moreover, the AIDS virus is different from contagious viruses (such as the influenza and poliomyelitis ones). It is different from other members of its family (HTLV-I, HTLV-II) as well, because "it takes a lot of virus to get a fully infectious agent" (p. 2870). A lot of virus means, of course, a lot of sexual contacts. It also means that the virus could go undetected for a long time, making antibody-positive persons into a "time bomb" (p. 2868). At the same time, AIDS can be gotten from a single sexual encounter or a single blood unit (p. 2870).

The assertion that the virus cannot become effective without multiple sexual contacts (expressed here in the metaphor of hard work) was of course consistent with the (by now) familiar notion that "homosexuals" were an extremely promiscuous group. This, in turn, was consistent with the thesis of widespread STDs in this group. Hence the explicit contrast with "contagious viruses which can spread like wildfire." But, paradoxically, a single sexual contact may suffice to contract the disease. How does this fit in with the low-contagion view? This observation, inserted more or less as an afterthought, apparently contradicts the previous statements: if multiple sexual contacts are needed for the virus to enter the body ("to make a hit"), then these must be contacts with persons who already carry the virus; otherwise there would be no "hit." What the article actually does is construct single-contact (contagion-like) transmission as the exception to the rule of "working hard to get it": cases of single-contact transmission are presented here as the exceptions that confirm this rule. The "fully infectious agent" means thus "a lot of virus" getting into the body through multiple contacts, which amounts to characterizing the retrovirus on the grounds of its risk.

Another thesis that relied on "clusterings" and on similarity with sexually transmitted diseases is that HTLV-III is more readily sexually transmitted than its supposed predecessor, HTLV-I. HTLV-I (the first human retrovirus identified by Dr. Robert Gallo) is a leukemia retrovirus, and Dr. Gallo's initial, paradoxical thesis (also embraced by other scientists) was that the AIDS and the leukemia retroviruses were closely related, although very different. If HTLV-I was not readily sexually transmitted, whereas HTLV-III was, the differences in their prevalence in the AIDS population, as well as in their effects, could be explained (*The Lancet*, September 1, 1984, pp. 481, 483). Thus we encounter once again the strategy of comparing two entities that, depending on context, are either similar or different. The criterion used for such a comparison (rate of transmission) is introduced post hoc in order to justify empirical differences in the prevalence rates. The differences established according to this post hoc criterion make the entities similar, by virtue of their being compared. Dr. Robert Gallo's team argued that weak correlations between serum antibodies to HTLV-I and AIDS were actually an argument for HTLV-III being the causal agent of AIDS, because the latter had "limited cross-reactivities with the known HTLV subgroups" (*Science*, May 4, 1984, 224, p. 506). They also argued that (1) a genomic modification could account for intra-family viral differences and (2) the HTLV virus causing AIDS is, unlike other HTLV viruses (which induce leukemia), mainly sexually transmitted. There were, however, further aspects of this virus that had to be explained away: HTLV-I was endemic in southern Japan, where AIDS had not yet been reported. Besides, Japan was far away from Africa. These facts seemed to undermine the causal role of HTLV-III. Robert Gallo discounted them in a few sentences: the virus had undergone a genomic modification on its way from Japan to Africa and, concomitantly, Japanese people had become immune to it (*Science*, May 20, 1983, 220, p. 865). We should remember here that "Africans" – whose continent was also an endemic AIDS space – had never been represented as immune to AIDS.

Dr. Gallo also reversed the significance of transmission means, so that they could lend more support to his thesis: for him, transmission through blood products or IV drug use was the most common. Nevertheless, the "high incidence of AIDS in homosexuals who apparently have not received blood transfusions or used intravenously administered drugs" meant that the virus was to be found in sperm and saliva too. Because the causal agent of AIDS was sex-related and distinct from other HTLV viruses, it would be transmitted through sexual contact. Therefore, it would not be (1) immediately identifiable in blood, as were the other HTLV viruses, and (2) in the places where other HTLV viruses are identified.

Other articles by Dr. Gallo stated that "HTLV-III is clearly distinguishable from HTLV-I and HTLV-II but is also significantly related to both viruses. HTLV-III is thus a true member of the HTLV family" (*Science*, May 4, 1984, 224, p. 503). The strategy was to assert first that "viruses of the HTLV family have been detected in some patients with the acquired immunodeficiency syndrome (AIDS) or with pre-AIDS." Then, "an involvement of viruses of the HTLV family" was suggested by the findings, but that alone appeared doubtful; "instead, it seemed likely that another member of the HTLV family might be involved in the etiology of AIDS" (*Science*, May 4, 1984, 224, p. 503). In a certain sense, the discovery of HTLV-III happened before it was actually discovered; because the retroviral family caused AIDS, it was only a matter of identifying a new member that was different, but not that different. Besides, this family argument made it possible to present the "French" retrovirus as just one genetic variety of HTLV-III, or as a member of the HTLV-III family, which in turn was a member of the larger "causal" family. A paper coauthored by Dr. Gallo argued exactly this, by transferring causality to a retrovirus family and re-defining HTLV-III as a subfamily within it. In this construction, LAV was just a member of the HTLV-III subfamily. This concept, among others, served to explain away the strong similarities between them, counteract suspicion, establish a clear hierarchy, and reinforce Gallo's priority claim with respect to the discovery of the virus:

Perhaps because of the rapid replication [...] there is a noteworthy diversity in the restriction-endonuclease cleavage patterns seen among HTLV-III iso-lates from different patients to date, indicating a genetic polymorphism not found in other viruses within the HTLV family. Therefore, we believe that HTLV-III really represents a set of closely related but varying genetic forms, and that lymphadenopathy-associated virus is one of these forms. (*NEJM*, November 15, 1984, 311/20, pp. 1294–5)

The arguments of the competition took pretty much the same turns, only in the opposite direction: LAV was presented as an agent similar to those of sexually transmitted diseases, and associated with STDs. It was also presented as a member of the HTLV family, but its "clear distinctness" was stressed. The first report on LAV published in *Science* by Dr. Montagnier's team presented AIDS primarily as a sexually transmitted disease, characteristic for certain risk categories. Because Montagnier did not have any HTLV family to defend, he did not need to explain why other retroviruses were found readily in blood, whereas the AIDS virus was not. True, his LAV was not isolated from blood either, but from lymph tissue. The best strategy for him was therefore to stick with the accepted view about the hierarchy of transmission means, in which sexual contacts occupied a prominent place (*Science*, May 20, 1983, 220, p. 868).

Dr. Montagnier reported "the isolation of a novel retrovirus from a lymph of a homosexual patient with multiple lymphadenopathies." The new virus was identified as a member of the human T-cell leukemia virus (HTLV) family. The patient was "a 33-year-old homosexual male" who had been treated several times for STD and had many sexual contacts: "During interviews he indicated that he had had more than 50 sexual partners per year and had traveled to many countries, including North Africa, Greece, and India. His last trip to New York was in 1979" (*Science*, May 20, 1983, 220, p. 870).

The association (and similarity) with sexually transmitted diseases frames the presentation of laboratory findings and the genetic analysis, so that when it comes to discussing the causal role of LAV at the end of the paper, its sexual transmission is emphasized. Montagnier did not claim that LAV is the causal agent, but rather that it is one possibility among many, including immune overload by repeated infection, some other virus, and some bacteria. Subsequent medical papers made use of the same frame, ignoring any connection to the HTLV family. The task was, therefore, to argue for differences, and not for any similarities between HTLV-III and LAV. Presenting HTLV-III as a subfamily of LAV would not work, because this would have meant acknowledging some sort of similarities. Montagnier's laboratory results needed an adequate representational frame if they were to be made into empirical evidence for a distinct retrovirus. One way to emphasize distinction and difference from HTLV-III was to look for similarities with other syndromes. A paper written by Montagnier's team presented LAV as a family of retroviruses that "clearly differ from HTLV-I morphologically," and belonged "to a new group of viruses which have the usual characteristics of retrovirus" (*The Lancet*, June 9, 1984, I/8389, p. 1255). This family of retroviruses was involved in both AIDS and the lymphadenopathy syndrome (LAS), which was presented as a lesser variant of AIDS. The strategy was to present a syndrome (LAS) specific to the LAV family and to argue that the latter was involved in both AIDS and LAS and hence was different from HTLV. Referring to their first paper from *Science*, the authors reformulated its epistemic claims as:

We have isolated a new human retrovirus from cultures of T lymphocytes from the lymph-node of a homosexual man with lymphadenopathy syndrome (LAS). The virus has been named lymphadenopathy-associated virus (LAV). Other viruses, similar or identical to LAV, have been isolated from several patients with frank AIDS or at risk of AIDS. They include a virus isolated from a homosexual man with Kaposi's sarcoma (KS) and viruses isolated from two siblings with haemophilia B, one of whom had AIDS. (*The Lancet*, June 9, 1984, I/8389, p. 1253)

The claim about causal agency follows indirectly, by systematically showing the presence of members of the LAV family in the known risk categories: hemophiliacs, homosexuals, Haitians, Africans (*The Lancet*, June 9, 1984, I/8389, p. 1254). The controls meant to prove the association of AIDS with LAV were "44 homosexual men without LAS [and hence without AIDS] who visited a venereal disease clinic in Paris." The identification of LAV antibodies "in a considerable number of healthy homosexual men who had had multiple partners and venereal diseases – a group at high risk for AIDS" (*The Lancet*, June 9, 1984, I/8389, p. 1255) was also presented as proof of association. Another proof, published at about the same time, was that antibodies to LAV were identified in serum samples "from homosexual men, 18 years of age or older, who sought medical care at the San Francisco City Clinic" (*Science*, July 20, 1984, 225, p. 322) and in "apparently normal homosexuals":

Since we also find antibodies to LAV p25 in apparently normal homosexuals, the results of the study on the distribution of antibodies to LAV have to be interpreted with caution. For example, in the case of adult T-cell leukemia (ATL) in Japan, there is a clear etiological relation between the disease and HTLV-I. Even though nearly 25 percent of the population in the endemic area have antibodies to HTLV-I, only a minor percentage of the population gets ATL. Thus, as with ATL in Japan, other cofactors in addition to viruses may be involved in the causation of AIDS. (*Science*, July 20, 1984, 225, p. 323)

The similarity to the situation in Japan (also discussed by Robert Gallo) is not used as a substitute for the similarity between the two retroviruses; rather, it is an argument for the similarity between two transmission models. In both cases, additional risk factors are needed to trigger AIDS. The strategy is to create dissimilarity through similarity to argue for the causal role of LAV: because antibodies are also found in "apparently normal" members of risk categories, a similar situation ("as with ATL") can guide their interpretation. This similar situation shows that the causal agent acts in the presence of cofactors; hence, LAV as a causal factor may also act in the presence of cofactors. At the same time, a dissimilarity between HTLV-I and LAV emerges: they have different effects. The formal similarity of the two causal chains (HTLV-I-ATL and LAV-AIDS) emerges as a difference that supports LAV as the distinct causal agent of AIDS.

The Gallo–Montagnier contest about the identity of the viral agent did not necessarily match standard scientific controversies: the identical genomic structure of the two retroviruses did raise questions about how they were obtained; neither Dr. Gallo nor Dr. Montagnier tried to discredit the other's version of the virus directly. It was never claimed that the competition's virus did not cause anything at all. Rather, the debate was about the relationship between HTLV-III and LAV, framed as a debate about how a human retrovirus can cause immune deficiency. Not only did participants in this debate mobilize laboratory probes and diagnoses in their attempts to construct viral hierarchies, but they also needed to provide narratives of where the virus was coming from and how it had traveled to North America and Europe. They also needed to show how it acted with respect to the various risk categories. In this respect, constructing a viral hierarchy (with HTLV-III or LAV, respectively, as a subfamily of a more important viral family) required a reordering of risk categories and of the relationship between them.

Recent studies have emphasized the role of rhetorical resources in scientific controversies (e.g., Cole 1996; Lewenstein 1995; Picart 1994), where such resources are used by the parties involved to define the object of controversy according to their own epistemic claims. The use of these resources delineates the zone where clashes take place and where the contested objects are situated. In our case, the contested zone was that of the HTLV–LAV hierarchy (see Figure 3). As stated at the opening of this chapter, each party in the controversy needed to show that HTLV-III and LAV were distinct, yet somehow related. As we know now, they were the same exemplar of the same retrovirus. The opponents had to construct a representational frame in which to show

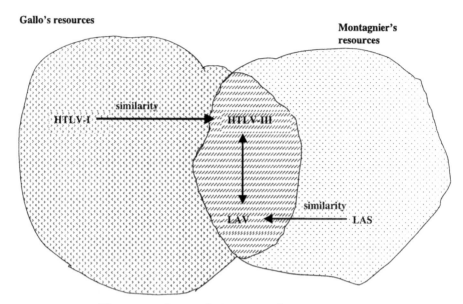

FIGURE 3. The contested zone of HTLV-III and LAV.

that their respective retroviruses (1) were related to STDs; (2) were associated with risk groups; (3) had originated in Africa at some point in time and had been disseminated around the globe; and (4) were related to each other. Because both parties had successfully argued (1)–(3), the decisive element was (4). The relationship between HTLV-III and LAV stood at the core of the contested zone.

Both Dr. Gallo and Dr. Montagnier had access to resources that lay outside this zone: Dr. Gallo's were tied to HTLV-I, whereas Dr. Montagnier's were based on the lymphadenopathy syndrome (LAS). Each of the disputants tried to bring his own resources into the contested zone and exclude the resources of the competition on the grounds that they were not relevant. For Montagnier, the relationship between HTLV-I and III was not of any interest because AIDS was not a form of cancer. For Dr. Gallo, LAS was not a topic of interest because both HTLV-I and III were human retroviruses. Thus, (1) the continuous reformulation of what counts as a relevant topic (Prelli 1989), (2) the redefinition of the syndrome, (3) the reordering of risk categories in transmission chains, and (4) the creation of narratives of the origins and travels of the virus were among the main rhetorical strategies by means of which both competitors tried to occupy this contested area.

In this sense, they tried to rearrange the resources at hand according to their aims rather than bring in new ones. In the process of reshuffling, two elements occupied a central place: showing how the virus traveled and where it came from. Consequently, travel narratives had to enter the scene at this point.

Social Spaces and the Retrovirus

A rather common strategy that was used to account for how the virus moved around was to transform simple networks or agglomerations of people into spatially determined statistical correlations between the retrovirus and risk factors. The argument of Dr. Gallo was based on the premise that a statistically significant correlation of HTLV-III with spatially deployed lifestyle factors (also named "determinants" of the virus) would be a proof of causality. This argument aimed at statistically connecting clinically-identified opportunistic diseases, numbers of blood cells, and laboratory-identified antibodies with the infectious agent and with "lifestyle risk factors." "Lifestyle" meant here the number of sexual partners and "homosexual-specific" sexual practices, which were in turn associated with "homosexual men in New York City, a group at high risk for AIDS" (*The Lancet*, September 29, 1984, II/8405, pp. 712–3). With spatial location defining not only the "groups at highest risk," but also the riskiest sexual practices, a statistical association between the retrovirus and one of these elements would mean evidence for the causal role of HTLV-III (*The Lancet*, September 29, 1984, II/8405, p. 712). Sexual practices (called "homosexual lifestyle exposures" and "lifestyle variables") were classified according to the criteria of "insertive/receptive," the number of sexual contacts in the previous year, and "intercourse act" (*The Lancet*, September 29, 1984, II/8405, p. 714). Subjects were drawn from Manhattan STD medical practices. The "lifestyle risk factors," "practices," or "determinants" were classified along a continuum from "strong correlation" to "weaker correlation." Statistical correlations were presented as an important argument for (1) HTLV-III as the etiologic agent of the syndrome; (2) implicitly, HTLV-III and not LAV being the etiologic agent, at a time when the two were seen as different; (3) evidence of the "carrier state" – that of an individual who already had antibodies for the infectious agent, but was otherwise free of any symptoms; and (4) the view that men were at a lower risk for being infected through sexual intercourse with women than with men:

This study of homosexual men at high risk for AIDS shows that the presence of HTLV-III antibodies is an important risk factor for three AIDS-related clinical conditions (lymphadenopathy, lesser AIDS and fully fledged AIDS). The presence of antibodies is also associated with a low helper T-cell level, the salient immunological characteristic of AIDS. We have also shown that the prevalence of HTLV-III antibodies correlates best with numbers of homosexual partners and frequency of receptive anal intercourse [...] Thus, epidemiologically HTLV-III could be the putative AIDS agent. (*The Lancet*, September 29, 1984, II/8405, p. 714)

Characteristically, the paper argued not on biological but on epidemiological grounds. These "epidemiological grounds" were produced first by selecting a risk group, and secondly, by statistically constructing risk factors such as "group lifestyle" in a way that is universal and exclusive. As Clatts and Mutchler (1989) have argued, the "group" produces the "factors" and the "factors" produce the "group." The infectious agent is presented here first as "risk" for clinical conditions; "lifestyle variables" are "risk" for HTLV-III. In turn, HTLV-III is the "putative agent" for AIDS and initiates "immune destruction" (*The Lancet*, September 29, 1984, II/8405, p. 715). Risk acquires a double status: on the one hand, it is a set of conditions that favor the occurrence of something (in this case, transmission of the infectious agent). On the other hand, risk determines this occurrence. In the second case, because risk is group-specific, the transmission of the infectious agent is also group-determined. In this line of argument, "lifestyle variables" or risk factors presented as group- and place-specific sexual acts support the view that HTLV-III is the retroviral agent. With respect to the genetic identities of HTLV-III and LAV, we can see that the authors of the paper quoted above (Robert Gallo and his team) construct a legitimate identity for their retrovirus by associating it with types of sexual acts and with frequency of sexual contacts. At a time when it was debated whether the virus had a high or a low virulence (a key question with respect to how it attacks the immune system), the simple copresence of antibodies and of "group-specific" sexual acts made a risk category into the best proof of causality.

Gender distinctions were also employed here. "Receptive anal intercourse" means that "rectal mucosa may be unusually vulnerable to passage of this lymphocytotoxic agent," and "insertive anal intercourse seemed to be relatively protective, a finding that may correspond to the low risk of transmission of AIDS from women to men" (*The Lancet*, September 29, 1984, II/8405, p. 715). These assertions dovetailed with the thesis of genetically determined differences between the male and the female body with respect to AIDS. They contradict the idea that it takes lots of the virus in order "to make a hit." It is exactly this thesis which supports the argument of very frequent anal intercourse as a relevant (if not the most relevant) risk factor. If certain sexual acts imply an "unusual vulnerability" of bodily membranes, you do not need lots of the virus to induce the immune deficiency. The strategy is to stress the receptor's role: once recipients are vulnerable, this vulnerability defines how the retrovirus acts. Although the paper discussed only risk factors pertaining to the "homosexual" risk group, it legitimized extrapolations by mentioning intravenous drug users and their sexual partners, for whom different male/female infection ratios had been statistically constructed. The number of sexual contacts ("partners") and the types of sexual acts are brought together, generating a risk constellation coextensive with the risk group.[2]

Spatial agglomerations as an argument for the causal role of the retrovirus were also present in subsequent papers, which used the acronyms HTLV-III/LAV or HIV. Some studies on "risk factors in homosexual men," which aimed to prove the causal role of HIV under the action of certain cofactors, selected their cases according to neighborhood; they correlated types of sexual acts with seropositivity, constructing statistical differences between frequencies of sexual acts, according to whether they were practiced in the same neighborhood or not. A study conducted in San Francisco selected "a six square-block area" and then investigated the differences in sexual act types and frequencies of the residents with AIDS-related clinical conditions (*AJE*, 1987, 125/6, p. 1037). This approach followed the argumentative pattern used for contagious diseases, because it clearly associated distribution of the virus with social space. Yet the aim could not be to provide an

---

[2] The paper stresses the "apparent synergistic interaction between these two activities" (p. 711).

overview of how the virus traveled (after all, sexual contacts must not be restricted to one's immediate residential area). Rather, this distribution was taken as proof of the virus's causal role: because it was there, it was the causal agent of AIDS.

From these spatial differences the thesis of a "sexually active subculture which was infected early with HIV" (*AJE*, 1987, 125/6, p. 1046) was advanced.[3] If the transmission of the retrovirus had a spatially determined pattern, an explanatory model would need to account for the geographical origins of the retrovirus. A story of its origins would thus be a strong causal argument.

The Story of the Origins

One of the strategies in arguing for HTLV-III as the cause of AIDS was to identify a retrovirus family from Africa, to derive from it the origins of HTLV-III, and to derive afterwards from these origins the causal role of HTLV-III. But the first members of this retrovirus family had been identified in southern Japan; bringing them from there to Africa might have seemed a difficult enterprise. One of Dr. Gallo's papers ("A Pathogenic Retrovirus [HTLV-III] Linked to AIDS") argued that a variety of HTLV-I had been identified in Africa, and that related retroviruses were known in African primates. The conclusion was that:

The wide distribution of HTLV-I in Africa and the presence of a closely related retrovirus in troops of Old World monkeys support the hypothesis that the HTLV family originated in Africa and that at least one member arrived in the Americas by way of the slave trade. Moreover, the presence of HTLV-I in Japan and the identity of this virus with the HTLV-I in Africa, the United States and the Caribbean is consistent with the speculation that HTLV-I arrived in Japan relatively recently, perhaps brought there by 16th century Portuguese mariners who had contacts with Africa and Japan during the same period. (*NEJM*, November 15, 1984, 311/20, p. 1294)

This meant that somewhere – "in an exceedingly remote portion of Central Africa" – there was a reservoir of the (HTLV-III) virus,

---

[3] After discussing briefly the argument about inhaled drugs (a secondary factor in sexual contacts, which "may increase intolerance to rectal abrasions"), the paper formulated the thesis of the "sexual subculture" without apparent relationship to neighborhood. This subculture is defined by its "engaging in extensive and traumatic rectal sex, accompanied by the use of nitrites."

which had recently migrated to urban centers through population shifts or through some other process (*NEJM*, November 15, 1984, 311/20, p. 1296). This explanation has a certain cinematic quality: at the darkest heart of Africa resides the unknown/the dangerous virus, which is spread over the world by sailors/merchants/the slave trade, only to be discovered centuries later by a scientific expedition. The "reservoir" metaphor, which was also present in the description of prostitutes as "reservoirs of infected semen," introduces here a distinction between the known and the unknown/the dangerous. It traces the limits of medical knowledge but, at the same time, opens a program of research. We should remember here that other articles had called for flying squads to be sent to Central Africa (and Manhattan too) to investigate the origins of AIDS.

The reservoir metaphor was taken over by other articles following a different line: carriers of the HTLV family in the US were unusual and found mostly in marginal populations, like rural African Americans or natives of Alaska. In healthy Caucasians from Europe and North America, "HTLV infection seems to be very rare, except perhaps in patients with the acquired immunodeficiency syndrome" (*The Lancet*, October 22, 1983, II/8355, p. 962). This led to the conclusion that Central Africa is to be seen as a "reservoir of HTLV," and that the whole family of retroviruses was brought to North America via the Caribbean at several points in time (*Science*, May 20, 1983, 220, p. 862); hence, the earliest infection must have taken place in Africa. "Black Africans" were infected by monkeys and, in turn, infected people from the Caribbean (read: Haiti). From here, the virus came to North America. The explanation links together disparate elements: Africans, Haitians, monkeys, and North Americans, into an account of the virus transgressing the barrier between species *and* traveling from Africa to North America (*Science*, May 20, 1983, 220, p. 963).

The strategy employed here is to construct an origin before the origin: if the whole retrovirus family originated in Africa a long time ago, then one member must also have been present there; hence, this member is the causal agent. Moreover, if African Kaposi's sarcoma is associated with a retrovirus from the HTLV family and with AIDS, then AIDS is associated with the "African reservoir" of HTLV-III too. Earlier retroviruses arrived in America with the slave trade; later ones (and with them AIDS) arrived with population shifts. HTLV-III was thus presented, depending on the context, sometimes as a sexually transmitted retrovirus, different from other HTLVs, and sometimes as a tropical retrovirus, similar to other HTLVs. One strategy was thus to argue for an indirect "African" association of AIDS with HTLV-III via "African KS"; another was to argue for a direct association of the "African" AIDS cases with the retrovirus. As pointed out previously, clinical reports and articles on patients with Kaposi's sarcoma seen in Central Africa were used as an argument for the compatibility between the "African" and the "homosexual" KS. In most cases, Kaposi's sarcoma was described as the only disease observed; in some of them, it was combined with several other opportunistic infections and diseases. In all of them it was presented as the decisive evidence for (1) a diagnosis of AIDS in Central African patients, (2) the long-standing existence of the infectious agent of AIDS in Central Africa, prior to its presence in Europe and North America, and (3) the transmission of the said agent from Africa to North America and Europe. Also important in this context was the question of whether the retroviral agent was related to Kaposi's sarcoma; a relationship between the two was a clear argument for the long-standing presence (and effects) of the retrovirus in Africa.

The emphasis was placed on the "African" risk factors, taken, however, out of the KS context in which they originated. One of these characteristics was the lower male-to-female ratio. This served at different points as an argument for (1) the extraordinary character of the "homosexual" KS, (2) the similarity between "African" and "homosexual" KS, and (3) the African specificity of heterosexual transmission. The latter, in turn, was used as an argument for the long-standing presence of the retrovirus in Africa. Heterosexual transmission was actually the originaly form of transmission, preserved (almost) only in Africa. The basic structure of the argument was then:

> Heterosexual transmission is a long-standing African risk factor for AIDS.
> The retrovirus has a long-standing presence in Africa.
> The retrovirus (HTLV-III, LAV, HTLV-III/LAV, etc.) is associated with heterosexual transmission and other African risk factors.
> Hence, the retrovirus is the causal factor of AIDS.

Later on, the association between HTLV-III and KS lost its relevance, because it became possible to show directly (1) antibodies to HTLV-III in African populations, as well as (2) a direct association between these antibodies and Africa-specific risk factors. The rhetorical strategy with regard to (1) was to push the association between AIDS and HTLV-III further into the past by showing that antibodies to the retrovirus existed in Africans long before the syndrome was signaled in North America. Actually, the same construction was used in arguing for the association between AIDS and KS – i.e., showing that AIDS-like syndromes had been related to KS in Africa in the 1970s. One such study claimed to have identified antibodies to HTLV-III in Ugandan children's serum samples from before 1973; this was proof that "residents of the West Nile region of Uganda have been and continue to be exposed to the virus at a very early age." This, in turn, was a proof that "certain host or environmental factors may facilitate or enhance exposure, susceptibility, or immune responsiveness to both [HTLV-I and HTLV-III] or even other viruses" (*Science*, March 1, 1985, 227, p. 1037). Showing that the retrovirus had been present in "remote regions" of Central Africa well before the first manifestations of the syndrome in North America meant that the syndrome was "endemic and not newly introduced," that is, it was "present in the environment" (*NEJM*, Oct. 18, 1984, 311/16, p. 1051). An almost identical argument had been made about "endemic KS" as a proof of the long-standing existence of the AIDS agent in Africa. If the retrovirus was endemic and part of the environment (like KS), then it would either go unnoticed or cause milder forms of AIDS. The report on the Ugandan serum samples stated that:

If, as we suspect, the antibody reactivities found represent widespread exposure or infection by HTLV-III, then it must be asked why the incidence of AIDS in the Ugandan population (and neighboring Zaire) has gone unnoticed for so long. It is possible that AIDS existed in African populations without being recognized as a separate disease entity. The virus may have originated in Africa in the past and exposure to the virus may be much more common than AIDS itself in some populations. As with many other infectious diseases, host responsiveness may vary between severe and subclinical. (*Science*, March 1, 1985, 227, p. 1038)

Full-fledged AIDS appears then as an outcome of the interaction between the endemic retrovirus and certain "African" risk factors, which are spatially distributed. The retrovirus was dormant in "remote regions" and "active" in risk spaces[4]; it caused both a mild and an acute version of the syndrome, according to where it was seen. But, then, we would have to go back to how the virus had crossed the barrier between animals and humans. The culprits are wild African Green monkeys, which harbor a virus similar to that of AIDS. This virus crossed the species barrier and "may have mutated in man and acquired some destructive properties" (*Science*, December 6, 1985, 230, p. 1141). Also, the African Green monkeys "have been considered as reservoirs or vectors of certain other viruses that sometimes cause disease in humans including Ebola fever, Marburg disease, and African yellow fever" (*Science*, Nov. 22, 1985, 230, p. 954). The rural environment was the place where the retrovirus crossed the barrier; an urban space provides the risks necessary for developing the acute version of the syndrome. Other versions of this model asserted that various environments have different risk factors: the rural areas have rituals of traditional medicine, through which the virus is transmitted. In urban environments, the virus is transmitted through sexual contacts (*The Lancet*, July 14, 1984, II/8394, p. 63).

The same arguments were used by Dr. Montagnier with respect to LAV. If the "African" group was special and distinct from all other risk categories, then an early presence of LAV in this group constituted a strong argument for its causal role (*Science*, Oct. 26, 1984, 226, p. 455).[5] At the same time, the presence of LAV in "Africans" enforced their distinctiveness; conversely, distinctiveness was an argument for the role of LAV in the pathogenesis of AIDS. However, Dr. Montagnier's problem was that the serum used in laboratory analyses had come from African residents of Belgium and France, or from Africans who had come to Paris for medical treatment. (This latter fact makes it improbable that the patients were members of an underprivileged, rural population.) Nevertheless, the problem was to show that the infection with the virus had taken place in Africa, and not in Europe. Otherwise, the arguments for the causal role of LAV would be

---

[4] See also *The Lancet*, July 14, 1984, II/8394, pp. 64–5.

[5] The paper reported a case of "familial transmission" dating from 1977, in which antibodies to LAV were identified in a "Zairian mother" who died in 1978. The daughter was presented as "a healthy 7-year-old living in Belgium," whose serum was "weakly positive by RIPA for LAV antibody."

much weakened. Therefore, the authors proceeded to show the special connection between Africa, KS, and LAV:

There is strong evidence that AIDS is endemic in central and equatorial Africa. The report of Kaposi's sarcoma in Zambia with clinical and biological findings similar to those in AIDS and the likely underestimation of cryptococcosis in Zaïre are further evidence. Our patient 1 meets the criteria for the diagnosis of AIDS and his wife has the prodromal symptoms for the disorder or AIDS-related complex. They do not differ epidemiologically from other African patients and belong to none of the other AIDS risk categories. AIDS in non-Africans is thought to be caused by an agent transmitted sexually or, less commonly, through needles or blood. Several reports have suggested that a virus from the human retrovirus family might be the etiological agent. The hypothesis of LAV being the agent is supported by its isolation from this couple. In addition, antibodies to LAV have been detected in sera of AIDS patients in Zaïre and at a much lower level in a Zaïrian control population (unpublished). (*The Lancet*, June 23, 1984, I/8391, p. 1383)

The report continues:

A virus called HTLV-III with characteristics similar to those of LAV has been reported as a possible aetiological agent of AIDS. Whether or not HTLV-III and LAV are the same virus is now under investigation. Since the AIDS incubation period may be as long as four years, our patients may have acquired the disease in Zaïre. We cannot establish whether they acquired the AIDS causative agent through sexual relations or independently by other modes of transmission. However, heterosexual transmission is seldom documented in non-Africans. The African AIDS risk category is special because of the unknown mode of transmission of the disease and its endemic pattern in Africa. Inoculation of LAV to animals with the reproduction of an AIDS-like disease and seroepidemiological studies, particularly in Africa, will be needed as definitive proof that LAV has an aetiological role. (*The Lancet*, June 23, 1984, I/8391, p. 1385)

The first statement asserts "strong evidence" for the endemic character of AIDS in Central Africa, supported by reports on Kaposi's sarcoma and probable underestimation of cryptococcosis. Some evidence is positive (reports on KS); other evidence (likely underestimation) is negative. The implication is that reports on Kaposi's sarcoma with clinical features similar to those of AIDS are proof of the endemic presence of AIDS and "aggressive," endemic KS. More important are the statements that the patients examined in the Bicêtre Hospital in Paris met the criteria for AIDS and that they do not epidemiologically differ from other African patients and do not belong to other risk categories. Up to this point, the structure of the argument is as follows: (1) there is evidence for endemic AIDS in Africa; (2) patients examined have been diagnosed with AIDS; (3) they did not differ epidemiologically from other African patients (which amounts to saying that they are Africans and, indirectly, says that they were infected in Africa); and (4) they did not belong to other risk categories. A double substitution process is performed (*endemic AIDS in Africa* is replaced by *two African patients in Paris* who afterwards are replaced by *African patients*), concomitantly with the assertion of a distinct identity of "African patients."

The metonymy supports the thesis that the patients were infected in Africa, not in Europe. At the same time, it reiterates the endemic character of AIDS in Africa. The infection in an African setting cannot be proved empirically (after all, the patients could have become infected in Paris, or even in the Bicêtre Hospital); nevertheless, it is crucial to the narratives of the virus's origins.

What follows is: the retroviral nature of the agent is evidence that LAV is this agent; the detection of antibodies to LAV in AIDS patients in Zaire is further evidence; there is a relationship between HTLV-III and LAV. The structure of the argument is as follows: (1) a human retrovirus is a possible agent; (2) LAV is the agent because it is a retrovirus *and* because it has been isolated in this African couple; and (3) LAV is the agent because it has been isolated from African patients. Thus, the argument for the etiologic agent relies heavily on (1) the "African risk group" and (2) the substitutability of the patients belonging to this group who have been examined. What follows are statements that the patients *may* have been infected in Zaire and that the means of infection cannot be exactly established. The uncertainty expressed in the active voice is countered by the next statement in the passive: heterosexual transmission is seldom documented in non-Africans. Thus, heterosexual transmission is presented as Africa-specific, which makes "Africans" even more special. The "two patients from Zaire living in France" is transformed into the "African risk category," which is special because of the "unknown transmission mode" and its endemic pattern in Africa. On the whole, the "discussion" constructs "Africans" as a special category by substituting parts for the whole, transforming these parts into separate categories, and classifying and reclassifying them.

Other papers distinguished between the mere presence of the retrovirus in a "healthy population at risk for AIDS" (i.e., "Africans") and the copresence of AIDS and the retrovirus in AIDS patients: the two were a strong argument for LAV's causal role, in a manner similar to that of arguing for the dormant and active states of HTLV-III in "Africans." On the grounds of seropositive probes from two hospitals in Kinshasa, Zaire, it was argued that the number of AIDS cases was indicative of a much broader infection with the virus in the "healthy population at risk for AIDS," although the latter was not precisely defined:

The prediction that a single infectious agent is at the origin of AIDS implies that all those with proven AIDS show signs of infection. Failures to show infection by the agent should be rare or must be reasonably attributed to lack of sensitivity for demonstrating virus or antibody. In the case of a lymphotropic, lymphocytolytic agent such as LAV, failure to show antibody may also be due to eventual depletion of cells that are a necessary link in immune reaction. Evidence for secondary antibody failure in AIDS was presented earlier. The prediction does not imply that all those infected by the agent proceed to clinical AIDS but, unless additional factors outweigh the direct role of the agent in the causation of AIDS, it does imply that the agent is relatively infrequent in the healthy population at risk for AIDS, and the frequency of infection in that population parallels, at a lower level, the frequency of AIDS cases. The incidence of AIDS in Zaire has recently been found to be very high in Kinshasa, ranging from 15 to 20 cases per 100,000 population. Our data, showing LAV infection in 94 percent of Zairian AIDS cases and in at least 5 percent of control populations, support the hypothesis that retroviruses of the LAV type are universally involved in this disease. (*Science*, Oct. 26, 1984, 226, p. 455)

As "further evidence of the causal relationship between LAV and AIDS," the article cites the "high prevalence of LAV antibody in AIDS among Caucasian homosexuals, parenteral drug users, and Haitians, and its rarity in control groups"; this amounts to presenting "Africans" as the primary evidence for the causal agency of LAV and to detaching this evidence from additional evidence. Apparently, the argument of causality is primarily theoretical, with seroepidemiologic findings serving only as empirical "evidence." It simply asserts that, if LAV is the causal agent, then antibodies to LAV must be detected in all AIDS cases and, to a lesser extent, in "healthy populations at risk." The empirical evidence is that the frequency of AIDS in Kinshasa was very high; therefore, the frequency of infection with LAV also must have been high. Moreover, the frequency of infection with LAV in the AIDS cases was very high. All this constituted the proof that LAV was the causal agent. Let us first examine the statement that "the incidence of AIDS in Zaire has been found to be very high in Kinshasa": here there is (1) a synecdoche that substitutes Zaire for Kinshasa, and (2) a statistical construction by which this incidence is obtained by dividing the number of cases of AIDS seen in three Kinshasa clinics by the total population of the city. The article referred to as evidence (*The Lancet*, July 14, 1984, II/8394, p. 68) relied for its assertions on cases from the same hospital, as well as from two other smaller clinics. It calculated an incidence of 17 per 100,000 inhabitants, which becomes "ranging from 15 to 20 cases" here. Thus the same cases are presented once as general incidence and once as specific cases of LAV infection, both being offered as self-confirmatory proof of causality. As a consequence, the rate of LAV infection in the "healthy population at risk" must also be relatively high, and higher than "that observed in European countries" (*Science*, Oct. 26, 1984, 226, p. 455), which again stresses the special character of the "African" risk. Empirical evidence is represented both as special (i.e., different from non-African empirical data) and as general. It supports the theoretical model (and hence the assertion of causality) not as a specific, but as a generally valid proof. Otherwise, it would make little sense to ground general theoretical assertions in evidence that has specific, limited validity. "Africans" are very special and very general at the same time; in this double status, they constitute proof of LAV's causal role. In this sense, the theoretical assertions serve rather as a middle term through which "evidence for LAV infection in Africans with AIDS" is transformed into "evidence for the causal role of LAV in AIDS."

These arguments, as well as the narratives about how Portuguese sailors and slaves brought the viruses to Japan and North America, respectively, or the special character of "Africans," may seem unimportant compared to the identification of antibodies to HTLV-III or LAV in "African" serum samples. After all, the decisive role was played by laboratory results. Historically seen, the rhetorical construction of the African origin of the HTLV family preceded the laboratory data showing antibodies to HTLV-III, and it was also a permanent presence in medical papers that presented this laboratory evidence. Narratives of the African origins of the virus thus constituted the frame in which laboratory data became relevant as empirical, hard evidence for the causal role of the human retrovirus. Correspondingly, proof of antibodies to LAV was always presented in a frame that stressed the special character of the "African" risk category. This frame allowed the interpretation of laboratory results not as contingent on, but as relevant for, the causal role of the retrovirus; it made (evidence of) seropositivity appear as such – i.e., as proof of causality.

One consequence of these (by no means singular) rhetorical moves was that, among other things, ways of transmission became associated with ethnically or sexually defined categories: Africans are exclusively heterosexual and Africa is a reservoir of the virus. Homosexuals are promiscuous and practice too much anal sex. These associations provide a frame for interpreting particular cases – interpretations that may ignore the cases that do not fit easily or factors that are not usually ascribed to a category. For example, the strict association between "Africans" and heterosexual sex may ignore other sexual practices, patterns of sexual transmission, or the role of poverty and malnutrition. They have been highlighted only very recently in anthropological field research (Setel 1999).[6] In other words, the categorical treatment of risk factors necessarily leads to the ignoring of other factors not usually associated with the group but which may nevertheless play an important role. The strong association between risk factors and groups is also a problem for contemporary AIDS prevention, which targets (ethnic) groups by emphasizing factors considered to be group-specific (Cohen 1999).

The exclusive ascription of a risk behavior to a risk group, which is then defined through this behavior, led to the (still influential) notion that male–male sex defines homosexual risk, male–female sex defines heterosexual risk, and certain ethnic and racial groups (such as Africans) are exclusively heterosexual. Social research has consistently shown that sexual behavior is complex and not confined to such categories. Outreach and prevention approaches are confronted even today with the fact that many African American men with (more or less regular) same-sex contacts define themselves as heterosexuals (e.g.,

---

[6] Even in the late 1980s, however, experienced epidemiologists had reported that African children with anemia were susceptible to infection with HIV (Mann 1987, p. 133).

Lemelle 2003). Sexual identity cannot thus be isolated from social and cultural identity; prevention approaches operating with identity stereotypes prove to be ineffective in many cases.

We could have envisaged an alternative development here, in which means of transmission did not become associated with risk groups, an association that has proven to be specious, given the developments since then. This association, however, was employed as a central argument both for the causal role of a retrovirus and for establishing its identity. Through replication in many scientific articles, the association has moreover acquired a life of its own and has become very difficult to dismantle.

"Simian AIDS"

After the reports on HTLV-III and LAV, it became important to construct primate models of the syndrome, in order to argue that (1) the retrovirus has actually transgressed the barrier between animals and humans and (2) it was inducing a similar immunodeficiency in monkeys, being therefore the universal causal agent. After Dr. Robert Gallo published the first article about HTLV-III in *Science*, the similarity between human and animal leukemia viruses was brought out as a strong argument in favor of HTLV-III as the causal agent of AIDS. Virologists argued that HTLV was similar to mouse Moloney leukemia virus, belonging to a larger family of oncogenic viruses. This was seen as proof that the AIDS virus was a leukemia retrovirus (*Nature*, July 21, 1983, 304, p. 206).

The idea that monkeys may harbor retroviruses transmissible to humans had already been formulated with respect to what was considered to be the first member of the HTLV family, the human T-cell leukemia virus (*The Lancet*, Sept. 18, 1982, II/8299, p. 658).[7] This retrovirus was first reported in Japanese macaques, and then in African Green monkeys. The Japanese macaques were presented as "a natural reservoir for virus transmission to man," and the question was posed whether humans "living in the same regions as the ATLV-infected monkeys acquire signs of the disease." Reports dating from 1983 also signaled an "epidemic of acquired immunodeficiency" and "a syndrome closely

---

[7] See also *The Lancet*, January 29, 1983, I/8318, pp. 240–1.

resembling acquired immunodeficiency syndrome (AIDS)" in rhesus monkeys (*The Lancet*, February 19, 1983, I/8321, p. 388). The disease was characterized as "striking," with a mortality rate "seven times greater than that observed in other groups of rhesus monkeys of comparable age and sex distribution," and with a "clinical picture which parallels that observed in human AIDS" (*The Lancet*, February 19, 1983, I/8321, p. 390). Later papers called it "simian acquired immunodeficiency syndrome" or SAIDS (*Science*, March 9, 1984, 223, p. 1083); a retrovirus isolated from blood samples was successfully transmitted through inoculation, and therefore presented as the agent of SAIDS. The (1) identification of antibodies to HTLV-I (ATLV) in Japanese monkeys, combined with (2) the observation of immune deficiency in monkeys ("animal AIDS") and (3) the assertion that the retrovirus had transgressed the interreign barrier in Africa and (4) that this transgression was proof of its causal role, led to attempts to construct an "animal AIDS" that would mirror the human AIDS point by point. This was done by inoculating primates with the cultured retroviruses of both SAIDS and AIDS; they were expected to induce the "animal AIDS" in the same way in which they induced the "human" one. One of the main arguments was that inoculation would prove that the barrier had been transgressed. If the human retrovirus had transgressed the barrier from human to primate, then it must have been able to transgress it in the opposite direction too; this would make it possible to find "the ancestral origin of the virus," argued Robert Gallo (*The Lancet*, October 22, 1983, II/8355, p. 963). Another idea was that, by inoculating primates with the SAIDS agent, one could observe how this would be distributed in the respective population, how much it would take to develop the full syndrome, and which measures would be necessary for "controlling SAIDS in primates" (*Science*, March 9, 1983, 219, p. 1085). Ways of transmission could be observed, and different retroviruses (HTLV-III, LAV) could be compared. Hence, a "simian AIDS" would also be strong proof of the causal role of HTLV-III or LAV, respectively, and an important argument in the debate. As one paper by Dr. Luc Montagnier's team (reporting "successful transmission of LAV to two chimpanzees") put it:

This is the first report of LAV/HTLV-III infection of a non-human primate. The chimpanzees had no serological or culture evidence of retrovirus infection before inoculation but demonstrated both afterwards, and the retrovirus recovered after inoculation was indistinguishable from prototype LAV. [. . .] The identification of an animal model for LAV infection has implications for the study of AIDS: (1) It offers the possibility of proof that LAV/HTLV-III is the cause of AIDS. Time will show whether these two LAV-infected chimpanzees will acquire the tumours or opportunistic infections characteristic of AIDS, though the changes in T-cell population may be an indication. (2) It provides an opportunity to study the natural history of LAV/HTLV-III infection. (*The Lancet*, December 1, 1984, II/8414, p. 1277)[8]

"Simian AIDS" is relevant neither because the simian retrovirus was identical with the human one, nor because of the more or less recent evolution of the latter from the former. Of interest here is how the central claim of mirroring "human AIDS" point by point is the relationship thus established between simian AIDS and risk, and what this relationship resembles. With risk a central element in arguing for the identity of the retrovirus and for its causal role, as well as for transmission patterns, it could be expected that such a discourse would have to take into account simian "risks" that mirror the human ones, especially when it comes to "controlling SAIDS." For example, we could expect that studies of the transmission of "simian AIDS" through body contact, body fluids, or sexual acts are important and that more could have been learned from such studies about preventing "human AIDS."

It appears that, although distinctions such as seropositive vs. seronegative and sick or diseased vs. healthy, as well as sex ratios (*Science*, March 9, 1984, 223, p. 1083) and transmission from mother to infant chimpanzee (*NEJM*, September 15, 1988, 319, p. 722), were used extensively for simians, there was no use of risk in the economy of the SAIDS discourse. These same distinctions, especially the ones concerning sex ratios, occupied an important place in the risk constellation for "human AIDS," so one could expect that sex ratios in primates would be presented in terms of risk. In other words, the same topics that in the case of AIDS are interpreted in terms of "risk" seem to be ordered here in a different way, so there is no need for terms such as "high- and low-risk macaques," "macaque risk behavior," or "macaque promiscuity." How can it be, then, that key topics with respect to understanding the disease are sometimes interpreted in terms of risk and sometimes not?

---

[8] For the corresponding assertion of Dr. Gallo about HTLV-III, see *Science*, November 2, 1984, 224, p. 552.

If we take into account that the aim of "simian AIDS" was to mirror point by point "human AIDS," these aspects become puzzling.

Answering the question of how this can be done without the help of "risk" requires taking the following factors into account: first of all, the category "simians" is not subject to classification practices, but is itself a special category of a different classification, meant to confirm both the system as such (i.e., barrier transgression) and the abstract "human" category. In other words, the purpose of "simian AIDS" is to confirm that this retrovirus is the causal agent of "human AIDS." But, given this, "simian AIDS" depends on (and receives its meaning from) "human AIDS," which it is supposed to confirm. In this context, "human AIDS" is not subject to a determination through "risk": rather, it is an abstract category, whose meaning is given by the rhetoric of barrier transgression. It would be tautological to speak of "human AIDS" with respect to people with the syndrome.

A second factor is that SAIDS has a complex status: it is represented as an animal variety of AIDS (being simultaneously similar to and different from AIDS) and as a proof for the origins of AIDS, but at the same time it is not seen as a disease anymore. In this latter respect, it belongs to the same order as the macaques: they coexist rather than harm each other. Thus, monkeys were represented as "reservoirs" and "vectors" of the viruses, and not as a target of the infectious agent. When monkeys are not inoculated, "simian AIDS spontaneously occurs" (*Science*, June 7, 1985, 228, p. 1200). This "spontaneous occurrence" (however paradoxical it may seem) obscures any questions about transmission means and risk. Because a causal model is meant only for humans (being used in the classification discussed), there is no need for the concept of risk when presenting simians infected with SAIDS. Looking more closely at distinctions such as "diseased vs. healthy macaques," we can see that they actually do not indicate any future infection. There is no "macaque agency" for passing on the infection; this is either externally induced through injections in the laboratory, or it occurs "spontaneously." The classification system of "human AIDS" allowed the generation of two different orders: (1) that of the infectious agent and (2) that of the agency of infection, where (1) depended on and was produced by (2). This makes it possible to conceive the causal agent as a human-related retrovirus, for which primates are vectors, reservoirs, and so forth. Hence, the discourse about "simian AIDS" cannot operate with "simian risk," as this would mean changing the said conditions, by constructing the causal agent (i.e., the retrovirus) through a "simian agency," which would radically change its identity.

One might well think that the controversies about the endemic character of AIDS in Africa, the transgression of the interreign barrier, and "simian AIDS" now belong to the past and should be seen as characteristic of the incipient phase of AIDS research, when "hard" data were scarce and "wild" hypotheses were common. But this is not so. Even a cursory look at the main topics in contemporary AIDS research[9] shows that, on the contrary, all these themes are doing very well. For example, for more than a decade, research had been directed at investigating how monkeys harbor retroviruses (Kestler 2001, p. 45) and why among them there is no mass extinction due to immune deficiencies; and how African populations have developed a genetic resistance to retroviruses, or how these transgress the interreign barrier. Some of the explanations, such as the genetic resistance of African populations to retroviruses, rework old topics (remember that "homosexuals" were genetically different) and seem to be at odds with the high rates of infection in Africa. This, again, recalls the plea of cultural anthropologists (but not only them) to take factors such as dire poverty and malnutrition more seriously (Barnett and Whiteside 2002, p. 34). In any event, what this does show is that the issues discussed in this chapter plainly do not belong exclusively to the early history of AIDS research. They have marked its evolution and continue to play a significant role today.

Contested Zones and the Rhetoric of Discovery

My main argument in this chapter is that the controversy around the discovery of HIV has been carried on in a contested zone. A contested zone is a definitional arena where the identity of scientific objects is disputed. Participants in the dispute try to bring their own resources into this arena and to exclude those of their opponents. Consequently, the boundaries of the zone are not fixed; they may change their shape during the controversy. Participants try to move the boundaries of the contested zone as much as possible into their own territory.

---

[9] See, among others, Gina Kolata: "When HIV Made Its Jump to People." *The New York Times*, January 29, 2002, p. F1.

Peter Galison's notion of a trading zone (1996b, p. 119) designates an "arena in which radically different activities could be *locally*, but not globally coordinated." Out of this coordination emerge new objects of scientific inquiry, new projects, and cognitive tools. By contrast, a contested zone is an arena in which the identity of scientific objects is established through the mobilization of (rhetorical) resources, with which this space can be occupied.

With respect to how Robert Gallo and Luc Montagnier defended their discoveries, we can see that both tried to occupy the disputed zone by mobilizing different arrangements of the same cognitive and rhetorical resources. Rather than directly disputing each other's findings, they tried to define and present the debated topics in such a way that the other's arrangement became inapplicable. At the same time, this mode of disputing a cognitive zone had the effect of reinforcing a certain set of topics, which from then on were taken as given and of fundamental importance: how the virus acts in primates, how it built a reservoir in Central Africa, how it migrated to North America and Europe. In this, the debate set the directions for future research and gained a significance beyond the dispute about priorities in the discovery of the AIDS agent.

5

The Spatial Configurations of "AIDS Risk"

Scientific Knowledge, Space, and Rhetoric

Very recently, the notion of space has received increased sociological attention as part of a broader interest in artifacts and their role in the constitution of social order. Space is a key dimension of social life, which is structured around distinctions such as public vs. private spaces, spaces of production vs. consumption, natural vs. artificial spaces, and so forth. Space also lies at the core of the distinction between the natural and the social world, central for our self-understanding as social beings: according to this distinction, society occupies a space distinct from that of nature. The two realms do not overlap, nor are they completely disconnected, but rather they are contiguous.

The social world is spatially organized with the help of artifacts such as buildings, which stabilize social life and differentiate it according to classes of social activities (Gieryn 2000, 2002a, pp. 35–6; Prior 1992). The distinction between the social and the natural is spatially constituted. Therefore, the realm of the political has to operate with and refer to this distinction at the symbolic level: this happens in the case of state-built gardens and parks, which reconstruct nature in terms of political and cultural considerations (Mukerji 2002; Carroll-Burke 2002). Consequently, social institutions, as well as human agency, are seen as depending on these distinctions and on the social organization of space.

Against this background, it becomes relevant to explore the connections between space and the production of scientific knowledge. The traditional sites where scientific knowledge has been produced are the laboratory and the field, closely tied to experiment and observation, respectively, as paradigmatic scientific activities. Scientific laboratories work as normative landscapes (Gieryn 2002b, p. 128): they establish rules of behavior and norms of action. At the same time, laboratories reconstitute nature in a controlled environment, in which "wild" phenomena are tamed, observed, and measured. To a large extent, laboratories have become standardized, so that scientists can assume a minimal variability in architecture and local arrangements of instruments. This makes experiments easier to replicate and truth claims easier to circulate in the scientific community.

Thomas Gieryn distinguishes between place and space. Whereas places are concrete arrangements of artifacts and human actors, space is abstract and geometrical, detached from cultural interpretations. Consequently, it is place that plays a role in the production of scientific knowledge. Although Gieryn is concerned with the architecture of scientific buildings, the question remains whether space, as opposed to place, is indeed void of any cultural determination.

An example that comes to mind here is narratives of space: can we claim that they have no cultural determination whatsoever? Given that places (laboratories, fields of observation, and so forth) play a role in the production of scientific knowledge, what about representations of space? Thomas Gieryn's argument is that, due to the high degree of place standardization, scientists no longer need to include laboratory descriptions in their articles: it is widely assumed that spatial arrangements vary minimally from lab to lab. Therefore, scientists focus on other means of persuasion to convince their audience. If this is so, then the question arises: how is the object of inquiry represented in scientific articles in relation to space? If space is a central dimension of scientific knowledge, and representations of laboratory spaces are no longer a rhetorical resource, what other resources are needed to represent space? What are the cultural determinants of these representations?

In the case of AIDS, representations of space played a significant role: the narrative of the origins of AIDS relied on an "African" space, distinct from the "Western" one. The debates about contagion vs. infection, in turn, were grounded in differing assumptions about how the AIDS agent is transmitted in space. Therefore, the questions I examine here are complementary to those about material places: on the one hand, I argue that scientific representations of space and disease are influenced by broader cultural assumptions. On the other hand, I argue that the rhetoric of space plays a role in the constitution of scientific knowledge.

Explanatory models represented the causal agent according to two categories of risk factors. Those stressing the role of a "history of sexually transmitted diseases" emphasized an STD-like agent inducing the acquired immunodeficiency. Those with "lifestyle" factors at their core represented the agent as belonging to and emerging from the social environment. Environment was providing the opportunities for intense risk contacts and encouraged social relations conducive to infection. In the case of the "Haitian risk group," it was the agglomeration and poverty in the slums of Port-au-Prince, as well as the quasi-rural, primitive space where rituals took place. In the case of the "IV drug users risk group," it was the shooting galleries; in the case of the "homosexual risk group," it was the recreation facilities of an urban gay subculture. For "infants" and "steady female sexual partners," it was the household space that led to infection. The syndrome was like a contagious disease, whose transmission was determined in the first place by the place where it happened. The "hemophiliac" model, by contrast, presupposed dispersed and isolated spaces, which excluded all kind of contacts and agglomerations. The first reports presented patients as dispersed, isolated, and not traveling, which suggested a lack of mobility and resources, as well as a spatial configuration different from that of other risk groups.

Clinical reports endorsing the STD model stressed that the patients did not know each other and were not part of the same environment. Later, the emphasis was put on "clusterings" and on "contact tracing" – that is, on identifying constellations of patients who did have sexual relationships with one another. This was seen as an argument for the syndrome being transmitted in the same way as a sexual disease. If the syndrome is transmitted like a sexual disease, but past STDs are not instrumental in transmitting it anymore, it becomes possible to locate the syndrome – that is, to look for the environment where it takes place. The environmental model, which tied contagion to "lifestyle risk," intervened here. Medical papers endorsing environmental factors characterized the "homosexual" risk group mainly in terms of its shared social settings and not in terms of past clinical diagnoses. These papers stressed the fact that the patients had the same "lifestyle," frequented the same encounter places, and were part of "clusterings" or networks. The idea of the syndrome as an infectious disease was combined with that of the syndrome as a contagious one. This is only apparently paradoxical: presenting the syndrome as infectious (i.e., STD-like) implies that space does not count; what counts is the direct sexual contact with persons bearing the agent. On the contrary, presenting the syndrome as contagious implies that the environment bears the agent; contacts emerge from and are defined through this environment. Hence, what counts is not individuals, but the environment that defines them. The agent is, so to speak, in that place, or on the "epidemic streets" (Hardy 1993). The representation of AIDS as a hybrid between an infectious and a contagious disease was crucial with respect to how the epidemiology of the syndrome was conceived and prevention policies were shaped. The ways in which "risk" was quantified depended to a large extent on understanding it as a spatial distribution of sexual acts and/or contacts. To see how "risk" was translated into computable magnitudes (and to what effect), we have to understand first how risk spaces were constituted. In the following section on Spatial Arrangements and Transmission Models, I examine how discourses of transmission combined these elements with regard to risk, ascribing to each category a specific environment or space, which in turn defined the "transmission risk."

Spatial Arrangements and Transmission Models

One of the first spatial patterns was the "San Francisco model," according to which the "homosexual" risk group was clustered in certain neighborhoods of the city. These neighborhoods, arranged on the city map, determined incidence rates of the syndrome, transmission models, and the ratio of "homosexual" to "heterosexual" population (*The Lancet*, April 16, 1983, I/8330, p. 924). The "homosexual population" was defined by one article as the number of never-married men over 15, plus the number of past-married homosexuals minus the number of never-married heterosexual men; two areas were drawn on the map of San Francisco: area A, with the highest homosexual population level; and area B, surrounding area A. Reported cases from the city's clinics were identified according to residence, and the ratios of the number of cases to the total "homosexual" population in these areas were computed. The areas thus constructed served as an argument for the thesis that the infectious agent was mainly sexually transmitted:

If the proportion of gay men among all men in area B were about 40% of that in area A, the two sets of rates would be comparable. However, there is reason to suppose that incidence rates of AIDS are different among different groups of gay men, depending on aspects of lifestyle and previous exposure to infectious diseases. Thus the lower rates in area B may represent a combination of different lifestyles and the smaller proportion of gay men among all men in area B. [...] Although incidence rates are given by geographical area we are not saying that geographical proximity is associated with risk, or that area A is a focus of infection in the classical sense. We think that rates are high in area A and area B because they contain the principal gay neighborhoods of the city, and most San Francisco cases are among gay or bisexual men. Given the large number of cases among gay or bisexual men in these areas, the small number of reported cases among heterosexual men and among women suggests, perhaps, that AIDS is not easily transmitted by non-sexual personal contact. (*The Lancet*, April 16, 1983, I/8330, p. 924)

Differences in lifestyle and the history of sexually transmitted diseases are constructed according to neighborhoods and derived from a spatial arrangement. The last paragraph of the paper claims that the main risk is given by geographical proximity, from which other risk factors are to be derived; this risk model excludes non-sexual, at-a-distance contact as a transmission means. Although the authors explicitly state that they do not consider their "area A" as a classical focus of infection, they contradict themselves in the next sentence. Yes, this area – a gay neighborhood – is a focus of infection, because heterosexual men and women cannot easily transmit AIDS sexually. The implications here are multiple and paradoxical: (1) non-sexual direct contact does not count as a means of transmission as long as it is not confined to a specific space; (2) contact between "heterosexual men and women" is not sexual and is therefore not a means of transmission; and (3) area-defined sexual contact (i.e., "homosexual" contact) is a means of transmission and a risk. The "homosexual" risk group is statistically recomposed as neighborhoods; incidence rates are also constructed according to spatial proximity, and differences in "lifestyle" or in sexually transmitted diseases are differences in vicinity; therefore, risk is recomposed as neighborhood, and neighborhood now defines risk.

A similar risk map was produced by a report on the AIDS epidemic in New York City, which identified risk zones in each borough by zip code (*AJE*, 1986, 123/9, pp. 1019–21). Whereas the San Francisco maps ordered only "homosexuals" according to areas, the New York City study ordered several risk groups: homosexual/bisexual, not a drug user; homosexual/bisexual, non-IV drug user; IV drug user, heterosexual; female IV drug user; sex partner in at-risk group; other, male or female. Special maps located each risk group and showed differences in their spatial distribution. The report tied differences in diagnosis to "different exposures in the different environments inhabited by these groups" (*AJE*, 1986, 123/9, p. 1124). Although published in 1986, the paper made no reference to the retroviral infectious agent and closed with the statement that AIDS is "a condition whose etiology remains unknown." Its collection of cases was based only on the diagnosis of opportunistic infections and on the statistics of the New York City Department of Health. Each group was defined by zip codes. For example, the "homosexual" risk group was located in central and southern Manhattan, and in a Brooklyn neighborhood, whereas the IV drug users were located in northern Manhattan and the adjacent Brooklyn area, so that each space had its own risk factors. The spatial model of risk became internationalized. A report on HTLV-III in "patients and individuals at risk for Acquired Immunodeficiency Syndrome in Italy" picked "six Italian cities considered representative from a geographic and socioeconomic point of view" and discussed geographically determined differences between the risk groups of "homosexuals" and IV drug users (*AJE*, 1986, 123/2, pp. 308–15). Again, the geographically ordered findings (comparing cities from northern and southern Italy) were presented as an argument for HTLV-III as the infectious agent and for gradual stages in the development of the syndrome.

We encounter a similar situation in the more recent case of Severe Acute Respiratory Syndrome (SARS). In this case too, risk categories were spatially ordered according to whether they were present in a Hong Kong hotel (*MMWR*, March 28, 2003, 52/12, pp. 241–8), whether they resided in a specific Hong Kong condominium, and whether they had contact with the personnel of a Hong Kong hospital (*EID*, September 2003, 9/9, p. 1064). Maps were published in epidemiological reports, showing how SARS patients had visited the same spaces and traveled to the same cities. Screening and prevention measures were designed based on this spatial principle: closing off the Hong Kong condominium in question, monitoring passengers travel- ing from Asia, and screening airport lounges with infrared cameras. Moreover, explanatory models of the epidemic had a spatial model at their core: the sewage system of the Hong Kong condominium al- lowed the distribution of the virus throughout the entire building and the infection of the whole neighborhood (*EID*, September 2003, 9/9, p. 1064).

Risk maps as visualization instruments made surveillance possible (Foucault 1979, p. 195) in the sense that they allowed a monitoring of risks on a collective (and even international) scale. At the same time, they made comparisons possible; risk was given a concrete shape – as something that can be pointed to not only at the individual level but also at the abstract and general level. In this way, these instruments con- tributed to the standardization and circulation of "AIDS risk" across various contexts and situations (Latour 1999, pp. 24–80). This, in turn, reinforced the association of certain risk factors with specific categories of risk classification. The "gay neighborhoods" were the places where risky sexual behavior was practiced, in the same way in which northern Manhattan was the place of shooting galleries.

Spatial classification criteria were introduced into the statistics, along with other parameters that stood for "risk groups" or "factors." This led to spatially constructed "risk subgroups" and to new cate- gories; for example, "Haitian entrants" (in the US) were distributed in "Miami," "New York City," and "other US locations." The "ho- mosexual" risk group was reordered in New York City, New Jersey, the Manhattan boroughs, San Francisco, Los Angeles, and other U.S. locations (*JAMA*, January 11, 1985, 253/2, pp. 217–18). The same was done for intravenous drug users, women, infants, and children. Space was thus a risk factor and a criterion for identifying the presence of other risk factors at the same time, for distinguishing between the safe and the unsafe. Such statistical constructions supported epidemiologi- cal models that stressed transmission through sexual contact or blood. An argument in this respect was that, because shooting galleries were more common in New York City and New Jersey than in other parts of the country, incidence rates among intravenous drug users from New York City and New Jersey were higher. It was also argued that IV drug users travel less than homosexual or bisexual men and are area-bound

(*JAMA*, January 11, 1985, 253/2, p. 219). The spatialization of risk factors sanctioned the view that the infectious agent was more readily transmitted from male to female than vice versa: women were not being infected at the same pace as men because not all forms of sexual behavior had the same risk; some were riskier than the others, and some were safe. Because anal intercourse emerged from these space-bound statistics as the riskiest form of sexual behavior, it explained the existent male/female ratio. Heterosexual intercourse being equated with vaginal sex, and vaginal sex being equated with lower risk sexual behavior, women were less exposed than men (*The Lancet*, September 29, 1984, II/8405, p. 715). But forms of sexual behavior, as well as the ratio of infection, were spatially determined. Risky heterosexual intercourse (embodied by "female sexual contacts") was determined by the spaces and agglomerations within shooting galleries, whereas homosexual intercourse was determined by neighborhood. This combined with the view that female sexual organs tended to act as a kind of reservoir for the virus and that they were resistant to infection (being double-walled, a view formulated in the environmentalist discourse).

Because "homosexuals" were "men of extreme sexual activity" (which was also implied by the spatial distribution of risk), they became infected at a high rate. Women (with the exception of prostitutes) were much less sexually active than men, or were only "steady sexual partners," and thus became infected at a much lower rate and ratio (*NEJM*, February 21, 1985, 312/8, p. 522). The IV drug users had higher incidence rates in New York City and New Jersey (the third category of the classification was "United States") and did not travel; the male/female ratio for the two categories was an argument for transmission through frequent sexual intercourse. The corollary was that "there may be fewer females in the population capable of transmitting the disease" (*NEJM*, February 21, 1985, 312/8, p. 522), which was an additional argument for women not being affected by the syndrome.

Representations of sexual vulnerability (associated with transmission models) were reinforced through spatial distribution. It was now possible to link transmission means according to a spatial pattern. The links were constituted by the bisexual husband, the homosexual drug user, or the Haitian prostitute. Perhaps more importantly, this linkage reinforced the thesis that heterosexual transmission was much rarer than homosexual transmission and therefore should not be intensively targeted. It was also very difficult to conceive of prevention directed at heterosexual transmission according to this spatial ordering. The only space associated with heterosexuality (outside Africa) was that of the household, which in turn was associated with representations of AIDS as a contagious disease.

By 1984, scientific journals were already using etiologic and epidemiologic constructions of "risk" to sustain the thesis of HTLV-III as the viral agent. "Lifestyle" or "lifestyle risk factors" were thus presented as a certain form of sexual contact; they belonged to a "risk group" or "community," and to a certain space at the same time.

If the retrovirus was a contagious agent, immunodeficiency would spread in spaces of sexual contact that involved large numbers of sexual partners. The "baths debate," which dominated the discussions on adequate risk policy (among medical experts, as well as among local politicians) in the mid-1980s, can be seen as a direct consequence of this new risk model, which conceived risk factors spatially. The two sides in this debate were the defenders and adversaries of a single policy measure: that of closing public baths, which were represented as *the* major encounter places of the "homosexual" risk group. Defenders of this measure argued in essence that restricting the social spaces of risk would lead to better control of it, whereas opponents of the measure (arguing for an educational approach in these places) considered that restrictive measures would only open up other, even less controllable risk spaces (Bayer 1989; Pollak 1992). In a very similar way, the first detection and prevention policies aimed at stemming the spread of Severe Acute Respiratory Syndrome (SARS) in the spring of 2003 were grounded in a spatial notion of risk: airports were seen as the major encounter place of people carrying the virus.[1] Consequently, airports were closely monitored and policed (with infrared temperature cameras, for example) whereas other public concourses and means of transportation (railways, railway stations) were not.

The notion of policing space, along with the distinction between high- and low-risk cities, arose from the same reasoning being used to explain why the syndrome was not more evenly distributed, as

[1] The first intercontinental cases were detected in passengers flying back to Asia from North America via Europe. The first case was that of a physician traveling between Hong Kong and Southern China.

STDs were: it was argued that the homosexual population of large cities (such as New York) was a "hyperendemic population," characterized by "the fully developed syndrome"; the homosexual population of smaller cities developed AIDS later. An epidemiological study took a "high-risk subset" of the customers of a Pittsburgh, PA bathhouse (none of whom corresponded to the CDC definition of AIDS) and classified them according to history of venereal diseases, number of sexual partners, drug use, and frequency of travel to New York City. The aim was to construct a population comparable with that of big cities (i.e., bathhouse clients) with contacts to these "endemic areas," to argue for the thesis of a gradually developing syndrome (*AJPH*, March 1984, 74/3, pp. 259–60). Some epidemiological reports presented residence as a kind of risk in itself: "high-risk" subsets of the "homosexual" risk group came to be almost automatically identified with residents of big cities, which, subsequently, were called "high-risk cities" or "endemic areas." Medical and epidemiologic reports usually operate with metonymy, especially in their summaries and titles: the syntagms just mentioned were commonly used in clinical and epidemiologic studies that investigated small numbers of individuals, selected from very few clinical practices, mostly catering to STD patients. A study dating from 1985 ("Sexual Contact in High-Incidence Areas for the Acquired Immunodeficiency Syndrome"), which investigated 180 individuals from two Washington-based clinical practices, stressed space as a risk factor:

The data suggest that deficit of helper T-lymphocytes can be acquired by homosexual contact with men in cities where AIDS is common. This supports the hypothesis that low helper T-cell counts may be caused by a sexually transmissible agent and that frequent homosexual exposure to residents of high-risk areas for AIDS may be an important means of spread of this agent. (*AJE*, 1985, 121/5, p. 629)

The report used "high-risk cities" and "high-risk (exposed) areas" as synonyms, to support the thesis that there are several stages in the development of the syndrome. It did not mention either HTLV-III or LAV, and it referred constantly to an "infectious agent" or "sexually transmissible agent," without discussing its nature. The laboratory findings consisted only in cell counts, with no antibody identification, so the paper actually constructed a correlation between cell counts and spatially organized sexual contact, presenting it afterwards as "AIDS risk."

After asserting that "it was our a priori hypothesis that American homosexual men from an area at low risk of AIDS who had sexual contact with men from high-risk (endemic areas) would have lower helper T-cell counts than men without such exposure" (*AJE*, 1985, 121/5, p. 635), the article suggested that stages in the development of the syndrome are arranged in a spatial pattern, where the "high-risk areas" have the full-blown pattern, the "low-risk" ones have lesser stages, and the contacts between the two act as a kind of intermediary. Accordingly, "low-risk" areas gradually become "high-risk." This argument ignored previous reports that the spatial ordering of risk actually made the concept of a contagious agent problematic (*JAMA*, March 16, 1984, 251/11, p. 1441). The conceptual difficulty was that the infectious agent was transmitted through highly frequent "anonymous sex, such as in bathhouses and bars" and that this anonymity made tracing contacts almost impossible. Nevertheless, it was possible to trace "homosexual contacts between international travelers" (*JAMA*, March 16, 1984, 251/11, p. 1442) and thus to establish a spreading pattern of low risk becoming high risk.

Studies were aimed at demonstrating that high-risk sexual act types correlated strongly with high-risk cities and less strongly with low-risk ones (e.g., *AJE*, 1985, 121/5, pp. 629–36). And if part I of this particular report did not identify the infectious agent as a human retrovirus and referred only to a general agent, part II (immediately following part I in the same journal issue) made reference to HTLV-III in the introduction, stating that "in the absence of this discovery, epidemiologic studies of persons at high risk of AIDS relied on indirect indices such as the immunologic abnormalities that are characteristic of AIDS" (*AJE*, 1985, 121/5, pp. 637–8). The paper constructed three risk groups: 85 high-risk men from central Manhattan ("New York"); 96 intermediate-risk men from Washington, D.C., with area homosexual contacts ("Washington-exposed"); and 64 low-risk Washington, D.C. men, without such contacts ("Washington-unexposed"). "Exposure" meant "those who had sexual contacts in cities of high risk of AIDS" (*AJE*, 1985, 121/5, pp. 637, 639). "Homosexual-specific sexual acts," also called "lifestyle variables" (*AJE*, 1985, 121/5, p. 641), were statistically correlated to risk spaces and cell counts. The result was risk space–typical sexual acts: accordingly, lower cell counts specifically correlated more strongly with "New York homosexual" acts and gradually less strongly with intermediary or "Washington homosexual"–specific acts (*AJE*, 1985, 121/5, p. 639). This supported the thesis of a single infectious agent, located in a certain space (in this case, New York City) and spreading through other cities. The virus was transmitted through "risky" sexual acts associated with mucosal abrasions (such as anal sex). They had a higher frequency in central Manhattan and a lower one in the Washington area (*AJE*, 1985, 121/5, p. 643).

This risk distribution accounts for how the virus gets into the bloodstream, and it refutes previous arguments about the immunosuppressive effects of sperm and inhaled drugs. The spatial ordering is generated here through a series of uses of metonymy: relatively small numbers of cases are made to stand for large urban areas. In turn, the corresponding clinical and behavioral data (such as cell counts, sexual act types, and frequency of sexual acts) are taken as substitutes for these areas, with the effect that it becomes possible to compute correlations and probabilities that cover a whole territory.

Risk maps and the corresponding statistics were not without influence on health policy debates. The fact that reality did not always correspond to such maps has been shown since by studies such as Cathy Cohen's (1999), which argues that African Americans with AIDS did not make it onto the risk maps (and hence into prevention policies) simply because they did not frequent the STD clinics from which most clinical studies were drawn. Although they were a very real phenomenon from the beginning, African Americans were not part of the classification system (when they were, they were "IV drug users") and were left out of a cognitive frame based on collective categories. Consequently, later prevention approaches had to contend with denial and misapprehension: many African Americans flatly refused to believe that they could get AIDS, whereas others saw AIDS as a scientific conspiracy against them. Either way, they resisted prevention measures. This corroborates Rayna Rapp's (1999, p. 70) and Michael Bloor's (1995, p. 26) arguments that the cognitive frames in which we conceive and speak of "risk" are not limited to an abstract and general level but become enacted in everyday life, in the interactions between medical staff, patients, and their families, as well as in the decisions they make.

The configuration of "Haitian" risk factors followed a similar pattern: risk was presented as having its center in the red-light district of Port-au-Prince, where most of the Haitian patients came from, and which was frequented by "American homosexuals."[2] Later, "Haitians" were partially absorbed into the categories of bisexuals, prostitutes, and blood donors, so cases were reported under this double classification. But, as late as 1987, medical papers reported "Haitians" as a risk category, in spite of their being taken off the official CDC classification at the end of 1983. "Haitian" risk factors (1) were of an environmental nature, (2) explained the action of a viral agent, and (3) illustrated the transmission of the virus from risk group to risk group. At the same time, they supported a more complex viral model. Clinical reports suggested that "Haitians" have a double "lifestyle." The "Haitian lifestyle" factor was the male prostitution district in Port-au-Prince. In the beginning, this was constructed somewhat amorphously, as partially opposed to the North American "homosexual lifestyle." A clinical report claimed that "multiple sexually transmitted infections and frequent use of prescription or recreational drugs were generally absent in Haitians" (NEJM, January 20, 1983, 308/3, p. 127). Nevertheless, this did not mean that Haitians, both in Haiti and the United States, did not have "lifestyles," which had to be examined more closely. Such an examination could show that heterosexual Haitians and homosexual Americans have more in common than one thinks (NEJM, January 20, 1983, 308/3, p. 128).

Homosexual tourists in Haiti got the virus somehow from the "Haitian" risk group and spread it into the "homosexual community," whose drug addict members passed it to the "heterosexual addict population." The risk factors of "homosexual Americans" are therefore environmental: the encounter spaces of the "homosexual community" favor frequent anonymous sexual encounters and thus the transmission of the viral agent. In this context, the risk factors of the IV drug users are sexual contacts with "homosexual drug addicts." The viral agent was transmitted from the "Haitian" risk group to "vacationing homosexuals" through sexual contact. Risk categories were arranged in a daisy chain, each with its own risk spaces: on the one hand, they were mutually exclusive, because every one of them was the negation of the others. We have thus the "Haitians," who are non-homosexuals, the "homosexuals," who are "Americans" (and thus non-Haitians),

---

[2] NEJM, October 20, 1983, 309/16, p. 949; The Lancet, May 28, 1983, I/8335, p. 1187.

and the "heterosexual addict population," which is non-homosexual. At the same time, "homosexuals" are redefined as "homosexual drug addicts," and "Haitians" as "homosexual." The device allowing for these operations is that of "lifestyle." Risk categories are accorded a double status: they retain their initial mutual exclusivity but can be rearranged into common subcategories (which may negate the initial categories). This explains how the immune deficiency is caused by a single viral agent, which is transmitted from individual to individual through only two routes (the sexual and the blood ones). Although this model rejected the thesis of several infectious agents and multiple transmission routes, it brought together relatively few risk factors, a single agent, and various risk groups.

In this sense, neighborhood-based epidemiological maps were tied to statistical instruments producing thus not only standardization and comparability, but also area-specific levels of risk. The latter was disentangled from its person-related, idiosyncratic aspects and transformed into something objective, into a given. One could now expect to face the risk of AIDS not on an individual, person-related basis, but on an area-specific one. This way of seeing AIDS risk, of making it visible, was not without concrete consequences.

The "Household Risk"

"Risk factors" in children were presented as family- or household-specific, being defined as the presence of members of high-risk groups in the family or household. The notion of "household risk" implied that the causal agent could be transmitted through casual contact; this idea was discussed at length in the media in the early 1980s. Several reports about medical personnel, civil employees, and sales clerks refusing to touch or stay in the same room with people with AIDS received prominent media exposure. Conservative voices argued on this basis for tougher prevention policies, which contributed to the stigmatization of risk groups. In turn, this triggered emotionally laden public debates. The notion of "household AIDS risk," then, was grounded in the representation of the Acquired Immunodeficiency Syndrome as a contagious disease, defined through spatial distribution. Dating from the first clinical reports, there were two tendencies in presenting risk factors for children, and both tendencies relied on spatial notions of risk. A relatively short-lived one was to treat the household in which a member of the risk groups lived as risk. Mere spatial copresence transferred risk from the individual to the familial environment. Thus, one of the first clinical reports on children with AIDS used expressions such as "families with recognized risks for AIDS" and "high-risk households" and stated that "children living in high-risk households are susceptible to AIDS" and that "sexual contact, drug abuse, or exposure to blood products is not necessary for disease transmission" (*JAMA*, May 6, 1983, 249/17, p. 2345). The case presentation clearly suggested that the simple presence of a high-risk person in the household could lead to infection:

His mother has no known risk factors for AIDS and has normal immunologic function. His father is an IV drug user with recent weight loss and adenopathy. His paternal uncle, a household contact, is homosexual and a drug abuser who has been diagnosed as having AIDS. (*JAMA*, May 6, 1983, 249/17, p. 2346)

All cases "had in common household exposure to one or more persons with known risk factors" and "there was no evidence that our patients had been sexually abused or given illicit drugs." This showed transmission without sexual contact or drug abuse "to an otherwise 'normal' host" (*JAMA*, May 6, 1983, 249/17, pp. 2347, 2349). The implication was that the simple presence of the infectious agent in the risk space of the household was sufficient for transmission. Notions such as family and household also implied that AIDS could be vertically transmitted, from mother to newborn. The possibility of casual transmission, however, was judged to be more important (*JAMA*, May 6, 1983, 249/17, p. 2375).

The infectious agent was presented as similar to those inducing contagious diseases; a banal bodily contact or prolonged presence in the same room would suffice. Models of contagious diseases usually emphasize the decisive role of copresence in the same space; the space-oriented epidemiological models of AIDS did not ignore this analogy. They took it over and embedded it in various argumentation strategies, according to whether they supported a viral cause or not. In this respect, it was important to define the household or familial space not through the presence of a "person with known risk factors for AIDS," but through its integration in a larger risk area, where the transmission of the infectious agent was already occurring in known groups. The thesis of perinatal transmission (and later, that of postnatal transmission) was thus derived from established transmission means, such as sexual contact and intravenous drug use. A clinical report asserted that sexually promiscuous and IV drug–using mothers were transmitting the infectious agent to their babies in utero. The best proof was the cluster of immunodeficient children signaled in an area with a high frequency of AIDS infection among IV drug users (*JAMA*, May 6, 1983, 249/17, p. 2356).

Two central claims (about the viral nature of the infectious agent and about intrauterine transmission) were sustained here by classifying cases according to risk area: because "sexually promiscuous and drug addicted mothers may undergo reactivation of EBV . . . and transmit the virus in utero to the partially immunoincompetent fetus" (p. 2355) and because the cases appeared in an area where AIDS was occurring among IV drug users, it follows that there was a viral agent transmitted in utero in this risk zone. Later papers and reports on children and infants with the syndrome continued this practice.[3] As a result, the new category of "parental risk groups" appeared and stayed in use until 1988–9.

In these cases, "household risk" promoted a new (perinatal) means of transmission, integrating it at the same time into the transmission chain. However, because the household status was unclear (Were they IV drug users? Bisexuals? Promiscuous? Monogamous?), prevention policies never managed to target it in a coherent fashion. Advertising campaigns from the late 1980s targeted heterosexual singles, considered to be more promiscuous than married people (who by definition were both heterosexual and monogamous). Prevention policies targeting IV drug users stressed the importance of sterile needles and single-use injection kits but paid little attention to the issue of sex. This shows the (still persistent) difficulties of implementing prevention policies grounded in the association between risk factors and groups, according to which one has only to target a few, group-specific risk behaviors.

---

[3] See *JAMA*, August 3, 1984, 252/5, p. 642; *NEJM*, January 12, 1984, 310/2, p. 77. Such a classification was first presented by the report on "household risks were already available," analyzed above.

Intercontinental Connections

Spatial representations of AIDS were needed not only locally, but also at an intercontinental level. If Central Africa had known an endemic form of the syndrome long before it was reported in North America and Western Europe, and if the origins of the virus were to be found there, "African" risk factors should explain not only how the virus passed the barrier between the animal and the human realm, but also how it traveled from one continent to the next. The first clinical and epidemiologic reports on these risks were somewhat contradictory, presenting them as located in an urban and at the same time a rural environment. Urban risk factors were "relatively high income," "heterosexual promiscuity," and "contacts with prostitutes," whereas the rural ones were traditional medicine, ritual practices, and poor hygiene (*The Lancet*, July 14, 1984, II/8394, pp. 62–5). This traditional medicine was described by the first reports as scarification, "often done with metallic instruments heated to redness." The identification of the viral agent as HTLV-III or LAV reinforced the thesis that a retrovirus had passed the barrier between primates (identified as African Green monkeys) and humans. It was asserted that an HTLV-III–related retrovirus had been isolated from African Green monkeys and that this was more similar to the "African" retrovirus isolates than to the "North American" ones (*Science*, November 22, 1985, 230, pp. 949, 951). The African Green monkeys were presented as common in a rural setting (*Science*, November 22, 1985, 230, p. 954); other articles suggested that the virus had been isolated from prostitutes (*Science*, December 6, 1985, 230, p. 1141) and had rapidly expanded into the urban population, even before mutating. This was an argument for the thesis that "the monkey virus itself may not be pathogenic but it may have mutated in man and acquired some destructive properties" (*Science*, December 6, 1985, 230, p. 1141).

Epidemiological models explaining how AIDS had left Africa relied on a narrative about the distinct character of the "African" risk group. At the same time, this distinctiveness made it difficult to explain how the virus had come out of Africa. The missing link was "Haitians," a fact which can account again for why they were maintained as a risk group for such a long time. The first step was to compare "African AIDS" not only to "United States AIDS," but also to "Haitian AIDS," establishing similarities and dissimilarities that made "African AIDS" special *but* allowed the virus to spread to other groups:

Two important differences between AIDS in Zaire and the disease in patients of European or American origin merit discussion – namely, the sex distribution and apparent lack of risk factors among patients in Zaire. The 1.1:1 ratio of males to females is likely to be more representative of the endemic situation than the ratio in patients from Zaire seen in Europe, which probably represents those able to afford treatment in Europe. A similar ratio (1.5:1) has also been reported for patients without attributable risk factors in the USA. The essentially equal proportion of males and females would require that transmission occurs both male-to-female and female-to-male, since one-direction transmission would soon result in an imbalance of the ratio. (*The Lancet*, July 14, 1984, II/8394, p. 68)

The almost equal male-to-female ratio is considered intrinsic to the endemic character of disease, and thus Africa-specific; the two-way heterosexual transmission is also Africa-specific, a distinct epidemic pattern not seen in the rest of the world. Thus, the "African group" retains its exceptional nature by being older (endemic) and otherwise unclassifiable. The thesis of an equal rate of male/female and female/male transmission is formulated here as an argument for this exceptionality. For "North American and European AIDS" this thesis was not acceptable: on the contrary, it was constantly argued that due to considerable differences in the resistance to infection of the male and female sexual organs and bodies, the transmission ratio could only be uneven. This is made clear by the assertion that "heterosexual male-to-female transmission of AIDS has been suggested in the USA, although so far this has been infrequent" (*The Lancet*, July 14, 1984, II/8394, p. 68).

An account of how the infectious agent had left its African setting had to be anchored in the specificity of African heterosexual transmission. Although several narratives about how the virus went from monkeys to humans in a rural setting, and from there to urban centers via prostitution, were already available, a story of how it left Africa was still missing. The solution was reverse migration – that is, not from Africa to the Americas but the other way around. This story was about the migration of "several thousand professional people" (assumedly heterosexual) from Haiti to Zaire in the 1960s and 1970s; these people subsequently left for Europe and North America (*The Lancet*, July 14, 1984, II/8394, p. 68). This made it possible to explain both the distinct heterosexual pattern in Africa and the migration of the virus (although it required a conversion of "Haitians" from heterosexuality to homosexuality).

Risk Spaces and Prevention Policies

The overall implication was that AIDS emerged as an epidemic in Africa and the United States simultaneously, although it had existed in a dormant form in Central Africa for a long time. The "several thousands" of Haitians who migrated to Central Africa and back to the Western hemisphere were the missing link: they brought AIDS from Africa and transmitted it further in the Western world. As for the "African AIDS," its pattern of heterosexual transmission remained "different and important." It has to be "clarified" by studying the retrovirus "strongly associated with AIDS." The model of "AIDS leaving Africa" operates with the following elements:

1. Two-way heterosexual transmission has an exceptional character, can be encountered only here, and is marginal and unclassifiable in the Western world.
2. The syndrome must have somehow originated in Africa, where it remained dormant for a long time.
3. The syndrome, although clinically similar all over the world, has completely different forms according to different risk categories.
4. Consequently, these risk categories are not only mutually exclusive, but also incompatible. "African risk" is not compatible with other risk factors, and "Western" risk categories are also incompatible with heterosexual transmission.

Risk, as it appears here, involves a series of rhetorical operations, such as substituting parts for the whole, constructing abstract categories from actual cases, generalizing from a few concrete descriptions, eliminating complexity, and building up metaphors, to name only a few. All of these were embedded in the rhetorical structure of medical papers, as necessary elements in the construction of hypotheses and in making sense of clinical results. These devices were not put to work as simple formal structures, but always implied certain representations and tacit suppositions about the social world. It was the supposition of an incompatibility between homosexuality and "Africa" that allowed for the mutual exclusivity of the respective risk groups, while the exclusivity of the "African" heterosexual transmission relied on a certain view of the social world of "Africa."

This argument structure reinforced the idea that heterosexual transmission is something that is African and something prevention policies should address only in an African context. Indirectly, explanatory models such as this contributed to orienting prevention and health policies according to spatial distributions of risk, which in turn were tied to the categories of the classification system. This model dovetailed well with representations of different sexual vulnerabilities, according to which (Caucasian) women, for example, were less exposed to risk, provided they were not prostitutes, and hence less in need of prevention policies anyway. It also dovetailed with the notion that those absent from this classification system (such as African Americans) did not need such policies either. AIDS prevention policies did not question, but relied upon, the classification of risk. As Sue Scott and Richard Freeman put it, in the 1980s "prevailing AIDS prevention policies might best be understood as fateful attempts to cling on to conceptions of society rooted in progressivist understandings of modernity. This means that they are unresponsive to the shifting conditions which prevail in late modernity. They are intended as rational, extrinsic solutions to specific social problems and, as such, they lack reflexivity" (1995, pp. 153–4).

The presentation of "AIDS risk" as a spatial ordering and clustering had a significant impact on health and insurance policy. In the mid-1980s, one major policy debate in the United States was whether measures should be centered on controlling what were perceived as risk spaces (and thus whether bars and bathhouses should be closed) or on educating "risk groups" (Pollak 1992; Bayer 1989, pp. 20–72). In March 1988, a position paper jointly published by the Health and Public Policy Committee of the American College of Physicians and the Infectious Diseases Society of America made recommendations for two sensitive policies (testing and insurance) in terms that clearly posited a spatial ordering of risk (*AIM*, 1988, 108/3, pp. 460–9). In defining three types of testing (mandatory, routine, and voluntary), the position paper rejected the first on the grounds that "such an approach would only drive potentially HIV-infected persons away from the health care system" and argued against "further expansion of mandatory testing in low-risk populations," because "it is not in the public interest to require the testing of persons whose social or sexual lifestyles render them unlikely to have been exposed to the virus" (*AIM*, 1988, 108/3, p. 464). At the same time, it argued for selective routine testing according to risk areas:

We do not believe that all persons admitted to hospitals should be tested on a mandatory or routine basis. We do support, however, the concept of increased routine testing for HIV antibody in high-risk populations. It may be appropriate, therefore, for hospitals in certain geographic, high-prevalence areas to consider routine testing of selected subpopulations shown to have an increased prevalence of HIV infection. (*AIM*, 1988, 108/3, pp. 464–5)

"High-risk populations" are constructed here as "high-prevalence areas," where "selected subpopulations" have "increased prevalence": risk populations and risk spaces are mutually defining. This appears even clearer in the insurance policy proposals. The members of one category ("single men between the ages 20 and 40") are defined as "risk" or "non-risk" with respect to insurance depending on whether they come from "high-risk geographic areas of the country" or not; in this case, too, space defines high-risk groups:

Insurance carriers may have legitimated interests in the HIV-antibody status of persons applying for life insurance, particularly in high-risk geographic areas of the country, and if they are single men between the ages 20 and 40, for example, and are seeking insurance for large sums. (*AIM*, 1988, 108/3, p. 466)

Cultural representations of sexual organs, bodies, vulnerability, and pollution left their imprint on medical representations of AIDS as a contagious disease, characterized through spatial distribution; the circle was closed when these representations made their way into the public sphere, being taken as a justification for policies which (in an objectified, indirect form) reinforced these representations on the basis of their scientific soundness and the objective knowledge on which they were based. Participants and patients were selected for clinical trials and epidemiological studies, respectively, according to spatial criteria and risk spaces. Although in the case of clinical trials this focus on risk space provided scientists with access to valuable community knowledge (Epstein 1996, p. 249), it also left out ethnic and social groups (such as African Americans) who did not live in "risk areas" or "risk neighborhoods" and did not visit STD clinics (or any clinic at all).

In a very similar way, the prevention policies against SARS were based on the representation of risk categories as occupying certain social spaces and having specific travel patterns: similar to the risk category of "homosexuals," represented as very mobile, SARS risk groups were seen as traveling very often between continents (which led to the monitoring of airports but not of railway or bus stations). They lived in certain neighborhoods (which were closed off) and had certain occupations (health care professionals, business people). Direct contact with these risk groups had to be avoided: among other things, this led to the use of sanitary masks irrespective of their effectiveness. This, again, is reminiscent of the use of surgical gloves in public spaces in 1983–4, when it was believed that the HI-virus could be transmitted through casual contact. Needless to say, the effectiveness of using surgical gloves in public spaces was never questioned.

With that, I come to my second argument, namely that scientific knowledge depends not only upon place, but also upon space. Place is understood as the material, local conditions under which knowledge is produced. Place is crucial to science as a social institution and to scientific agency. Space is understood here as the set of rhetorical procedures and resources with the help of which the epistemic categories of disease are meaningfully ordered according to geographical and topographical distinctions. This ordering took the form of (1) geographic narratives of HIV origins and travels around the world; (2) classifications of social groups according to risk zones; and (3) classification of transmission means according to spatial categories. As I show in Chapter 6, spatial ordering made possible the quantification of AIDS risk. Quantities of risk, in turn, confirmed risk categories and were a strong argument for viral models of AIDS. In this sense, space is crucial for accounts of causality and agency and hence for scientific knowledge about the virus.

6

Who Is How Much?

From Qualities to Quantities of AIDS Risk

AIDS Risk, Quantification, and Rhetoric

As the word is commonly understood, risk is intrinsically related to computing the probability of undesirable events, along with their degree of harm. This operation requires quantifying, measuring, and comparing the consequences of events. Knowledge about AIDS risk, its prevention, and the transmission of HIV is expressed in quantities of risk: that is, in probabilities of infection, low cell counts, developing opportunistic infections, and the like. From a broader perspective, quantification is an intrinsic feature of the biomedicalization process discussed by Clarke et al. (2003): the permanent monitoring of health status and the transformation of everyday life activities into risk factors require the quantitative treatment of life features that we very often perceive as highly idiosyncratic, personal, and even unique. Yet features we view as pertaining to the quality of our lives are made computable and treated in terms of magnitudes. How does this happen?

With respect to AIDS, there are quite a few epidemiological papers computing the exact amount of risk for every risk category and for every type of risk behavior, and quantitative evaluations of risk are present in many clinical reports. Statistical figures seem to present us with an objective image of risk, based on precise mathematical operations and free of any rhetorical elements. How is such an objectivity obtained? How can we assert with such certainty that "doing X" or "doing Y" has such and such a risk probability? The problem here is how qualitatively defined categories are transformed into computable magnitudes and how a computable risk (relying on a probabilistic calculus) becomes possible. A second aspect of the problem is how qualities classified as incommensurable can be ordered from high to low on a risk scale. A third issue is how homogeneous categories are reordered from higher to lower risk according to "factors" or "behavior." Finally, a fourth, not less important, issue is the place occupied by qualities and quantities of risk in the economy of the discourse.

Although there are many studies about the role of statistics and quantification in science in general (e.g., Mackenzie 1981; Porter 1995; Hacking 1990) and in medicine in particular (e.g., Bartley, Smith, and Blane 1997, p. 130), the quantification of risk in medical articles on AIDS has not been examined until now. Yet, as I argue in Chapter 5, this quantification lent support to and justified prevention and health policy proposals. Its premises were given by the treatment of AIDS risk in spatial terms, a procedure which assigned each risk category a supposedly homogeneous concrete environment. In this way, heterogeneous data (such as frequency of sex acts and cell count) were brought together and could be statistically processed. What role did rhetoric play in this process?

Quantity and Metaphor

Among the rhetorical techniques used to transform qualities into quantities is metonymy, by which a number of cases (quantity) is postulated as representing a category, which is reconstructed in successive steps from this quantity. Consider how one of the first clinical reports on opportunistic infections performed these operations. The paper, published at the end of 1982, reported the identification of a mycobacterium in the lung, spleen, and lymph tissues of five patients seen in a Los Angeles university clinic. The paper opened by simultaneously presenting the unusual clustering of acquired immunodeficiency cases and making a classification of risk categories: "An unusual clustering of cases of acquired immunodeficiency has recently been described in New York and in California in homosexual and, rarely, heterosexual men" (*JAMA*, December 10, 1982, 248/22, p. 2980). Afterwards, the associated opportunistic infections are listed; after that, the report introduces the cases seen at the UCLA Center for the Health Sciences as "five patients dying with this syndrome" that "form the basis of this report" (and in whom mycobacterial infection is described). There is apparently no relationship between the category of the first line (five patients) and the category of the following lines (homosexuals). The "report of cases," however, reorders the above elements: the "five patients" are now "a 30-year-old homosexual man" (two such cases), "a 34-year-old homo-sexual man," "a 31-year-old homosexual man," and "a 35-year-old homosexual man" (*JAMA*, December 10, 1982, 248/22, pp. 2980–1). They stand for "homosexual men," and the technique of repetition re-inforces it. The "comment" starts by speaking of "five case reports in homosexual patients." It continues by alternately using the syntagms "homosexual patients," "homosexual men," and "homosexuals," and it ends by asserting that "we now vigorously seek evidence of mycobac-terial infection in homosexuals with unexplained lymphadenopathy, *P. carinii* infection, and Kaposi's sarcoma," and that "it may not be unreasonable to treat homosexual patients with acquired immunodefi-ciency who are seriously ill with an unexplained infection empirically, pending the results of mycobacterial cultures, even if acid-fast bacilli are not identified on smears and tissue sections" (*JAMA*, December 10, 1982, 248/22, p. 2982). The abstract category of the first opening ("ho-mosexual men") is thus recomposed several times in the course of the paper, reemerging at the end as an abstract category with a new prop-erty, namely mycobacterial infection. Thus, the report transformed its epistemic claim from an empirical, particular one (namely, describing one mycobacterium seen in five cases) into a general claim of broader theoretical and practical relevance: that of a new opportunistic infec-tion associated with immune deficiency, which necessitates appropriate clinical treatment.

Looking more closely at the rhetorical techniques of this recompo-sition, we can see that categories and quantities were first introduced separately; then, quantity was transformed into a risk category, which in turn took the place of the quantitative presentation. This was by no means a singly occurring rhetorical device, but a strategy constantly used for transforming quality into quantity and vice versa. A small number of patients from a specific clinic, however, are not identical with socio-medical categories such as "homosexuals," or "homosex-ual patients." The general socio-medical category is substituted for the concrete cases and made a vehicle for general theoretical claims. In this respect, litotes and metonymy work in a way similar to the way theory-constitutive metaphors, which structure the object of inquiry, work (Fleischman 2003, p. 484): we know that whole social categories are at risk on the grounds of these substitutions.

The "General Population" as a Quantifying Device

A second rhetorical device used for transforming qualities into quantities of risk was to build up abstract and universal reference categories, such as the "general population." The "general population" as a universal reference category is by no means restricted to AIDS; indeed, the majority of health factors and related risks are represented with the help of the "general population." This reference category can transform a qualitative, abstract distinction into a quantitative comparison and vice versa. If we take into account the insistence with which it was asserted in the early and mid-1980s that the "general population," the "we," was not at risk of contracting AIDS, its meaning becomes even more puzzling. The construction of this universal reference category, among others, shows how qualities and quantities of risk were translated from one medical report to another, the result being general, legitimate assertions about the quantity of risk for specific risk groups. The case examined here is that of two clinical reports published in January and July 1982, respectively, in two medical journals. The July report formulates a general assertion about a precise quantity of risk for Kaposi's sarcoma in "homosexual men," relying on and referring to operations performed for the January report.

The risk classification by which new categories were usually introduced did not allow transformations of this kind: the categories of "renal transplant recipients" or "men of Mediterranean origin" could not back up such operations, serving only to distinguish between the usual and the unusual. Abstract and universal reference categories cannot, apparently, be transformed into quantities; still, they allowed one-sided transformations. Consider how the "general population" category makes the transition from quantity to quality. The paper's introductory paragraph reasserts the classification of Kaposi's sarcoma that is no longer valid (i.e., the categories of "older men," of "Eastern European origins," and "renal allograft recipients") and then states the new "risk group" quantitatively, pitting it against an abstract category:

Kaposi's sarcoma is rare in the United States, occurring predominantly among older men of Eastern European descent and in renal allograft recipients receiving immunosuppressive drugs. Since 1979 the Centers of Disease Control have identified 89 cases of KS in homosexual men and have suggested that the risk of KS in this population is at least one hundred times greater than in the general population. (*The Lancet*, July 17, 1982, II/8290, p. 125)

How can we know so precisely that the risk for KS in "homosexuals" is exactly one hundred times greater than in the general population – which, statistically seen, includes women and children, who are at minimal risk of getting KS? First, KS has to be characterized for practical purposes. This characterization ("rare in the US") performs several functions: it reinforces the risk group as a category in itself; it excludes the group from the previous categories of KS; it excludes the group from the "general population"; it makes a quantitative assertion about risk; and it gives not absolute but relative magnitudes. The category of "homosexual men" is presented here ambiguously with respect to risk, once quantitatively ("89 homosexual men"), and once qualitatively ("this population"), so the comparison with the "general population" is made both qualitatively and quantitatively. At this point, a reference in the text sends us to a previous report (published in January 1982) as the source of this risk comparison and of the relative magnitude of "one hundred times." For the sake of clarity, the January report is called here "report A," and the July report, "report B." Report A was a "special report" of the Centers for Disease Control and Prevention, and it opened its "discussion section" with the paragraph:

The current outbreak of Kaposi's sarcoma, *P. carinii* pneumonia, and other opportunistic infections is highly unusual. Kaposi's sarcoma is a rare, malignant neoplasm, predominantly affecting elderly men and seldom causing death. Although precise rates are unavailable, the annual incidence in the United States has been estimated to be 0.021 to 0.061 per 100,000 population. In one large series, Safai et al. reported a 3:1 male-to-female ratio and a mean age of 63 years among patients with Kaposi's sarcoma. Precise incidence estimates specific for sexual preference are not available, because the number of homosexual men living in the cities where Kaposi's sarcoma has occurred is unknown. Nonetheless, the highly localized occurrence of 88 cases among men under 60 suggests at least a 100-fold increase in age-specific risk among homosexual men in the cities reporting cases, as compared with previous estimates of incidence. (*NEJM*, January 28, 1982, 306/4, p. 250)

The first sentence is the usual one about the unusualness of Kaposi's sarcoma, *Pneumocystis* pneumonia, and opportunistic infections; the second sentence defines both KS and the categories in which it can be seen. (Remember that "elderly men" becomes "older men of Eastern European descent" in report B.) The third sentence states that the incidence rates are unknown but afterwards presents a quantitative estimation of annual incidence rates. At this point, the text cites two studies published in a cancer journal in 1962. The way these rates are presented leads to reading them as numbers of cases per population unit (with a unit of 100,000); they are designated not as risk but as incidence rates. Through their statistical construction, they homogenize and disperse reported cases of Kaposi's sarcoma with respect to an abstract, quantitatively built category. The next sentence provides a specific male-to-female ratio and an average age, taken from a 1980 study (referenced in the text). After this, the paper states that there are no incidence estimates of occurrence of Kaposi's sarcoma with respect to sexual orientation; the cause of this absence is the unknown number of "homosexual men living in cities where Kaposi's sarcoma has occurred." No rationale is provided for why the relationship between incidence estimates and sexual orientation should be relevant here. The previous dermatologic literature did not claim that heterosexuals contract KS more easily than people with other sexual orientations. A connection is introduced at this point without any justification; once introduced, it can be quantified and processed. Perhaps even more to the point, the absence of data about this connection is transformed into a topic of note. Nothing is known about this topic because of lack of data. This is a good example of the perlocutionary force of an apparently simple, constative utterance – a force by which the opposite of what is said is achieved. In a most interesting manner, this assertion (i.e., estimates are not available) is negated as follows:

1. A quantified category is asserted ("88 cases among men under 60").
2. An event concerning this quantified category is asserted ("highly localized occurrence").
3. A subjectively formulated thesis is asserted ("suggests that").

4. This subjectively formulated thesis is objectified, magnified through minimization (metonymy), and quantified in two steps (first step – "at least"; second step – "100-fold increase").

The syntagm "100-fold increase in age-specific risk among homosexual men" has "the annual incidence in the United States" of Kaposi's sarcoma as its reference. Risk is given a double meaning here: on the one hand, it is treated as a simple statistical construct (incidence of cases per population unit); on the other hand, it is presented as the probability of exposure. Moreover, risk increase in the risk-specific group of "homosexual men" is constructed from non-risk, because it relates to the incidence in the general population. The category of "homosexual men" is synonymous with "general population" (in the past), and at the same time it is a special, distinct category (in the present); this makes it possible to compare quantities apparently ascribed to completely different categories. The result of this chain of operations is that the "highly localized occurrence of 88 cases among men under 60" is asserted as the legitimate basis of "a 100-fold increase in age-specific risk" for the category of "homosexual men in the cities reporting cases." The reader must herself perform a couple of operations to complete the deductive chain: first, she must recompose the "88 cases" as "homosexual or bisexual" with Kaposi's sarcoma, or with Kaposi's sarcoma and *Pneumocystis* pneumonia, from a table on the next page of the report; this can be done by adding and subtracting various quantities from various categories labeled "sexual preference." Second, the reader has to divide this quantity by the total number of cases reported by the paper (158 reported cases of Kaposi's sarcoma, *Pneumocystis* pneumonia, KS/PCP, KS/PCP, and other infections) to obtain a percentage that is 100 times greater than the incidence rate of Kaposi's sarcoma in the United States in 1962, as the text affirms. Therefore, the text presents the reader with two possibilities: (1) take the assertion about risk increase for granted; or (2) perform for herself the operations through which risk is constructed as an absolute quantity, thus legitimizing herself the assertion about the relative quantity (and dynamics) of risk.

The rhetorical strategy of the text is to leave deductive chains incomplete, attracting the reader into performing the text's own operations of transforming qualities into quantities. As shown above, this relative quantity of risk (a "100-fold increase in age-specific risk among homosexual men") is taken by report B as the basis for performing a comparison between the risk for Kaposi's sarcoma in the general population and in the category of "homosexual men." The conclusion is an "at least one hundred times greater risk" for "homosexual men." Through references in the text, the assertion of report B is presented as an already legitimate one, which does not require additional empirical evidence or statistical computation. Report B thus translates the assertions in report A as follows:

1. A relative quantity designating a change with respect to the past is transformed into an ordinal number that allows different categories to be compared.
2. Complex descriptions such as "homosexual men under 60 in cities reporting cases" are transformed into general categories, such as "homosexual men."
3. The past–present relationship (which allowed qualities to be transformed into quantities and vice versa) is translated into a present–present relationship, based on distinctions between general categories.
4. A referential population unit (hence: a convention) is translated into a universal reference category ("general population") which also plays the role of an absolute reference point, allowing quantitative orderings of distinct categories.

The introduction of a universal reference category allows a couple of apparently paradoxical operations: namely, constructing the general quantitative risk of a skin cancer form presented as unusual, rare, problematic, and rarely seen before, and comparing it with the quantitative risk of a specific population, for whom this rare skin cancer form was claimed to be specific. The paradox lies in that the category of "general population" was presented simultaneously as a non-risk and a risk category, as instrumental in performing classifications, and as a low-risk category (i.e., as the reference point from which risk begins to grow). Its use was generalized by further medical reports, so it has become commonplace.

How Sexual Acts Came To Be Quantified and Compared

As shown in Chapter 5, a third way of transforming qualities into quantities of risk was provided by the spatial presentation of risk itself. Risk was represented as urban areas, zones, or agglomerations; risk classifications differentiated between high- and low-risk cities, urban areas, or neighborhoods, which (by virtue of their definition) could be transformed from qualities into quantities. With high-risk areas defined as cities where risk categories agglomerated, quantities of risk were constructed as estimates of such agglomerations. For the "homosexual" risk category, these estimates were constructed on the basis of the number of single and never married men in the respective areas. This was a central instrument in distinguishing between areas with different risk degrees in San Francisco and New York. Numbers of AIDS cases diagnosed in a certain time span were divided by numbers of single and never married men, or IV drug users. The results were presented as "incidence rates in selected population groups in the United States in 1984."[1] Through the identification of "homosexual men" with "single and never married men," a distinct risk group was quantified according to space; a similar process took place for other risk categories.[2] For example, "Haitian entrants" were divided by total population (before and after 1977); the result was distinct risk rates for "Haitians." The same operation was performed for the categories of "persons with hemophilia," "sexual contacts with male IV drug users," and "transfusion recipients," without time or space distinctions.

The spatial organization of risk as agglomerations or "densities" opened the possibility of constructing not only frequencies, as shown above, but also means, medians, and similar statistical instruments. Comparing the risk degrees of different spaces according to "incidence rates" became usual (*AJE*, 1985, 121/5, p. 633). This comparison was (and continues to be) common in epidemiologic reports. I refer here only to a couple of such reports, which I analyzed at length in

---

[1] James W. Curran et al.: "The Epidemiology of AIDS: Current Status and Future Prospects," *Science*, September 27, 1985, 229, pp. 1352–7.

[2] A risk category that remained unquantified until the 1990s in this process of organizing risk spatially was that of infants and children; although they were distributed according to the parents' risk, the usual rhetorical strategies of quantification were not applied here.

Chapter 5; they presented the distribution of risk in New York City by risk group and borough, whereby risk was defined not only by group, but also by mean age, which allowed comparison with risk for sexually transmitted diseases (*AJE*, 1986, 123/6, p. 1025). Another report on high- and low-risk cities distinguished them by the construction of mean number of sexual partners, which was correlated with the mean number of helper T-cells. In this context, risk became primarily frequency or density of a category in a certain area, from which the probability of transmission was derived. At the same time, the quantification of risk categories as frequencies or densities reinforced and reproduced the spatial model of risk and hence the qualitative distinction between high- and low-risk areas and urban spaces. Risk spaces or cities (also termed "endemic areas") were those with a lower mean of helper T-cell count; cities with a high helper T-cell count were low-risk (*AJE*, 1985, 121/5, pp. 629, 637). Statistical constructions thus defined qualitative differences, which in turn served as bases for creating such constructions.

Sexual contact and, more importantly, sexual act types were defined as risk factors for the "homosexual" risk category, which in turn was defined through these spatially arranged risk factors. In the absence of any self-sustaining "heterosexual" risk category, sexual contact and sexual act types in "low-risk populations" (including women) were not defined as risk factors; they were seen rather as dependent or collateral risk (*JAMA*, September 9, 1983, 250/10, p. 1312). Sexual contact as a risk factor for women enjoyed the paradoxical status of leading to the transmission of the etiologic agent from male to female without actually being a proper risk factor. "Low-risk populations" (which included women) were populations without "obvious risk factors," which nonetheless acquired the virus. Therefore, even if heterosexual contact was proved to be a means of transmission, this did not change its risk status much; this status was always presented as "intimate heterosexual contact directly or indirectly with persons in a high-risk group," thus depending on homosexual contact or IV drug use. Moreover, heterosexual act types were not even the object of a classification, as in the case of "homosexual" risk. When they were presented as risk factors (as in the case of "African AIDS") they were ordered spatially. Initially, heterosexual contact enjoyed an ambiguous status, being presented as a risk factor and at the same time as a non-factor (*The Lancet*,

July 14, II/8394, 1984, p. 68). It is notable in this context that sexual act types in "African AIDS" began to be classified (and therefore to be presented as risk factors) very late, at the beginning of the 1990s.

Risk factors defining other categories, such as intravenous drug users, were not quantified.[3] Those associated with blood transfusions were systematically presented as donor-related; this required identifying distributions of high-risk donors in a "general donor population" (*NEJM*, January 12, 1984, 310/2, pp. 70–1), which mirrored the comparison between "homosexual" risk and the "general population." On this basis, the number of transfusion units necessary to transmit the etiologic agent was computed. Perhaps not surprisingly, the result was one unit. In this frame, the first category for which risk factors were quantified was the "homosexual" risk group. This operation relied on distinguishing between types of sexual acts, and it generated a scale ranging from the riskiest to the least risky sexual act types. Many epidemiological studies used this ordinal scale, indicating which sexual act types are riskier than which others (on the basis of numerical comparisons), which is the riskiest, and so forth (see, e.g., *AJE*, 1985, 121/5, pp. 640–2). Frequencies of sexual act types and of sexual partners (obtained through interviews) were statistically correlated with diagnoses of opportunistic infections; the result was a specific risk of AIDS for each sexual act type. Later studies began to correlate frequencies of sexual act types and of sexual partners directly with the diagnosis of seropositivity, regardless of whether a diagnosis of opportunistic infections had been made.

Toward the end of the 1980s, studies began to compute and present this scale numerically, with clear differences in the quantities of risk induced by the frequency of each sexual act type (*AJE*, 1987, 125/6, pp. 1039–41, 1053–5). This meant that one could quantitatively compare the risks of performing, say, sexual act types A and B and see that the risk of performing A was 1.5 greater than that of doing B; conversely, this also meant that one could practice B 1.5 times more with the same risk as practicing A. To give just one example, an article on "Risk Factors for AIDS and HIV Seropositivity in Homosexual

---

[3] They were continuously presented as "sharing of contaminated needles," and they were often characterized as being only the "presumed mode of transmission"; see *NEJM*, January 12, 1984, 310/2, p. 69.

Men" (*AJE*, 1987, 125/6, pp. 1035–47) published in 1987 by several authors, including a team from the Institut Pasteur in Paris, found a risk magnitude of 0.5 for oral insertive sexual acts, and a magnitude of 1.5 for oral receptive sexual acts (*AJE*, 1987, 125/6, p. 1040). This was presented as evidence that insertive sexual acts were less risky than receptive acts. This evidence could also mean that practicing oral insertive sexual acts three times more than oral receptive acts would amount to the same quantity of risk. Evidently, three times more oral insertive sexual acts for one person could also mean three times more partners practicing oral receptive sexual acts, which would make oral insertion riskier by the standards of this risk scale.

Studies from the early 1990s computed statistical correlations between the number of T-helper cells and variables such as "early ejaculation" or "erectile dysfunction," without specifying how delayed ejaculation, for example, reduced the risk of infection. Clinical and epidemiologic studies from the late 1980s adopted a full-fledged quantification of risk factors, relating them directly to the diagnosis of seropositivity.[4] The starting point in quantifying risk factors was provided by the selection of a risk group; frequently used criteria were area of residence and attendance at a clinic for sexually transmitted diseases. The population thus obtained was then quantified according to results of serological tests, diagnosis of opportunistic infections, and sexual history. This last factor meant classifying through interviews along "scales of homosexual behavior."[5] "Sexual histories" were classified as "life histories": the subjects were asked to recall their total lifetime number of sexual partners and sexual act types. Another version of "sexual histories" was "study year histories," in which case the subjects had to recall numbers of partners and sexual act types in the year preceding the onset of symptoms. Additional classifications were used for histories of drug use, sexually transmitted diseases, "history of recent medical occupation, Italian or Eastern European ancestry, smoking or alcohol consumption," and "washing shortly after sex" (*AJE*, 1987,

---

[4] There is no essential difference between earlier and later epidemiological studies in the quantification of risk factors; the only differences were provided by (1) the correlation of quantified risk factors to the diagnosis of seropositivity and (2) the more refined statistical computing techniques.

[5] Many studies used Kinsey's scale (*AJE*, 1987, 125/6, pp. 1037, 1050) or self-constructed scales (Meyer-Bahlburg et al. 1991).

125/6, p. 1043). Secondary classifications (according to criteria such as food, ancestry, profession, tobacco use, and the like) were already present in clinical and epidemiological reports in 1983–4. The usual rhetorical strategy was to show that they were not significant, in contrast to the main risk classifications. They acted as a contrastive means, for showing that, say, Kaposi's sarcoma was not due to Mediterranean origins (as in usual KS). These contrast factors were often put in the text under the rubric "other exposures." The results were absolute and relative frequencies of sexual act types for each class of partner frequencies. The frequencies were statistically correlated with the diagnosis of seropositivity, as well as with that of opportunistic infections, obtaining quantities of risk for different sexual act types. Not surprisingly, sexual act types had greater quantities of risk than factors under the rubric "other exposures"; moreover, the sexual act type–related risks were also quantitatively differentiated.

This leaves out the statistical techniques employed for obtaining numerical values for correlations; these techniques were made possible by several means of classifying and reclassifying risk. The first was to build up a category through metonimy: a selected group (such as the patients of a clinic) was taken to represent a general risk category. In a subsequent step, subcategories were set up for each risk factor; the patient's life history was structured along a few quantifiable dimensions. Once the life history became quantifiable, subcategories of risk could be expressed as precise quantities.

A consequence was that sexual act types that seemed incommensurable were made compatible; they could now be ordered, compared, and weighed against one another. It thus became possible to assert not only that A was, say, riskier than B, but also how much riskier it was. This, in turn, had the effect of consolidating the categories already produced, which were confirmed in their distinctiveness. Distinctiveness, in turn, reinforced the abstract category of "AIDS risk." Quality was again produced from quantity. Here is one example from a study that calculated comparable quantities of risk; after presenting numerical correlations between seropositivity and sexual act types at length, it produced in the "discussion" a new quality, namely "AIDS risk." The paper concluded:

AIDS risk was strongly associated with number of sexual partners, doubling with every 20–30 partners when cases were compared with antibody-negative neighborhood controls. Risk of seropositivity doubled with every 30–40 partners when antibody-positive and antibody-negative neighborhood controls were compared. [...] Rectal receptivity was clearly the primary sexual behavior leading to the transmission of HIV. Men rectally receptive with most or all their partners were at a four- to sevenfold risk compared with those receptive with few or some. (*AJE*, 1987, 125/6, p. 1045)

Several qualities of risk emerge here from quantification: (1) a category of men with several sexual partners, transformed later in the section into a "sexually active subculture ... defined by its engaging in extensive and traumatic rectal sex"; (2) the category of "AIDS risk" as a confirmed and predictable, very concrete probability; (3) the same category as a causal chain, through which a specific sexual behavior "clearly" acts as a transmission means; and (4) "AIDS risk" as a cause of the syndrome. A second consequence of quantification was that it generated subcategories of risk according to the frequencies of the sexual act types performed. Thus, when "AIDS risk" doubles with every 20–30 partners and "risk of seropositivity" with every 30–40, this means not only quantitative comparisons, but also clear, qualitatively differentiated risk classes: it shows broader classes for seropositivity than for AIDS, and it also shows that being ordered in a lower class means being at, say, only half the risk.

A closer look, then, reveals that the quantification of AIDS risk is not as rhetoric-free as one may think. Not only does it presuppose a whole series of preliminary rhetorical operations that ensure the comparability of otherwise incommensurable categories, but the process of quantification itself produces (and requires) rhetorical figures such as the "general population," without which quantitative assertions about risk would lose their meaning. Quantification standardizes "AIDS risk" and provides this otherwise abstract, unclear entity with a concrete shape, so that it can be processed according to the existent epidemiological rules. It allows comparisons across wholly different contexts and homogenizes the field of expert AIDS knowledge, in the sense that it creates common reference points for all participants in epidemiologic research.

In terms of prevention policies, quantification according to risk factors (which are strictly ascribed to groups) can achieve unintended effects: for example, it might reinforce the idea that it is safe to practice less risky sexual acts with a greater number of partners, for whom these acts are actually riskier. More generally speaking, it appears that

the notion of risk is inextricably tied to that of groups or categories;
the rhetorical practices in which the quantification of risk is embedded
have solidified these ties in such a manner that it becomes impossible
to speak of "AIDS risk" without associating it with a classification
system. This remains valid today, even if "risk factors" are apparently
individual. The point I am making is that these factors become significant by being ascribed to specific groups. Therefore, the question is
whether prevention approaches based on "risk" can be effective in the
long run. Recent observations suggest that they do not reach those who
do not perceive themselves as belonging to a clear-cut group and that
they wear out in time. In Western Europe, recent prevention campaigns
have shifted from stressing "risk" to representing condoms as objects
of fun and pleasure, used not because they diminish dangers, but because it is cool and enjoyable to use them. In the same vein, those who
create prevention policies in developing countries (where the incidence
of AIDS is especially high) could reflect more on the effectiveness of
approaches based exclusively on quantified "risk." Cultural anthropologists (Setel 1999, pp. 53–5) have recently suggested that risk-based
approaches are bound to fail because they do not take into account
the extent of concrete practices and the silent rules regulating sexual
relationships in various contexts. They argue that these rules, which
are beyond quantification, should be taken as the starting point for any
preventive policies.

7

In Lieu of a Conclusion

Do Rhetorical Practices Matter?

How Rhetorical Practices Work

The aim of this book is to examine the relationship between the rhetoric of risk and medical knowledge pertaining to the Acquired Immuno-deficiency Syndrome. The idea of "AIDS risk" rests on the assumption that there is a necessary relationship between retroviral entities entering the human body and affecting its immune system (a natural process), on the one hand, and certain social characteristics, on the other hand. Here, the term "characteristics" covers a wide range of features: belonging to a social or ethnic group, pursuing a specific "lifestyle," being male or female, performing certain sexual acts, performing very many sexual acts, and inhabiting certain areas. In other words, performing a certain sexual act (or too many), embracing a certain "lifestyle," and belonging to a certain ethnic group are risks because they necessarily trigger a biological process with negative outcomes. Necessity, as well as "facts," can take many forms here: they both can be conceived as collective or individual and as behavior- or group-related. It is because of this necessity that "AIDS risk" exists in the world.

This logic obliges us first to learn more about how retroviruses (or indeed any agents or entities) enter the body and affect the human immune system, to be able to see which kinds of social "facts" constitute risk. Knowledge about rare opportunistic infections and about a new immunodeficiency syndrome underlying them allows one to develop knowledge about the etiologic agent, how this enters the body, and consequently, which acts or facts of social life lead to this process. In this sense, knowledge of risk is derived from medical knowledge about the natural facts of retroviruses or about their means of transmission.

One of the main questions posed in the present inquiry is whether the rhetoric of risk can be said to co-constitute the medical knowledge about rare opportunistic infections, the immunodeficiency syndrome underlying them, etiologic agents, and means of transmission. The answer is yes. The rare and new opportunistic infections are "rare," "new," and "previously unseen" only with respect to a classification that provides the frame for deciding when a disease or infection is usual and when it is unusual, when it is known and when it is unknown. Rhetorical devices were central in establishing the existence of a new syndrome with its own etiology, a specific means of transmission, and its own risks.

The frame for conceiving the etiological agent as being similar to the etiological agents of sexually transmitted diseases, or as environmental, household contact, viral, or "lifestyle factors," was given by classification practices. In this context, the thesis of a retrovirus as the etiological agent of AIDS imposed itself not in spite of, but because of and via previous theses about, STD-like viral agents and environmental factors.

If the ways in which the syndrome, its etiologic agent, and its means of transmission are seen to depend on particular, contextually defined frames of risk, then there can be no unitary, homogeneous, and serial biomedical discourse on AIDS, no line of uninterrupted progress from modest beginnings up to the complexities seen today. Rather, there are several disparate streams constituting what is called the "medical AIDS discourse" and providing only an ostensible unity, if any. The picture of steady progress and expansion of medical knowledge of the syndrome, interrupted only intermittently by accidents, minor errors, corrected misconceptions, and so forth, proves to be inadequate. It is not that medical knowledge has not substantially changed between the first reports in June 1981 and now; it has, dramatically. But these changes are not brought about by steady progress and enlargement; rather, it is this multiplicity of rhetorical frames that generates change. Old discourses are not replaced by new and better ones; they simply run in different directions and intersect, compete, borrow from each other, and become intermingled.

As shown in this book, a medical discourse on "women's risk of AIDS," an enduring mystery for social scientists, simply does not exist. Instead, we encounter several narratives and representations of "spouses," "female sexual partners," "prostitutes," and "African women," promoting different, and to a certain extent incompatible, views on the etiological agent and its transmission, as well as on the susceptibility of the female body to infection.

Another example is the thesis of immunosuppressive sperm: apparently long forgotten, it is one more curiosity, a misconception belonging to a past era. Besides the fact that it was still referred to in epidemiological papers on "homosexual risk" in the 1990s and is therefore not as forgotten as one might think, it has produced arguments central to the depiction of the action of the retrovirus and the body's immune defenses. In the mid-1990s, AIDS scientists called for more research on the immunity of mucosal linings, considering it crucial for understanding the immune defenses of the human body (Grady 1995, p. 94). The idea that mucosal linings played an important role in the virus entering the human body was part and parcel of the immunosuppressive sperm thesis. All these examples (and many others could be produced) show that medical knowledge of AIDS did not simply follow a linear pattern of progress, but has consisted of a variety of different and rather contradictory theses, arguments, and representations.

"AIDS risk" is analyzed here as a rhetorical practice that determines what passes as medical knowledge and what does not. As such, "AIDS risk" is a rule for communicating knowledge shared by the (medical) community. The rule as such would appear to be both negligible and crucial at once; it is negligible because it does not actually determine the production of (medical) knowledge. It only determines how things ought to be presented if they are to be accepted as "knowledge" in the community. It is crucial precisely because of the role it plays in persuading, that is, in making the community accept a given body of knowledge as legitimate. Rhetoric, it seems, is not something authors merely append to their texts according to mood, whim, or imagination, but rather something determined by community rules. Nor is it the case that some authors choose to adorn their texts, whereas others prefer not to do so, presenting instead a stark, honest account. If the community has such rules of communicating (and there is no reason why a community should not), according to which something is accepted or rejected as convincing or not, and if knowledge must be shaped according to these rules in order to pass as knowledge at all, it follows that knowledge will always be shaped according to such rules, and that in practice knowledge and rules of persuasion are indistinguishable.

This is, however, not the full story. I argue in the Introduction that the context of production (discovery) and the context of justification (communicating knowledge) cannot be separated. Therefore, community-shared rules of persuasion are intrinsic to the production of (scientific) knowledge. Rhetorical practices are not only relevant with respect to how the (scientific) community becomes persuaded or convinced that something is the case. They are relevant with respect to how knowledge is produced too.

This brings us back to the initial question of how rhetorical practices work. Two arguments are central throughout this book: the first is methodological, the second, conceptual. The methodological argument is that rhetorical practices cannot be analyzed at an abstract level; they cannot be separated or distilled from their concrete products. They cannot be conceived as abstract rules of persuasion or talk; this would mean that they are external with respect to the social action they determine (Turner 1994, p. 6). In other words, if rules of persuasion can be separated from instances of persuasive speech, we should be able to formulate abstract rules in such a way that they are (1) co-extensive with every instance of persuasive speech and (2) formulated in a language distinct from that of concrete instances of persuasive speech. This means that we should be able to formulate rules of persuasive speech in a formal language, for instance. More generally speaking, these are the two conditions every kind of abstract rule of social action should fulfill (Arrington 1993, p. 58).

Both conditions, however, are impossible to fulfill: we cannot exclude misapplications of the rules of persuasion, and we cannot formulate them in a language distinct from and irreducible to natural language. It follows from this that we cannot formulate abstract rules of persuasion as isolated from their concrete applications (see also Pleasants 1999, p. 16). Methodologically speaking, what we can do is provide an analytical reconstruction of the rules of persuasion-in-action.

Rhetorical practices are closely imbricated with the production of knowledge. The two cannot be separated, in the same sense in which methods of practical action cannot be separated from what is achieved with them. Rhetoric, understood as social practice, is not merely an assemblage of devices vegetating on the periphery of hard factual statements, or impinging now and then upon the readers. It is the very condition under which it becomes possible to express, order, and legitimate epistemic claims. The rhetorical practice of "risk" produces an epistemic order of the Acquired Immunodeficiency Syndrome: that is, it shows what it is possible to know about the syndrome and how it is possible to know it.

The conceptual argument, related to the methodological one, is that rhetorical practices do not work as rigid, unchangeable rules. They do not automatically reproduce the same arguments. This, however, is not necessarily a disadvantage. An important analogy I used in Chapters 1 and 2 is the one between classification practices and changes in the protein surface of viruses. Classifications (as a variety of rhetorical practice) do not work with fixed categories: rather, they effect local changes, adapt, expand, engulf contradictory cases, and reproduce in a changed shape. To push the viral analogy further, rhetorical practices work by using local change and non-identical replication.

What is, then, the import of all this for the sociology of scientific knowledge? First, rhetorical practices should not be understood as a kind of social fantasy – i.e., as something that exists only in the minds of social actors (in this case, scientists). Second, (scientific) texts are not "flat"; instead, they are social practices of expressing and organizing knowledge (although this statement is in itself tautological), and as social practices they say something to the sociologist. Third, rhetorical practices have concrete consequences. In this case, rhetorical practices have had consequences for AIDS prevention and outreach policies, for the organization and financing of research, and for democracy in advanced societies.

How Rhetorical Practices Matter for AIDS Prevention

My argument here is that rhetorical practices do have consequences for how AIDS prevention policies are conceived and organized. There are at least four aspects of AIDS prevention to be considered here: (1) the social groups targeted by prevention policies; (2) the self-perception of these groups with respect to risk; (3) the persuasion techniques for inducing behavioral changes; and (4) the interaction between medical practitioners and at-risk individuals.

Throughout the book, I show that what counts as an AIDS-relevant case depends on the risk categories that frame the meaning of the syndrome. Contrary to what is generally assumed, the notion of risk behavior has not replaced that of risk categories, but coexists with the latter in prevention policies. The thesis that certain forms of social behavior favor infection with HIV has been accompanied by the idea that these forms of behavior are characteristic for certain social groups. Consequently, prevention policies cannot but target these groups in a special manner. This is a direct outcome of the classificatory frame in which medical knowledge about AIDS was constituted. An important consequence is that cases of people with HIV and/or AIDS are treated as belonging to one of the risk categories in this classificatory frame. Cases that cannot easily be ascribed to a given category tend to be ignored; cases that belong to more than one risk category are simplified. Forms of behavior are considered to be exclusively category-specific and are treated as such when it comes to preventive measures. And so these measures fail, at least partly, to reach ethnic groups that do not fit into the classificatory scheme.

For example, same-sex sexual practices are taken to be characteristic of "homosexuals" as a risk category. Prevention measures focusing on same-sex sexual practices target this medical category, which is seen as overlapping with the socio-cultural category of "gays," almost exclusively, ignoring the fact that many individuals have same-sex sexual practices without identifying themselves as homosexual or gay (Alonso and Koreck 1993; Carrier and Magana 1992). This is true both for members of some ethnic groups (e.g., Turkish men in Europe, Latinos) and for members of the mainstream "general population." They perceive themselves as straight or "heterosexual" and resist prevention measures. Another case in point here is that of African Americans, who were ignored for a long time in regard to being at risk for AIDS. Throughout the late 1980s, for example, 9% of the subjects in AIDS clinical trials conducted in New York City were African American. The percentage of African Americans among AIDS cases in New York City was 35% (Institute of Medicine 1991, p. 83). Because cases of African Americans with HIV and/or AIDS did not neatly fit in with the categories of the classificatory scheme, they were left out of many clinical trials. Because AIDS was (and still is) defined as an STD, in many cases the subjects of clinical trials were recruited from venereal medical practices in certain middle class neighborhoods. Individuals who did not frequent these practices (or any medical practice at all) were left out of the trials. As social scientists now acknowledge, this has made AIDS prevention among African Americans very difficult: many do not perceive themselves as being at any risk or reject prevention as an attempt to undermine their sexual and social identity (Airhihenbuwa et al. 1992, p. 270; Icard et al. 1992, p. 441).

The orientation of AIDS prevention to certain "risk groups" correlates thus with the level of self-perception: social actors perceive themselves as being at risk or not at risk for AIDS according to whether they identify themselves as belonging to a risk category or not. Self-perception affects attitudes with respect to prevention (such as condom use) and to infection with HIV. Risk categories influence the ways in which social actors position themselves in relationship to AIDS and HIV as natural phenomena, as "things." At the same time, actors position these "things" in their social universe with respect to and by means of risk. It is the rhetorical practices of risk that shape (1) the subject of risk, as well as (2) the non-subject, (3) the relationships of the risk subjects (and those of the non-subjects too) to the disease, and (4) the relationships between subjects and non-subjects with respect to the disease. Moreover, they also shape a series of social entities, such as the AIDS patient, her family, and the relationship of the medical practitioner to AIDS patients.

The operation of classifying, that is, of generating social categories susceptible to the acquired immune deficiency, generates different social positions with respect to the disease. How social actors position themselves with respect to AIDS depends on the techniques of defining risk through which they do or do not become members of a category with a clear and definite position with respect to the syndrome. That is, one can become a member of a category such as "homosexual" or "African," in which case this position is clearly defined. It shows how a member has to "report" herself to the disease, how she becomes a subject in this relationship. Or, one becomes a non-member, which again defines the position with respect to the disease and to the members; the relationship of exclusion defines how non-members align themselves to the syndrome and to members of risk categories, and how they become non-subjects of risk. This, again, should have consequences for how prevention policies are conceived. We should ask ourselves whether campaigns based on "risk" can conceivably reach everybody, and whether we should look for new approaches. Consider the large-scale, mass-media publicity campaigns of the early 1990s, such as "AIDS concerns us all" in Germany, "grim reaper" in Australia, and those in Great Britain and the US: they all claimed that there should be no difference in the way people relate themselves to the syndrome. In other words, they tried to assert that everyone is a risk subject and everyone is at risk. This was their explicit message, and it failed. It did so because the rhetorical practice of risk is inherently classificatory and because it had already established a social cleavage, an ontology within which there were subjects and non-subjects. Claiming that everyone is at risk was self-negating. As I mentioned above, men may well have same-sex relationships without perceiving themselves as gay. Consequently, they will not perceive sexual acts such as anal intercourse as risky, because this is not "gay sex." They see themselves as non-subjects, engaging in non-risk activities.

If one takes into account the enormous diversity of individuals – and of their sexual practices – risk categories do not say much. They cannot function normatively. But as part of a classificatory system, such categories transform abstract qualities into quantities and vice versa. It becomes possible to count types of sexual acts, their frequency, their environment, their history, and so forth, and thus to provide such a risk category with a post hoc norm by showing what a "homosexual" does, how many times, where, and so on – in short, to normatize it as a category. Therefore, it becomes possible to find and occupy a position with respect to normalized risk, a process that requires appropriate discursive techniques. "Becoming a member of a risk category" means that there are discursive techniques, grounded in the rhetorical practice of risk, by which one is positioned and/or by which one positions oneself with respect to the categories of the classification. It is through this process of positioning that someone becomes a subject or non-subject of risk. Membership is not given but rather appears as a discursive construction. Correspondingly, subjects and non-subjects of AIDS risk are not given but made, by means of these techniques.

This is not without consequences for the techniques of persuasion designed to induce behavioral changes. Worldwide, prevention strategies have promoted condom use as a measure providing relatively efficient protection against infection with HIV. To get people to use condoms, there needs to be some sort of persuasive strategy. Very frequently, this has involved playing on people's fears: regular condom use is induced, campaign planners have reasoned, by instilling fear of infection with HIV and its consequences. Many mass campaigns for condom use have used this strategy. Although it was considered effective in the 1980s, especially in the gay communities, there are indications that it does not work well with the generation now becoming young adults. On the one hand, a persuasion strategy based on fear may achieve the opposite: defiance of risk in order to show lack of fear. On the other hand, the rising generation does not have a direct experience of the impact of AIDS on social communities. Therefore, it has been argued that it would be a better persuasive strategy to create the idea that using condoms on a casual basis is cool and fun. With this approach, presumably, using condoms would no longer be perceived as "preventive" (that is, special), but as habitual behavior.

A further and perhaps deeper level at which rhetorical practices have made an impact is that of the interactions between medical practitioners and individuals seeking counseling, diagnosis, or treatment. In many cases, medical practitioners have to identify patients as risk or non-risk, sometimes even before looking more closely at the symptoms or making a diagnosis of seropositivity. This happens as a rule in STD clinics, because (1) AIDS has the double role of being a sexually transmitted disease and of being induced by STDs and (2) a great number of epidemiological studies are drawn from patients in STD clinics in inner cities. The identification requires a series of discursive techniques through which the patient positions herself with respect to risk categories and has to acknowledge having done "things" – i.e., has to admit that she is a risk subject. Until the mid-1980s, it was a real problem for medical practitioners to achieve this positioning by having the patients acknowledge "things," because of poor discursive techniques, as they themselves admitted. Those in many studies complained about poor sampling or about the difficulties in identifying cases and constructing relevant cohorts. A good technique makes the interviewee talk about and recognize the things she did as "risky things" and therefore acknowledge herself as a subject of risk. Counseling manuals and instructions on how to pose good questions, both directed at medical practitioners, have flourished since the mid-1980s. I give just two examples here. Complaining that physicians from STD clinics lack knowledge about "homosexual lifestyles," a medical article described the following discursive techniques for gaining information from adolescents:

The physician may determine the sexual orientation of the patient by asking directly. Since many patients feel uncomfortable with the clinical term "homosexual," phrasing the question as "Are you gay or straight?" may convey to the homosexual adolescent a sense of empathy and understanding. Another way the physician may approach this question is to ask the patient "Have you ever had sex with guys, women, both, or neither?" Still another way to inquire about sexual orientation is to include it with other questions about personal lifestyles: "Is there anything in your lifestyle, such as recent travels, sexual practices, diet, or use of drugs that might help me to diagnose your medical problem?" (*JAHC*, July 1985, 6/4, p. 278)

Once this knowledge has been gained, the physician may proceed to ask questions about sexual acts or "risk factors," which, in turn, necessitate a very specific kind of conversation, as in the following:

If the physician feels comfortable using colloquial terms for these practices, then he or she should use them. If not, the physician may ask, for example, "When having sex, does your partner's penis come in contact with your anus?" or "Does your mouth ever come in contact with your partner's anus?" (*JAHC*, July 1985, 6/4, pp. 278–9)

A more complex *AIDS. Guide to Clinical Counseling*, published in 1989 in London at the Science Press by Riva Miller and Robert Bor, recommended discursive techniques in which the patient first had to define what risk is, then to acknowledge the things she does, and finally to classify them as risky. It recommended that physicians put the following questions in this order:

What is your understanding of how the HIV is transmitted, or passed on? What do you mean by "sex"? Is it kissing, hugging etc...? What do you understand about the risk of transmission of HIV from woman to man, and man to woman? Through intercourse, which body fluids are most likely to carry the virus? What sexual activities do you consider to be "risky"? What is it that makes them "risky"? How many sexual partners have you had in the last year? What do you know about the number of sexual partners and the risk of transmission of HIV? (p. 43)

After the patient has gone through them, there are questions for transfusion recipients, intravenous drug users, people who have traveled to Africa, and many more. A specific line of questioning is required here, so that the patients become subjects or non-subjects of risk. Moreover, the patient may acknowledge herself as a risk subject even before seeking out a medical practitioner. Members of well organized urban gay cultures are an example in this sense: immersed as they are in the medical discourse on AIDS risk (through community medical information services, newsletters, meetings, or counseling) to an extent which makes them "better" than virologists or immunologists, they are able to transform themselves into risk subjects. Steven Epstein (1996) shows how the gay community has developed its own medical counter-expertise – i.e., how it has thematized itself as a risk group in order to defend itself as such. Having already acknowledged the "risky things" one has done provides a frame for seeing symptoms and bodily signs "right," as signs and symptoms of the risk one already has.

The direction taken by the conversation may be reversed, in that the patient gives the medical practitioner the clues to make the latter recognize him as a subject of risk. As a consequence, self-acknowledged risk subjects may cope better with the news of seropositivity. People who perceive themselves as non-subjects of risk, and who are reconstructed as subjects through discursive techniques, are the ones who have to endure the greatest shock. In an interview, a physician from an established AIDS research clinic with about 4,000 patients annually described self-identification as follows:

It changes, it's very different . . . mostly yes . . . mostly yes, because the patients, most patients belong to a risk group, and they know their risk group. This has become a very popular idea, has become well known, and therefore people know behavior related to infection with HIV, and naturally they do have an idea that it might be possible that it's an infection with HIV. That's why people already for themselves . . . well, perhaps they do not count on it, but they take it as possible, possible to a high degree. Other patients, who have no risk at all, well, the ones who have no risk at all, it's very difficult for them, they cannot believe it. They are shocked. . . . (Interview with clinical AIDS specialist)

Knowing one's risk category makes it "natural" that one's bodily signs are signs of infection with HIV (i.e., signs of being at risk; correspondingly, having no risk category at all, that is, having "no risk at all"/being a non-subject of risk makes it equally "natural" that bodily signs are signs of not being at risk). Moreover, knowing one's risk category means that one has to know it with certainty – that is, one must construct one's identity as a risk subject with respect to one, clear-cut category which is then adopted as "my risk," "my identity," and the identity of "my bodily signs." A similar phenomenon has been recently described by Rayna Rapp with respect to the genetic counseling of pregnant women. Rapp shows (1999, p. 70) that genetic counseling sessions interactively construct pregnant women as subjects or non-subjects of risk according to given statistical categories. The result is that women represent more general, pregnancy-related problems and anxieties in statistical and genetic terms, acknowledging themselves in this way as members of a risk category.

When devising persuasion techniques for behavioral change, outreach programs, or strategies of coping with seropositivity, we should never forget that rhetorical practices do matter. We should also keep in mind that using risk categories inevitably means not only inclusion, but also exclusion: prevention policies and outreach programs anchored in classificatory systems will automatically leave some relevant cases and groups out. Knowing the epistemic history of AIDS – the role played by classifications, by narratives of origins, by representations of sexual difference – can help us devise better persuasion techniques and policies.

How Rhetorical Practices Matter for Scientific Research

Do rhetorical practices affect the ways in which scientific research is organized and funded? My argument is that they do. At a first, basic level, rhetorical practices play a role in the writing of grant proposals. Research grant proposals are quintessential instruments of persuasion: reviewers and grant-giving institutions must be persuaded to invest sometimes considerable sums of money in a long research process with an uncertain outcome. The authors' skills in presenting their argument play an important role here: successful applicants take grant proposals very seriously and invest a considerable amount of time in writing them.

At another level, rhetorical practices play a role in controversies about research funding: I have analyzed such a case in Chapter 3. After two years of underfunding, in 1983 AIDS research received federal funds of over $14 million, diverted from other research programs. This decision was discussed in medical journals, with arguments about how these funds should be spent. Although it cannot be argued that funding decisions were influenced solely by the arguments formulated during the controversy, these arguments created a legitimating frame for funding decisions: in other words, decisions to invest the money in a particular program (e.g., in retroviral research vs. research on amyl nitrites) had to be justified with respect to these arguments.

A third level at which rhetorical practices influence the organization of research is the distribution of research activities across various research centers and institutes. Federal AIDS research, for instance, has never been centralized in an already existing or newly created institute, but rather it has been distributed across several National Institutes of Health, in addition to the research done at the Centers for Disease Control and Prevention. The argument was that decentralization would ensure better coordination of AIDS research with fundamental research done at the NIH, putting resources and competencies to better use. (It also made it easier to shift funds from other programs to AIDS research.) In the 1980s, the bulk of AIDS research activity was concentrated at two NIH institutes: the National Institute of Allergy and Infectious Diseases (NIAID) and the National Cancer Institute (NCI). In 1991, for example, 53.8% of the AIDS research funding at the NIH was channeled into the NIAID and 20% into the NCI. In the same year, 47.7% of the total NIAID funding and 9.4% of the total NCI funding were devoted to AIDS research (Institute of Medicine 1991, p. 120). The NIAID was also the institute where federal research on sexually transmitted diseases was concentrated. Federal research on viruses and vaccine programs was concentrated at the NCI. In 1982, federal research at the NIH was done only by the NCI, with a staff of 20. A year later, research began at the NIAID too, with a staff of 12, compared with the NCI's 31 (Institute of Medicine 1991, p. 126). Between 1982 and 1991, AIDS research staff at the NCI grew 15-fold. Between 1983 and 1991, research staff at the NIAID grew over 28-fold.

If we compare this growth pattern in research staff (and hence funding) with the life cycle of the various theses about the causal agent, we can see that in 1982 Kaposi's sarcoma topped the list of candidates. KS was a skin cancer with a viral cause. However, 1982 was also the year of the amyl nitrites thesis, according to which AN caused cancer (possibly even KS, along with immune suppression). The NCI was the federal research institute that did research on the connection between cancers and viruses: Dr. Robert Gallo, who worked at the NCI, had identified HTLV-I in the 1970s as a retrovirus causing a cancer form. The NCI also hosted vaccine research and in the 1970s had been at the forefront of the fight against cancer (which included vaccine research). Between 1989 and 1991, the NCI spent a total of $224,582,000 on AIDS vaccine research (Institute of Medicine 1991, p. 122). These funding efforts were preceded by ample discussions of vaccine benefits in the medical press. Between 1986 and 1989, for instance, *Nature* and *Science* alone published 26 features about a vaccine against AIDS, including interventions from the respected polio vaccine pioneer Jonas Salk and the announcement that the Soviets were preparing a vaccine against AIDS (*Nature*, 1987, 330, p. 414).

In 1983, the association between AIDS and sexually transmitted diseases became prominent. Since then, AIDS had been represented as an STD and/or a contagious disease. Both infectious and contagious diseases were the preserve of the NIAID. In 1985, the NIAID was designated the leading institute in federal AIDS research. The NIAID director was designated the NIH AIDS coordinator (Institute of Medicine 1991, p. 22). At that time, it had become clear that AIDS was not a cancer form and that HIV was not associated with HTLV-I.

Whatever the advantages of a decentralized research structure and the synergies between various research institutes (Institute of Medicine 1991, p. 37), the organization of AIDS research at the NIH level closely follows the life cycle of the theses about the AIDS causal agent: when the causal agent was believed to be a carcinogenic agent (virus), research was concentrated at an institute specializing in cancer and viruses. When this thesis faded and the definition of AIDS as an infectious and contagious disease gained prominence, research was started at an institute where STD research is done. When it became clear that the virus is not carcinogenic, the institute where STD research is done took the lead.

There is, however, a further level at which rhetorical practices influence research organization and funding – that of determining what counts as important, legitimate research that is worth funding. In the 1980s, at the National Institutes of Health, AIDS research was funded either externally, through contracts with third parties (research centers, university departments, and the like), or internally. Externally funded research was done either through peer-review grant proposals or through designated contracts. In the first case, grant applications for external funding passed a multi-stage review process which, in the late 1980s, took nine months on average (Institute of Medicine 1991, p. 104). External research contracts were awarded by the NIH without a peer-review process, on the basis of NIH research interests, that could not be pursued with internal resources.

In the 1980s, the proportion of AIDS research that was internal to the NIH declined steadily; compared with other areas of biomedical research at the NIH, AIDS research relied less on project grants and more on research contracts. In 1986, for example, $22.7 million was spent on research grants, compared with $64.1 million spent on research contracts (Institute of Medicine 1986, p. 242). The Committee on AIDS Activities of the National Academy of Sciences stated twice, in 1986 and 1991, that "with contract funding, the scope of work and approaches used tend to be specified by federal scientists... emphasis on the contract mechanism for the channeling of funds for AIDS and HIV research means that a lower proportion of the total funding is available for investigator-initiated proposals. The influence of the non-federal research community in setting the national research agenda is substantially diminished" (Institute of Medicine 1986, p. 242).

Therefore, if we examine the research projects funded through research contracts and grants at the federal level in the 1980s, we can see which topics are worth investigating and which not, and which categories of knowledge are taken for granted and as legitimations of research funding. In the first two years of the AIDS epidemic, federal funding of AIDS research was negligible. In 1983, the Public Health Service decided to appropriate over $14 million for AIDS research from other research activities. Afterwards, federal funding at the NIH increased steadily, reaching over $800 million in 1991. This amounted to 9.7% of the NIH's overall research operations budget (Institute of Medicine 1991, p. 119). Between 1982 and 1991, the NIH spent $3.149 billion on AIDS research; 68.18% of this sum was spent in the fiscal years 1989–91. In the same period of time, the NIH spent only $12.401 million on AIDS-related mechanisms of behavior and behavioral change. This is 0.57% of the NIH AIDS research budget for 1989–91. Although mechanisms of human behavior and behavioral change are crucial for AIDS prevention and are still little understood, they were not deemed worth knowing about. Instead, the NIH structured its social research according to known risk categories: the funding tables used by the National AIDS Program Office break down total sums according to money spent on sexual transmission (i.e., homosexuals), IV drug users, hemophiliacs, blood recipients, infants, and mothers. These categories are used to make sense of both the disease and funding for research on the disease simultaneously.

Deficits in research on social behavior and behavioral change were systematically signaled by the National Academy of Sciences throughout the 1980s and the early 1990s (Institute of Medicine 1991, p. 69, 1988, p. 247, 1986, p. 193). Yet, in the classificatory system of AIDS risk categories, behavior did not appear to be worth any more rigorous investigation. Quite the contrary: it was the known element that allowed the direction of the investigation of the etiologic agent to be established. As I have shown in the preceding chapters, the behavior of "homosexuals" was considered to be characterized by excessive sex and promiscuity, and that of "Africans" by exotic sexual practices and so on.

During the August 1983 AIDS hearings before the Subcommittee on Intergovernmental Relations and Human Resources of the U.S. Congress, the Public Health Service (PHS) laid bare the research projects financed by the NIH either through grant applications or through contracts. 1983 was a crucial year because it marked a sevenfold increase in federal financing of AIDS research. One of the questions asked at the hearing was whether the PHS had "a plan or a set of guidelines that are used to set priorities for studying these or other groups affected by AIDS." The answer was that "investigative priorities have been based upon surveillance data and epidemiologic evidence that a new group may appear to be at risk for AIDS. Accordingly, investigations have been conducted of AIDS in homosexuals, intravenous drug abusers, hemophiliacs, children, heterosexually exposed, and transfusion-related cases" (Federal Response to AIDS 1983, p. 590). This shows that far from being seen as uncharted territory worth investigating, behavior was viewed as being well understood and indeed as the factor underlying the given lines of investigation. Among the epidemiological studies financed by the NCI in 1983 was a survey of a "new high risk population in Hawaiian Oriental gays" at a cost of $300,000 (Federal Response to AIDS 1983, p. 593). This study came at a time when HTLV-III, Dr. Robert Gallo's retrovirus, was the favorite for the title of causal agent of AIDS (Gallo, incidentally, worked at the NCI). A key element in the HTLV-III model was accounting for how the virus could have come from Japan to the US. Hawaii (and "Oriental gays") appeared to be good candidates. The NCI spent another $300,000 on the "investigation of the household and sexual contact of heterosexual IV drug using cases," which fit the model of agent transmission through casual contact that was in vogue at that time in medical articles.

In September 1983, the NCI received a grant application from Ohio State University, called "Development of Laboratory Models for AIDS and KS." It was one of several research projects on AIDS animal models (funded by the NCI and the NIAID). Animal models were regarded as crucial for understanding how the virus works and for developing a vaccine. The Ohio State University's grant application was summarized as follows: "homosexual behavior is common between both male and female hogs housed in communal facilities. Researchers at Ohio State have observed the spontaneous development of a tumor with pathologic similarities to Kaposi's sarcoma in a single boar so maintained. Unfortunately, no data documenting concomitant immunosuppression exist for this particular animal, and data from other animals (who have not developed tumors) are quite weak" (Federal Response to AIDS 1983, p. 566). What we encounter here is a research grant proposal postulating homosexual behavior in hogs, which purports to investigate a KS-like tumor and immunosuppression in one (presumably homosexual) hog. In April of the same year, the thesis of a connection between viruses in Haitian pigs and AIDS had been published in *The Lancet*. Although this grant proposal (and the thesis it supported) were not followed by further research, it shows that topics such as "KS and homosexuality in hogs" were seen as perfectly legitimate funding requests and worthy of investigation.

Hence, my argument is that rhetorical practices do have consequences for how research money is distributed, for which research topics are seen as legitimate and worth funding, and for the organization of scientific research. This, of course, is not to say that rhetorical practices are the only factor influencing the funding and organization of research: interests, social relationships, and the scientific and social prestige of the grant seekers, among other factors, may play here a role. Nevertheless, rhetorical practices set up distinctions (known/unknown, legitimate/illegitimate) that frame the funding process. In the case of AIDS research, behavior and behavioral change were almost non-topics, due to the classificatory system that associated risk categories and forms of behavior. We are still feeling the consequences of these associations today.

Rhetorical Practices and "Expert Democracy"

On October 9, 2003, the defense ministers of the North Atlantic Treaty Organization, meeting in Colorado Springs, Colorado, decided to change the rules of the game. In the future, they decided, whether or not to intervene militarily in a non-NATO country would be decided not by the parliaments of the NATO member countries, but by a committee of military and technology experts, along with the defense ministers.[1] If this decision is put into practice, waging war will be transferred from the domain of purely political decisions to that of expert knowledge. This is just an example of the crucial role played by expert and/or scientific knowledge in almost all domains of political, social, and personal life.

Another example is the extent to which monitoring and prevention of the SARS epidemic relied on sophisticated technology: infrared cameras installed in airport lounges and at passport control booths were thought to reliably detect passengers with higher body temperatures, an indication of susceptibility to infection with the SARS virus. Wearing surgical masks in public places was expected to filter the virus and prevent its spread. Contemporary society is dominated by expert and scientific knowledge; the democracy of advanced societies is, to a large extent, an "expert" or "technological" democracy.

In the "world risk society," science and technology necessarily expand their influence in all domains of social life: we expect an expert answer to all the problems, challenges, and risks we encounter (Drori, Meyer, Ramirez, and Schofer 2003, p. 295). The increasing reliance on expert and scientific knowledge makes policy more and more

---

[1] See, for example, Thom Shanker, "NATO Officials Play Out Terrorism Scenario at Colorado Talks," *New York Times*, October 9, 2003, p. A10.

dependent on this kind of knowledge (which is not to say that this is the only factor determining policy-making). Because it affects the values, situation, and interests of various social groups, or the society as a whole, policy-making should be accompanied by public debate and discussion as intrinsic features of the democratic process. The very notions of civil society and democracy require informed public debate as part of the decision-making process. But, and here the paradox arises, how can informed public debate take place when expert (i.e., specialized, largely inaccessible) knowledge defines the issue at stake? How can the public debate and decide on something only experts and/or scientists can understand? How is democratic participation in policy and decision-making compatible with expertise? How, then, is "expert democracy" possible?

Apparently, we have to deal with a gap between two kinds of knowledge. Scientific knowledge, on the one hand, becomes more and more complex and difficult to access. Fewer and fewer social actors have access to it: how many of us can claim to really understand particle physics or molecular biology in detail? Yet this understanding becomes crucial when it comes to policy-making on reproductive and fertility issues, or on therapy issues, for example. On the other hand, everyday knowledge is broadly shared and easily accessible. But can the intricacies of scientific knowledge be translated into everyday knowledge, so that all members of society can take part in informed debates? Or, can broad social groups acquire such a level of expert knowledge as to be able to participate in these debates? The inaccessibility of expert and/or scientific knowledge is compounded by doubts about neutrality and objectivity. Is expert knowledge really neutral, or is it biased towards certain social interests? Because this knowledge is not easily accessible, we cannot assess its neutrality and objectivity. Stephen Turner considers this to be an unintended legacy of liberalism, with its stress on knowledge and democratic participation:

These two problems, the problem of the character of expert knowledge, which undermines liberalism, and the problem of the inaccessibility of expert knowledge to democratic control, thus combine in a striking way. We are left with a picture of modern democratic regimes as shams, with a public whose culture and life world is controlled or "steered" by experts whose actions are beyond public comprehension and therefore beyond intelligent public discussion, but whose "expert" knowledge is nothing but ideology, made more powerful by virtue of the fact that its character is concealed. This concealment is the central legacy of liberalism. (2003, p. 23)

Again, if we take into account the ubiquity and relevance of scientific knowledge in advanced societies, we should not underestimate these questions.

Rhetorical practices play a central role here: persuasion, argument, and public debate go hand in hand. At the same time, the problem is whether scientific argument can be translated into accessible knowledge, or whether social groups can acquire enough scientific knowledge to participate in informed debates. Either way, rhetorical practices are at the center of the picture.

With respect to the possibility of a true "expert democracy," we encounter three kinds of answers: two of them are more optimistic, and the third is more skeptical. The optimistic answers are formulated by Steven Epstein and Michel Callon, while the more skeptical comes from Stephen Turner.

Steven Epstein's (1996, pp. 336–7, 1997, p. 717) argument is that a high level of education, combined with high motivation and group cohesion will enable social groups and communities to acquire the scientific knowledge required to dialogue with scientists on their own terms. Epstein's examples are the gay communities which, during the AIDS crisis of the 1980s and early 1990s, did not despair or resign. Instead, they studied medical articles and textbooks and acquired enough scientific knowledge to have an informed dialogue with AIDS researchers, make their voices heard, and have a say in clinical trials and therapy. Community activists are thus not simply external observers of a scientific experiment or a clinical trial, but an intrinsic part of that trial or experiment. At the same time, the experiment itself unfolds as a dialogue between the scientific community and that of the activists. Social scientists should not despair either, argues Epstein, because democracy is not lost: higher education combined with high motivation and high social solidarity mobilizes communities and enhances the democratic process.

A slightly different version of this argument is put forward by Michel Callon, who also argues that contemporary societies are dominated by big technical systems (Callon, Lascoumes, and Barthe 2001). These systems, along with the expert knowledge accompanying them, pose a true challenge to democratic policy-making. Saving democracy, however, does not imply demonizing scientists and going back to policy-making explicitly based on the agendas of narrow interest groups. Science is irreplaceable in the social fabric. Democracy, argues Michel Callon, is grounded in access to knowledge: this access is ensured not only by higher education but also by debates in the public sphere. Open controversies and debates between the (lay, but informed) public and scientists are characteristic of vigorous democracies. Therefore, expert democracy is saved by (1) increasing access to scientific and technical education and (2) simultaneously encouraging and organizing public debates between scientists and the public. Discussion, argues Michel Callon, should be taken out of the back room and moved to the open plaza. "You don't understand this" is not a viable argument. Similar with Steven Epstein, Michel Callon sees the informed, educated public as a participant in scientific research. Scientific research projects or experiments thus involve several communities (scientists, subjects of clinical trials, the informed public). Dialogue and debate in the public sphere become intrinsic features of the research process.

Stephen Turner's argument is more skeptical: expert democracy has a translation problem and hence an authority problem too. We have to translate scientific theories into accessible language at minimal loss, but at the same time, scientists and experts undeniably exert a charismatic authority over the public, one which goes hand in hand with the difficulty of accessing their knowledge (Turner 2003, pp. 50–51). When lay groups attain a high level of scientific knowledge, the charismatic authority of the scientist loses part of its hold over the public: the mobilization of the gay community against AIDS is a case in point. Nevertheless, the problem of translation remains.

A possible solution is the purposeful organization of knowledge communities: groups of citizens that organize themselves around knowledge issues, so as to be able to sustain an informed dialogue with experts and scientists. This organization would not be reactive (that is, responding only to a rising problem) and isolated, but proactive and systematic. Knowledge communities would not rely on media popularizations of science, but would seek to acquire firsthand knowledge. Some of these knowledge communities could then work as "boundary organizations," in which scientists and lay people together produce knowledge and intervene in the policy-making process without being part of a bureaucratic apparatus.

But even so, the problem of persuasion remains: assuming that educated lay people can and will acquire the knowledge they need to sustain a dialogue with scientists, does this not then enlarge the gap between highly educated, knowledgeable lay people and the rest of the public? It would seem that narrowing one knowledge gap entails a concomitant widening of another, and this might lead in turn to closed knowledge communities, separated from the less educated public. All the authors discussed here highlight a set of key elements that have to be put in place if expert democracy is to work: broad access to higher education, less reliance on media popularizations, direct access to scientific information, community-building, and public debate.

My argument is that a further element has to be added to the above, to bridge the gap between the broad public and scientific communities. We have to deal here with two distinct kinds of knowledge (scientific and everyday knowledge), which, at their core, do not touch upon each other. Scientific knowledge may be anchored in the everyday practices of scientific communities, but these are not shared with the public at large. These two different kinds of knowledge form the basis for different kinds of rhetorical practices, with different arguments and different persuasive devices. This is what makes dialogue and translation so difficult.

The picture just sketched is one of rhetorical practices as closed systems, confined to a certain kind of knowledge. Yet I have argued the opposite in this book. Rhetorical practices are not closed systems: the scientific arguments about the origins of AIDS, its causal agent, and its means of transmission made use of narratives, representations, and classifications systems that are shared with the broader culture. It can hardly be argued that narratives of traveling in Africa are specific to biomedicine, for instance. These cultural elements were adopted, transformed, and adapted to the specific persuasive aims of the scientific discourse. Rhetorical practices do not work through closure: they work through openness, transformation, and adaptation. It follows, then, that a clear distinction between scientific persuasion and lay persuasion cannot be sustained. Scientific persuasion adopts, integrates, and adapts elements of rhetoric that are employed by the lay public in everyday life. Science is indeed irreplaceable in the social fabric; but it is not an isolated element in this fabric. Rather, what makes science so vital and dynamic is its capacity to adapt and integrate elements from the broader socio-cultural fabric. With respect to the dialogue between scientists and non-scientists in the public sphere, this has the following consequence: knowledge communities should operate as mediators between scientific communities and the wider public. This is why they are boundary communities: they bring together different people with different interests and with different levels of knowledge. First and foremost, knowledge communities acquire the knowledge necessary for an informed dialogue with scientists.

These communities, however, should also bring to light and discuss the broader cultural and social assumptions present in the rhetoric of science. They could (and should) make both scientists and the lay public aware of these assumptions. If knowledge communities are to work as mediators, acquisition of scientific knowledge is not enough: this acquisition alone does not suffice to open a dialogue with the broader public. It has to be accompanied by reflection on (and discussion of) the broader cultural assumptions of the rhetoric of science, precisely because these assumptions are common to scientific and popular rhetoric alike. This means a different understanding of the task of translation that knowledge communities should fulfill. In the narrow sense, knowledge communities should translate scientific discourse into broadly accessible, simple arguments. This is doomed to failure from the outset, however, because by acquiring scientific knowledge, such communities distance themselves from the general public. What I suggest here is a different, more complex task: knowledge communities should bridge the gap by uncovering common cultural presuppositions and by fostering the discussion of these presuppositions.

There are many domains where such knowledge communities could meaningfully intervene in this way: previously, I gave the example of military intervention decided by expert committee, which is bound to become a reality. Shouldn't the public have a voice in this kind of decision? Decision by committee is usually justified by pointing out the sophistication of high-tech wars, which preclude lay understanding. Is a knowledge community not a dire necessity here – a community that would not only acquire the necessary technological knowledge, but also lay bare the cultural assumptions of the "science of war"? This uncovering and reflection could provide the basis for the dialogue in the public sphere. Such a knowledge community could also supplement popular media representations of advanced war technologies; question rhetorical terms such as "precision," "infallibility," and "accuracy," and make the public aware of not only the issues at stake but also the assumptions underlying these issues.

In a similar way, knowledge communities could promote public examination and discussion of the cultural assumptions and rhetorical practices underlying prevention policies such as the use of infrared cameras or surgical masks: such a public examination could show, for example, that the use of risk categories in prevention policies inevitably entails social stigmatization and diminishes the effectiveness of prevention efforts.

From this perspective, rhetorical practices are not an obstacle but rather a necessary ingredient of expert democracy. Bridging the gap between science and the general public has become crucial to the public sphere and democracy. This means we must acknowledge that rhetorical practices do matter and act accordingly.

References

Airhihenbuwa, Collins, Ralph Diclemente, Gina Wingood, and Agatha Lowe. 1992. "HIV/AIDS Education and Prevention Among African Americans: A Focus on Culture." *AIDS Education and Prevention* 4/3:267–76.

Albert, Edward. 1986. "Illness and Deviance: The Response of the Press to AIDS," pp. 163–94 in Douglas A. Feldman and Thomas M. Johnson (eds.): *The Social Dimensions of AIDS. Method and Theory.* New York: Praeger.

Alonso, Ana Maria, and Maria Teresa Koreck. 1993. "Silences: 'Hispanics,' AIDS and Sexual Practices," pp. 110–26 in Henry Abelove, Michèle Aina Barale, and David M. Halperin (eds.): *The Lesbian and Gay Studies Reader.* New York: Routledge.

Arno, Peter S., and Karyn L. Feiden. 1993. *Against the Odds. The Story of AIDS Drug Development, Politics, and Profits.* San Francisco: Harper Collins.

Arrington, Robert L. 1993. "The Autonomy of Language," pp. 51–80 in John V. Canfield and Stuart G. Shanker (eds.): *Wittgenstein's Intentions.* New York: Garland.

Ashmore, Malcolm. 1989. *The Reflexive Thesis. Writing the Sociology of Scientific Knowledge.* Chicago: University of Chicago Press.

Atkinson, Paul, Claire Batchelor, and Evelyn Parsons. 1997. "The Rhetoric of Prediction and Chance in the Research to Clone a Disease Gene," pp. 101–26 in Mary Ann Elston (ed.): *The Sociology of Medical Science and Technology.* Oxford: Blackwell.

Austin, John Langshaw. 1976 [1962]. *How to Do Things with Words.* Oxford: Oxford University Press.

Austin, John Langshaw. 1970. *Philosophical Papers.* Oxford: Oxford University Press.

Baker, Andrea J. 1986. "The Portrayal of AIDS in the Media: An Analysis of Articles in The New York Times," pp. 179–96 in Douglas A. Feldman and

Thomas M. Johnson (eds.): *The Social Dimensions of AIDS. Method and Theory*. New York: Praeger.

Bakhtin, Mikhail. 1986. *Speech Genres and Other Late Essays*. Austin: University of Texas Press.

Barnett, Tony, and Alan Whiteside. 2002. *AIDS in the Twenty-First Century. Disease and Globalization*. Basingstoke, UK: Palgrave Macmillan.

Barnes, Barry, David Bloor, and John Henry. 1996. *Scientific Knowledge: A Sociological Analysis*. Chicago: University of Chicago Press.

Bartley, Mel, George Davey Smith, and David Blane. 1997. "Vital Comparisons: The Social Construction of Mortality Measurement," pp. 127–52 in Mary Ann Elston (ed.): *The Sociology of Medical Science and Technology*. Oxford: Blackwell.

Bayer, Ronald. 1989. *Private Acts, Social Consequences. AIDS and the Politics of Public Health*. New York: The Free Press.

Bazerman, Charles. 1994. *Constructing Experience*. Carbondale, IL: Southern Illinois University Press.

Bazerman, Charles. 1989. "Introduction to the Symposium: Rhetoricians on the Rhetoric of Science." *Science, Technology and Human Values* 14/1:3–6.

Bazerman, Charles. 1988. *Shaping Written Knowledge: The Genre and Activity of the Experimental Article in Science*. Madison: University of Wisconsin Press.

Beck, Ulrich. 2000. "Risk Society Revisited: Theory, Politics and Research Programmes," pp. 211–29 in Barbara Adam, Ulrich Beck, and Joost Van Loon (eds.): *The Risk Society and Beyond. Critical Issues for Social Theory*. London: Sage.

Beck, Ulrich. 1992. *Risk Society. Towards a New Modernity*. London: Sage.

Beck, Ulrich, Wolfgang Bonss, and Christoph Lau. 2003. "The Theory of Reflexive Modernization. Problematic, Hypotheses and Research Programme." *Theory, Culture & Society* 20/2:1–33.

Becker, Gary. 1986. "The Economic Approach to Human Behavior," pp. 108–22 in Jon Elster (ed.): *Rational Choice*. New York: New York University Press.

Berg, Marc. 1997. *Rationalizing Medical Work. Decision-Support Techniques and Medical Practices*. Cambridge, MA: MIT Press.

Berkenkotter, Carol, and Thomas N. Huckin. 1995. *Genre Knowledge in Disciplinary Communication. Cognition/Culture/Power*. Hillsdale, NJ: Lawrence Erlbaum.

Bernheimer, Charles. 1989. *Figures of Ill-Repute: Representing Prostitution in 19th Century France*. Cambridge, MA: Harvard University Press.

Berridge, Virginia. 1992a. "The Early Years of AIDS in the United Kingdom 1981–1986: Historical Perspectives," pp. 302–28 in T. Ranger and P. Slack (eds.): *Epidemics and Ideas*. Cambridge: Cambridge University Press.

Berridge, Virginia. 1992b. "AIDS, the Media and Health Policy," pp. 13–25 in Peter Aggleton, Peter Davies, and Graham Hart (eds.): *AIDS: Rights, Risks and Reasons*. London: The Falmer Press.

Berridge, Virginia, and Philip Strong. 1991. "AIDS in the UK. Contemporary History and the Study of Policy." *Twentieth Century British History* 2/2:150–74.

Bersani, Leo. 1988. "Is Rectum a Grave?" pp. 197–222 in Douglas Crimp (ed.): *AIDS: Cultural Analysis/Cultural Activism*. Cambridge, MA: MIT Press.

Bloor, Michael. 1995. "A User's Guide to Contrasting Theories of HIV-Related Risk Behavior," pp. 19–30 in Jonathan Gabe (ed.): *Medicine, Health and Risk. Sociological Approaches*. Oxford: Blackwell.

Bourdieu, Pierre. 2001. *The Science of Science and Reflexivity [Science de la science et réflexivité]*. Paris: Raisons d'agir.

Bowers, John, and Kate Inei. 1993. "The Discursive Construction of Society." *Discourse and Society* 4/3:357–93.

Bowker, Geoffrey, and Susan Leigh Star. 1999. *Sorting Things Out. Classification and Its Consequences*. Cambridge, MA: MIT Press.

Brandt, Allan M. 1990. "The Cigarette, Risk, and American Culture." *Daedalus* 119/4:155–75.

Brandt, Allan M. 1988. "AIDS and Metaphor: Toward the Social Meaning of Epidemic Disease." *Social Research* 55/3:413–32.

Brandt, Edward. 1983. Statement of Dr. Edward Brandt, Assistant Secretary for Health, Department of Health and Human Services, accompanied by Dr. William Foege et al, pp. 292–391 in *Federal Response to AIDS. Hearings Before a Subcommittee of the Committee on Government Operations, House of Representatives, 98th Congress, First Session*. Washington, DC: U.S. Government Printing Office.

Brint, Steven. 1994. *In an Age of Experts. The Changing Role of Professionals in Politics and Public Life*. Princeton, NJ: Princeton University Press.

Brown, Judith E., Okako Bibi Ayowa, and Richard C. Brown. 1993. "Dry and Tight: Sexual Practices and Potential AIDS Risk in Zaire." *Social Science and Medicine* 37/8:989–94.

Butler, Judith. 1997. "Sovereign Performatives in the Contemporary Scene of Utterance." *Critical Inquiry* 23:350–77.

Callon, Michel. 1991. "Techno-Economic Networks and Irreversibility," pp. 132–64 in John Law (ed.): *A Sociology of Monsters. Essays on Power, Technology and Domination*. London: Routledge.

Callon, Michel. 1986. "Some Elements of a Sociology of Translation: Domestication of the Scallops and the Fishermen of St. Brieux Bay," pp. 196–223 in John Law (ed.): *Power, Action and Belief: A New Sociology of Knowledge?* London: Routledge.

Callon, Michel, Pierre Lascoumes, and Yannick Barthe. 2001. *Action in an Uncertain World. Essays on Technical Democracy* [Agir dans un monde uncertain. Essais sur la démocratie technique]. Paris: Seuil.

Calvez, Marcel. 1990. *Composing with a Danger. An Examination of the Social Responses to HIV-Infection and AIDS [Composer avec un danger. Approche des réponses sociales á l'infection au VIH et au SIDA]*. Rennes: IRTS de Bretagne.

Carricaburu, Danièle, and Janine Pierret. 1995. "From Biographical Disruption to Biographical Reinforcement: The Case of HIV-Positive Men." *Sociology of Health and Illness* 17/1:65–88.

Carricaburu, Danièle, and Janine Pierret. 1992. *Everyday Life and Reconstruction of Identities around Seropositivity [Vie quotidienne et recompositions identitaires autour de la séropositivité].* Paris: CERMES.

Carrier, Joseph M., and Raul J. Magana. 1992. "Use of Ethnosexual Data on Men of Mexican Origin for HIV/AIDS Prevention Programs," pp. 243–58 in Gilbert Herdt and Shirley Lindebaum (eds.): *The Time of AIDS. Social Analysis, Theory and Method.* London: Sage.

Carroll-Burke, Patrick. 2002. "Material Designs: Engineering Culture and Engineering States – Ireland 1650–1900." *Theory and Society* 31:75–114.

Ceccarelli, Leah. 2001. *Shaping Science with Rhetoric. The Cases of Dobzhansky, Schrödinger, and Wilson.* Chicago: University of Chicago Press.

Champagne, Patrick. 1991. "The Construction of Social Diseases in the Media" [La Construction Médiatique des Maladies Sociaux]. *Actes de la Recherche en Sciences Sociales* 90:64–75.

Chirimuuta, Richard C., and Rosalind Chirimuuta. 1989. *AIDS, Africa and Racism,* revised ed. London: Free Association Books.

Clarke, Adele. 1990. "Controversy and the Development of Reproductive Sciences." *Social Problems* 37/1:18–37.

Clarke, Adele, Laura Mamo, Jennifer Fishman, Janet Shim, and Jennifer Ruth Fosket. 2003. "Biomedicalization: Technoscientific Transformations of Health, Illness, and U.S. Biomedicine." *American Sociological Review* 68:161–94.

Clatts, Michael C., and Kevin M. Mutchler. 1989. "AIDS and the Dangerous Other. Metaphors of Sex and Deviance in the Representation of Disease," pp. 13–22 in Ralph Bolton (ed.): *The AIDS Pandemic. A Global Emergency.* New York: Gordon & Breach.

Cohen, Cathy. 1999. *The Boundaries of Blackness. AIDS and the Breakdown of Black Politics.* Chicago: University of Chicago Press.

Cole, Simon. 1996. "Which Came First, the Fossil or the Fuel?" *Social Studies of Science* 26/4:733–66.

Collins, Harry. 1992. *Changing Order. Replication and Induction in Scientific Practice.* London: Sage.

Collins, Harry. 1988. "Public Experiments and Displays of Virtuosity: The Core-Set Revisited." *Social Studies of Science* 18:725–48.

Compas, Jean-Claude. 1983a. Statement of Dr. Jean-Claude Compas, Vice President, Haitian Medical Association Abroad, pp. 41–3 in *Federal Response to AIDS. Hearings Before a Subcommittee of the Committee on Government Operations, House of Representatives, 98th Congress, First Session.* Washington, DC: U.S. Government Printing Office.

Compas, Jean-Claude. 1983b. Prepared Statement of Dr. Jean-Claude Compas, Vice President, Haitian Medical Association Abroad, New York Chapter,

Chairman, Haitian Coalition on AIDS, pp. 44–9 in *Federal Response to AIDS. Hearings Before a Subcommittee of the Committee on Government Operations, House of Representatives, 98th Congress, First Session.* Washington, DC: U.S. Government Printing Office.

Connor, Steve, and Sharon Kingman. 1988. *The Search for the Virus.* London: Penguin.

Connors, Margaret M. 1992. "Risk Perception, Risk Taking and Risk Management Among Intravenous Drug Users. Implications for AIDS Prevention." *Social Science and Medicine* 34/6:591–601.

Conrad, Peter. 1986. "The Social Meaning of AIDS." *Social Policy* 16:51–6.

Conrad, Peter, and Joseph W. Schneider. 1985. *Deviance and Medicalization. From Badness to Sickness.* Columbus, OH: Merrill.

Crystal, Stephen, and Margaret Jackson. 1992. "Health Care and the Social Construction of AIDS: The Impact of Disease Definitions," pp. 163–80 in Joan Huber and Beth Schneider (eds.): *The Social Context of AIDS.* Newbury Park, CA: Sage.

Curran, James W., and W. Meade Morgan. 1987. "AIDS in the United States: Future Trends," pp. 127–30 in J. C. Gluckman and E. Vilmer (eds.): *Acquired Immunodeficiency Syndrome.* Paris: Elsevier.

De Certeau, Michel. 1988. *The Writing of History.* New York: Columbia University Press.

De Man, Paul. 1983. *Blindness and Insight. Essays in the Rhetoric of Contemporary Criticism.* Minneapolis: University of Minnesota Press.

De Man, Paul. 1978. "The Epistemology of Metaphor." *Critical Inquiry* 5:13–31.

de Saussure, Ferdinand. 1959 [1916]. *Course in General Linguistics.* New York: MacGraw-Hill.

De Vault, Marjorie. 1990. "Novel Readings: The Social Organization of Interpretation." *American Journal of Sociology* 95/4:887–921.

Derrida, Jacques. 1979. *On Grammatology.* Baltimore, MD: Johns Hopkins University Press.

Derrida, Jacques. 1972a. *The Margins of Philosophy* [*Marges de la philosophie*]. Paris: Gallimard.

Derrida, Jacques. 1972b. *Positions* [*Positions*]. Paris: Editions du Minuit.

Dillon, George L. 1986. *Rhetoric as Social Imagination. Explorations in the Interpersonal Function of Language.* Bloomington: Indiana University Press.

Dobrovolskij, Dmitrij. 1997. "Metaphors and Idioms in Oral Scientific Communication on AIDS. An Exemplary Analysis" [Metaphernmodelle und Idiome in muendlichen Fach- und Vermittlungstexten. Eine exemplarische Analyse zum Thema AIDS], pp. 148–79 in Bernd Ulrich Biere and Wolf-Andreas Liebert (eds.): *Metaphors, Media, Science. The Presentation of AIDS Research in Print and Radio* [*Metaphern, Medien, Wissenschaft. Zur Vermittlung der AIDS-Forschung in Presse und Rundfunk*]. Opladen, Germany: Westdeutscher Verlag.

Douglas, Lawrence. 1995. "The Force of Words: Fish, Matsuda, MacKinnon, and the Theory of Discursive Violence." *Law & Society Review* 29/1:169–90.

Douglas, Mary. 1992a. *Risk and Blame. Essays in Cultural Theory*. London: Routledge.

Douglas, Mary. 1992b. "Rightness of Categories," pp. 239–71 in Mary Douglas and David Hull (eds.): *How Classification Works*. Edinburgh: Edinburgh University Press.

Douglas, Mary. 1985. *Risk Acceptability According to the Social Sciences*. New York: Russell Sage Foundation.

Douglas, Mary. 1967. *Purity and Danger*. London: Routledge & Kegan Paul.

Douglas, Mary, and Aaron Wildavsky. 1982. *Risk and Culture. An Essay on the Selection of Technical and Environmental Dangers*. Berkeley: University of California Press.

Drori, Gilis., John W. Meyer, Francisco O. Ramirez, and Evan Schofer. 2003. *Science in the Modern World Polity. Institutionalization and Globalization*. Stanford CA: Stanford University Press.

Duesberg, Peter. 1996. *Inventing the AIDS Virus*. Washington, DC: Regnery.

Durkheim, Émile. 1965 [1915]. *The Elementary Forms of the Religious Life*. New York: The Free Press.

Durkheim, Émile, and Marcel Mauss. 1963. *Primitive Classifications*. Chicago: University of Chicago Press.

Elster, John. 1986. "Introduction," pp. 1–33 in Jon Elster (ed.): *Rational Choice*. New York: New York University Press.

Epstein, Steven. 1997. "Activism, Drug Regulation, and the Politics of Therapeutic Evaluation in the AIDS Era: A Case Study of ddC and the 'Surrogate Markers' Debate." *Social Studies of Science* 27/5:691–726.

Epstein, Steven. 1996. *Impure Science. AIDS, Activism, and the Politics of Knowledge*. Berkeley: University of California Press.

Epstein, Steven. 1992. "Gay Politics, Ethnic Identity: The Limits of Social Constructionism," pp. 239–94 in Edward Stein (ed.): *Forms of Desire. Sexual Orientation and the Social Constructionist Controversy*. London: Routledge.

Epstein, Steven. 1988. "AIDS and the Medicalizing of Gay Identity." *Research in Law, Deviance and Social Control* 9:3–36.

Estep, Rhoda, Dan Waldorf, and Toby Marotta. 1992. "Sexual Behavior of Male Prostitutes," pp. 95–114 in Joan Huber and Beth Schneider (eds.): *The Social Context of AIDS*. Newbury Park, CA: Sage.

Fahnestock, Jeanne. 1999. *Rhetorical Figures in Science*. New York: Oxford University Press.

Fairclough, Norman. 2001. "The Discourse of New Labor: Critical Discourse Analysis," pp. 229–66 in Margaret Wetherell, Stephanie Taylor, and Simeon J. Yates (eds.): *Discourse as Data. A Guide for Analysis*. London: Sage.

Fairclough, Norman. 1992. "Discourse and Text: Linguistic and Intertextual Analysis within Discourse Analysis." *Discourse and Society* 3/2:193–217.

Federal Response to AIDS. 1983. *Hearings Before a Subcommittee of the Committee on Government Operations, House of Representatives, 98th Congress, First Session.* Washington, DC: U.S. Government Printing Office.

Fish, Stanley. 1989. *Doing What Comes Naturally. Change, Rhetoric and the Practice of Theory in Literary and Legal Studies.* Oxford: Clarendon Press.

Fleischman, Suzanne. 2003. "Language and Medicine," pp. 470–502 in Deborah Schiffrin, Deborah Tannen, and Heidi E. Hamilton (eds.): *The Handbook of Discourse Analysis.* Oxford: Blackwell.

Foucault, Michel. 1989. *Course Summary [Résumé des Cours].* Paris: Julliard.

Foucault, Michel. 1979. *Discipline and Punish. The Birth of the Prison.* New York: Vintage.

Foucault, Michel. 1966. *The Order of Things [Les Mots et les Choses].* Paris: Gallimard.

Fuller, Steve. 1993. *Philosophy, Rhetoric, and the End of Knowledge. The Coming of Science and Technology Studies.* Madison: University of Wisconsin Press.

Galison, Peter. 1996a. "Introduction: The Context of Disunity," pp. 1–36 in Peter Galison and David Stump (eds.): *The Disunity of Science. Boundaries, Contexts, and Power.* Stanford, CA: Stanford University Press.

Galison, Peter. 1996b. "Computer Simulations and the Trading Zone," pp. 118–57 in Peter Galison and David Stump (eds.): *The Disunity of Science. Boundaries, Contexts, and Power.* Stanford, CA: Stanford University Press.

Gallo, Robert C., M. G. Sarngadharan, S. K. Arya, and F. Wong-Staal. 1987. "Human Retroviruses with Emphasis on HTLV-III/LAV: Now and Future Perspectives," pp. 23–9 in Jean-Claude Gluckman and E. Vilmer (eds.): *Acquired Immunodeficiency Syndrome.* Paris: Elsevier.

Geertz, Clifford. 1988. *Works and Lives. The Anthropologist as Author.* Stanford, CA: Stanford University Press.

Gieryn, Thomas. 2002a. "What Buildings Do." *Theory and Society* 31:35–74.

Gieryn, Thomas. 2002b. "Three Truth-Spots." *Journal of History of the Behavioral Sciences* 38/2:113–32.

Gieryn, Thomas. 2000. "A Space for Place in Sociology." *Annual Review of Sociology* 26:463–96.

Gieryn, Thomas. 1999. *Cultural Boundaries of Science. Credibility on the Line.* Chicago: University of Chicago Press.

Gilman, Sander. 1998. *Love + Marriage = Death. And Other Essays on Representing Difference.* Stanford, CA: Stanford University Press.

Gilman, Sander. 1993: "Plague in Germany, 1939/1989: Cultural Images of Race, Space, and Disease," pp. 54–82 in Timothy F. Murphy and Suzanne Poirier (eds): *Writing AIDS. Gay Literature, Language, and Analysis.* New York: Columbia University Press.

Gilman, Sander. 1988. *Disease and Representation. Images of Illness from Madness to AIDS*. Ithaca, NY: Cornell University Press.

Grady, Christine. 1995. *The Search for an AIDS Vaccine. Ethical Issues in the Development and Testing of a Preventive HIV Vaccine*. Bloomington: Indiana University Press.

Gragson, Gay, and Jack Selzer. 1993. "The Reader in the Text of 'The Spandrels of San Marco,'" pp. 180–201 in Jack Selzer (ed.): *Understanding Scientific Prose*. Madison: University of Wisconsin Press.

Grmek, Mirko D. 1990. *History of AIDS. Emergence and Origin of a Modern Pandemic*. Princeton, NJ: Princeton University Press.

Gross, Alan. 1996. *The Rhetoric of Science*, revised ed. Cambridge, MA: Harvard University Press.

Grover, Jan Zita. 1992. "Visible Lesions: Images of PWA in America," pp. 23–51 in James Miller (ed.): *Fluid Exchanges. Artists and Critics in the AIDS Crisis*. Toronto: University of Toronto Press.

Gusfield, Joseph. 1976. "The Literary Rhetoric of Science. Comedy and Pathos in Drinking Driver Research." *American Sociological Review* 41/1:16–34.

Hacking, Ian. 1996. "The Disunities of the Sciences," pp. 37–74 in Peter Galison and David J. Stump (eds.): *The Disunity of Science. Boundaries, Contexts, and Power*. Stanford, CA: Stanford University Press.

Hacking, Ian. 1990. *The Taming of Chance*. Cambridge, UK: Cambridge University Press.

Hak, Tony. 1989. "Developing a Text-Sociological Analysis." *Semiotica* 75/1–2:24–42.

Halliday, Michael A. K., and John R. Martin. 1993. *Writing Science. Literacy and Discursive Power*. Pittsburgh, PA: University of Pittsburgh Press.

Hardy, Anne. 1993. *The Epidemic Streets. Infectious Disease and the Rise of Preventive Medicine, 1856–1900*. Oxford: Clarendon Press.

Hell, Bertrand. 1999. *Possession and Shamanism. The Masters of Disorder [Possession et chamanisme: Les maîtres du désordre]*. Paris: Flammarion.

Herzlich, Claudine, and Janine Pierret. 1989. "The Construction of a Social Phenomenon: AIDS in the French Press." *Social Science and Medicine* 29/11:1235–42.

Hilgartner, Stephen. 1985. "The Political Language of Risk," pp. 25–66 in Dorothy Nelkin (ed.): *The Language of Risk. Conflicting Perspectives on Occupational Health*. Beverly Hills, CA: Sage.

Hooper, Edward. 2000a. *The River. A Journey Back to the Source of HIV and AIDS*. London: Allen Lane.

Hooper, Edward. 2000b. "Genesis of AIDS: Mother Nature, or Hand of Man?" *Science as Culture* 1/9:73–101.

Horton, Meyrick, and Peter Aggleton. 1989. "Perverts, Inverts and Experts: The Cultural Production of an AIDS Research Paradigm," pp. 74–100 in Peter Aggleton, Graham Hart, and Peter Davies (eds.): *AIDS: Social Representations and Social Practices*. Barcombe, UK: The Falmer Press.

Icard, Larry, Robert F. Schilling, Nabila Bassel, and Dale Young. 1992. "Preventing AIDS Among Black Gay Men and Black Gay and Heterosexual Male Intravenous Drug Users." *Social Work* 37/5:440–5.

Institute of Medicine. 1991. *The AIDS Research Program of the National Institutes of Health*. Washington, DC: National Academy Press.

Institute of Medicine. 1988. *Confronting AIDS. Update 1988*. Washington, DC: National Academy Press.

Institute of Medicine. 1986. *Confronting AIDS. Directions for Public Health, Health Care, and Research*. Washington, DC: National Academy Press.

Iser, Wolfgang. 1993. *The Fictive and the Imaginary: Charting Literary Anthropology*. Baltimore, MD: Johns Hopkins University Press.

Jaffe, H. W., A. M. Hardy, T. J. Bush, R. M. Selik, and W. Meade Morgan. 1987. "AIDS Within Population Groups in the United States," pp. 137–40 in Jean-Claude Gluckman and E. Vilmer (eds.): *Acquired Immunodeficiency Syndrome*. Paris: Elsevier.

Jones, James W. 1992. "Discourses on and of AIDS in West Germany: 1986–1990." *Journal of the History of Sexuality* 2/3:439–68.

Kane, Stephanie, and Theresa Mason. 1992. "'IV Drug Users' and 'Sex Partners': The Limits of Epidemiological Categories and the Ethnography of Risk," pp. 199–224 in Gilbert Herdt and Shirley Lindebaum (eds.): *The Time of AIDS. Social Analysis, Theory and Method*. London: Sage.

Kestler, Harry W. 2001. "Animals," pp. 44–6 in Raymond A. Smith (ed.): *Encyclopedia of AIDS. A Social, Political, Cultural, and Scientific Record of the HIV Epidemic*. New York: Penguin.

Kinsella, James. 1989. *Covering the Plague. AIDS and the American Media*. Rutgers, NJ: Rutgers University Press.

Kitzinger, Jenny, and David Miller. 1992. "'African AIDS': The Media and Audience Beliefs," pp. 28–51 in Peter Aggleton, Peter Davies, and Graham Hart (eds.): *AIDS: Rights, Risk and Reason*. London: The Falmer Press.

Klatzmann, Daniel, and Jean-Claude Gluckman. 1987. "The Pathophysiology of HIV Infection: A Complex Pathway of Host–Virus Interaction," pp. 77–85 in Jean-Claude Gluckman and E. Vilmer (eds.): *Acquired Immunodeficiency Syndrome*. Paris: Elsevier.

Knorr, Karin. 1981. *The Manufacture of Knowledge: An Essay on the Constructivist and Contextual Nature of Science*. Oxford: Pergamon.

Knorr Cetina, Karin. 1999. *Epistemic Cultures: How the Sciences Make Knowledge*. Cambridge, MA: Harvard University Press.

Lachmund, Jens, and Gunnar Stollberg. 1992. "The Doctor, His Audience, and the Meaning of Illness. The Drama of Medical Practice in the Late 18th and Early 19th Centuries," pp. 53–66 in Jens Lachmund and Gunnar Stollberg (eds.): *The Social Construction of Illness. Illness and Medical Knowledge in Past and Present*. Stuttgart: Steiner.

Lash, Scott. 2000. "Risk Culture," pp. 47–62 in Barbara Adam, Ulrich Beck, and Joost Van Loon (eds.): *The Risk Society and Beyond. Critical Issues for Social Theory*. London: Sage.

Latour, Bruno. 1999. *Pandora's Hope. Essays on the Reality of Science Studies*. Cambridge, MA: Harvard University Press.

Latour, Bruno. 1988. *The Pasteurization of France*. Cambridge, MA: Harvard University Press.

Latour, Bruno, and Steve Woolgar. 1986. *Laboratory Life: The Construction of Scientific Facts*, 2nd ed. Princeton, NJ: Princeton University Press.

Law, John (ed.). 1986. *Power, Action, and Belief. A New Sociology of Knowledge*. London: Routledge.

Lay, Mary M., Laura J. Gurak, Clare Gravon, and Cynthia Myntti. 2000. "Introduction. The Rhetoric of Reproduction Technologies," pp. 3–26 in Mary M. Lay, Laura J. Gurak, Clare Gravon, and Cynthia Myntti (eds.): *Body Talk: Rhetoric, Technology, Reproduction*. Madison: University of Wisconsin Press.

Lemelle, Anthony J. 2003. "Linking the Structure of African American Criminalization to the Spread of HIV/AIDS." Paper presented at the 2003 ASA Annual Meeting, Atlanta, GA.

Lemert, Charles. 1990. "The Uses of French Structuralisms in Sociology," pp. 230–54 in George Ritzer (ed.): *Frontiers of Social Theory: The New Synthesis*. New York: Columbia University Press.

Letvin, Nicholas L., M. D. Daniel, N. W. King, L. O. Arthur, M. Kiyotaki, M. Kannagi, and R. C. Desrosiers. 1987. "An HIV-Related Virus from Macaques," pp. 71–4 in Jean-Claude Gluckman and E. Vilmer (eds.): *Acquired Immunodeficiency Syndrome*. Paris: Elsevier.

Levy, Jay A., L. Evans, C. Cheng-Mayer, L.-Z. Pan, A. Lane, C. Staben, D. Dina, C. Wiley, and J. Nelson. 1987. "Biologic and Molecular Properties of the AIDS-Associated Retrovirus that Affect Antiviral Therapy," pp. 31–41 in Jean-Claude Gluckman and E. Vilmer (eds.): *Acquired Immunodeficiency Syndrome*. Paris: Elsevier.

Lewenstein, Bruce. 1995. "From Fax to Facts: Communication in the Cold Fusion Saga." *Social Studies of Science* 25/3:403–36.

Locke, Simon. 2002. "The Public Understanding of Science – A Rhetorical Invention." *Science, Technology, & Human Values* 27/1:87–111.

Luhmann, Niklas. 1990. *Risk and Danger [Risiko und Gefahr]*. St. Gallen, Switzerland: Hochschule St. Gallen.

Lupton, Deborah. 1993. "AIDS Risk and Heterosexuality in the Australian Press." *Discourse and Society* 4/3:307–28.

Lupton, Deborah, Sophie McCarthy, and Simon Chapman. 1995. "'Panic Bodies': Discourses on Risk and HIV Antibody Testing." *Sociology of Health and Illness* 17/1:89–108.

Lynch, Michael. 1992. "Extending Wittgenstein. The Pivotal Move from Epistemology to the Sociology of Science," pp. 215–65 in Andrew Pickering (ed.): *Science as Practice and Culture*. Chicago: University of Chicago Press.

Maasen, Sabine, and Peter Weingart. 2000. *Metaphors and the Dynamics of Knowlegde*. London: Routledge.

Mackenzie, Donald. 1981. *Statistics in Britain, 1865–1930: The Social Construction of Scientific Knowledge.* Edinburgh: Edinburgh University Press.

MacKinnon, Catharine A. 1993. *Only Words.* Cambridge, MA: Harvard University Press.

Mane, Purnima, and Peter Aggleton. 2001. "Gender and HIV/AIDS: What Do Men Have to Do with It?" *Current Sociology* 49/6:23–37.

Mann, Jonathan. 1987. "The Epidemiology of LAV/HTLV-III in Africa," pp. 131–6 in Jean-Claude Gluckman and E. Vilmer (eds.): *Acquired Immunodeficiency Syndrome.* Paris: Elsevier.

Maticka-Tyndale, Eleanor. 2001. "Twenty Years in the AIDS Pandemic: A Place for Sociology." *Current Sociology* 49/6:13–21.

McCloskey, Donald. 1998. *The Rhetoric of Economics.* Madison: University of Wisconsin Press.

McCloskey, Donald N. 1994. *Knowledge and Persuasion in Economics.* Cambridge, UK: Cambridge University Press.

McCloskey, Donald N. 1990. *If You're So Smart. The Narratives of Economic Expertise.* Chicago: University of Chicago Press.

McGovern, Theresa, and Raymond Smith. 2001. "Case Definition of AIDS," pp. 32–6 in Raymond Smith (ed.): *Encyclopedia of AIDS. A Social, Political, Cultural, and Scientific Record of the HIV Epidemic.* New York: Penguin.

McGrath, Judith, Debra A. Schumann, Jonnie Pearson-Marks, Charles B. Rwabukwali, Rebecca Mukasa, Barbara Namande, Sylvia Nakayiwa, and Lucy Nakyobe. 1992. "Cultural Determinants of Sexual Risk Behavior for AIDS Among Baganda Women." *Medical Anthropology Quarterly* 6/2:153–61.

McMullin, Ernan. 1987. "Scientific Controversy and Its Termination," pp. 49–91 in H. Tristram Engelhardt, Jr. and Arthur L. Caplan (eds.): *Scientific Controversies. Case Studies in the Resolution and Closure of Disputes in Science and Technology.* Cambridge, UK: Cambridge University Press.

Meyer-Bahlburg, Heino F. L., Theresa M. Exner, Gerda Lorenz, Rhoda S. Gruen, Jack M. Gorman, Anke A. Ehrhardt. 1991. "Sexual Risk Behavior, Sexual Functioning, and HIV-Disease Progression in Gay Men." *The Journal of Sex Research* 28/1:3–27.

Miller, James (ed.). 1992. *Fluid Exchanges. Artists and Critics in the AIDS Crisis.* Toronto: University of Toronto Press.

Mills, Sara. 1997. *Discourse.* London: Routledge.

Mirowski, Philip (ed.). 1994. *Natural Images in Scientific Thought: "Markets Read in Thought and Claw."* Cambridge, UK: Cambridge University Press.

Montgomery, Scott L. 1996. *Inventing the Scientific Voice.* New York: The Guilford Press.

Mukerji, Chandra. 2002. "Material Practices of Domination: Christian Humanism, the Built Environment, and Techniques of Western Power." *Theory and Society* 31:1–34.

Murray, Stephen O., and Kenneth W. Payne. 1989. "The Social Classification of AIDS in American Epidemiology," pp. 23–36 in Ralph Bolton (ed.): *AIDS Pandemic. A Global Emergency*. New York: Gordon & Breach.

Myers, Greg. 1991. "Stories and Styles in Two Molecular Biology Review Articles," pp. 45–75 in Charles Bazerman and James Paradis (eds.): *Textual Dynamics of the Professions. Historical and Contemporary Studies of Writing in Professional Communities*. Madison: University of Wisconsin Press.

Myers, Greg. 1990. *Writing Biology. Texts in the Social Construction of Scientific Knowledge*. Madison: University of Wisconsin Press.

Nash, Walter. 1989. *Rhetoric. The Wit of Persuasion*. Oxford: Blackwell.

Nelkin, Dorothy. 1991. "AIDS and the News Media." *The Milbank Quarterly* 69/2:293–307.

Nelkin, Dorothy. 1985. "Introduction: Analyzing Risk," pp. 11–24 in Dorothy Nelkin (ed.): *The Language of Risk. Conflicting Perspectives on Occupational Health*. Beverly Hills, CA: Sage.

Nelkin, Dorothy, and Sander Gilman. 1988. "Placing Blame for Devastating Disease." *Social Research* 55/3:361–77.

Nickles, Thomas. 1995. "Philosophy of Science and History of Science," pp. 139–63 in Arnold Thackray (ed.): *Constructing Knowledge in the History of Science*. Chicago: University of Chicago Press.

Nickles, Thomas. 1992. "Good Science as Bad History: From Order of Knowing to Order of Being," pp. 85–129 in Ernan McMullin (ed.): *The Social Dimensions of Science*. Notre Dame, IN: University of Notre Dame Press.

Norris, Christopher. 1990. *What's Wrong with Postmodernism. Critical Theory and the Ends of Philosophy*. New York: Harvester Wheatsheaf.

Ochs, Elinor, and Lisa Capps. 1996. "Narrating the Self." *Annual Review of Anthropology* 25:19–43.

Oppenheimer, Gerald M. 1992. "Cause, Cases and Cohorts. The Role of Epidemiology in the Historical Construction of AIDS," pp. 49–83 in Elizabeth Fee and Daniel M. Fox (eds.): *AIDS. The Making of a Chronic Disease*. Berkeley: University of California Press.

Oppenheimer, Gerald M. 1988: "In the Eye of the Storm: The Epidemic Construction of AIDS," pp. 267–300 in Elizabeth Fee and Daniel M. Fox (eds.): *AIDS. The Burdens of History*. Berkeley: University of California Press.

Patton, Cindy. 1993. "From Nation to Family. Containing African AIDS," pp. 127–38 in Henry Abelove, Michèle Aina Barale, and David M. Halperin (eds.): *The Lesbian and Gay Studies Reader*. New York: Routledge.

Patton, Cindy. 1990. *Inventing AIDS*. London: Routledge & Kegan Paul.

Patton, Cindy. 1989. "The AIDS Industry: Construction of "Victims," "Volunteers" and "Experts," pp. 113–26 in Erica Carter and Simon Watney (eds.): *Taking Liberties. AIDS and Cultural Politics*. London: Serpent's Tail.

Patton, Cindy. 1985. *Sex and Germs*. Boston: South End Press.

Pêcheux, Michel. 1990. *The Restlessness of Discourse* [*L'inquiétude du discours*]. Paris: Editions des Cendres.

Pêcheux, Michel. 1975. *The Truths of La Palice: Linguistics, Semantics, Philosophy*. Paris: Maspéro.

Pels, Dick. 2000. *The Intellectual as Stranger. Studies in Spokespersonship*. London: Routledge.

Pera, Marcello. 1994. *The Discourses of Science*. Chicago: Chicago University Press.

Perrow, Charles, and Mauro F. Guillen. 1990. *The AIDS Disaster: The Failure of Organizations in New York and the Nation*. New Haven, CT: Yale University Press.

Peters, John Durham. 1990. "Rhetoric's Revival, Positivism's Persistence: Social Science, Clear Communication, and the Public Space." *Sociological Theory* 8/2:224–31.

Picart, Caroline Joan. 1994. "Scientific Controversy as Farce: The Benveniste-Maddox Counter Trials." *Social Studies of Science* 24/1:7–37.

Pickering, Andrew. 1995. *The Mangle of Practice*. Chicago: University of Chicago Press.

Piot, Pierre, and Michael Mann. 1987. "Bidirectional Heterosexual Transmission of Human Immunodeficiency Virus (HIV)," pp. 149–56 in Jean-Claude Gluckman and E. Vilmer (eds.): *Acquired Immunodeficiency Syndrome*. Paris: Elsevier.

Pleasants, Nigel. 1999. *Wittgenstein and the Idea of a Critical Social Theory*. London: Routledge.

Poirier, Richard. 1988. "AIDS and Traditions of Homophobia." *Social Research* 55/3:461–75.

Pollak, Michel. 1992. *AIDS: A Problem for Sociological Research*. London: Sage.

Porter, Theodore M. 1995. *Trust in Numbers. The Pursuit of Objectivity in Science and Public Life*. Princeton, NJ: Princeton University Press.

Potter, Jonathan. 1988. "What is Reflexive About Discourse Analysis. The Case of Reading Readings," pp. 37–52 in Steve Woolgar (ed.): *Knowledge and Reflexivity. New Frontiers in the Sociology of Knowledge*. London: Sage.

Potter, Jonathan, Margaret Wetherell, and Andrew Chitty. 1991. "Quantification Rhetoric – Cancer on Television." *Discourse and Society* 2/3:333–65.

Prelli, Lawrence A. 1989. *A Rhetoric of Science. Inventing Scientific Discourse*. Columbia: University of South Carolina Press.

Pressman, Jack D. 1990. "AIDS and the Burdens of Historians." *Journal of the History of Sexuality* 1/11:137–43.

Prims, Gwyn. 1989. "But What Was the Disease? The Present State of Health and Healing in African Studies." *Past and Present* 124:159–79.

Prior, Lindsay. 1992. "The Local Space of Medical Discourse. Disease, Illness, and Hospital Architecture," pp. 67–84 in Jens Lachmund and Gunnar Stollberg (eds.): *The Social Construction of Illness*. Stuttgart: Steiner.

Rapp, Rayna. 1999. *Testing Women, Testing the Fetus. The Social Impact of Amniocentesis in America*. New York: Routledge.

Rawling, Alison. 1994. "The AIDS Virus Dispute: Awarding Priority for the Discovery of the Human Immunodeficiency Virus." *Science, Technology and Human Values* 19/3:342–60.

Sarup, Madan. 1988. *An Introductory Guide to Poststructuralism and Postmodernism.* New York: Harvester Wheatsheaf.

Sauer, Beverly A. 1996. "Communicating Risk in a Cross-Cultural Context. A Cross-Cultural Comparison of Rhetorical and Social Understandings in US and British Mine Safety Training." *Journal of Business and Technical Communication* 10/3:306–29.

Schatzki, Theodore. 1996. *Social Practices. A Wittgensteinian Approach to Human Activity and the Social.* Cambridge, UK: Cambridge University Press.

Schatzki, Theodore, Karin Knorr-Cetina, and Eike von Savigny (eds.). 2001. *The Practice Turn in Contemporary Theory.* London: Routledge.

Scollon, Ron. 2001. *Mediated Discourse. The Nexus of Practice.* New York: Routledge.

Scott, Alan. 2000. "Risk Society or Angst Society? Two Views of Risk, Consciousness and Community," pp. 33–46 in Barbara Adam, Ulrich Beck, and Joost Van Loon (eds.): *The Risk Society and Beyond. Critical Issues for Social Theory.* London: Sage.

Scott, Sue, and Richard Freeman. 1995. "Prevention as a Problem of Modernity: The Example of HIV and AIDS," pp. 151–70 in Jonathan Gabe (ed.): *Medicine, Health, and Risk. Sociological Approaches.* Oxford: Blackwell.

Searle, John R. 1979. *Expression and Meaning. Studies in the Theory of Speech Acts.* Cambridge, UK: Cambridge University Press.

Searle, John R. 1970. *Speech Acts. An Essay in the Philosophy of Language.* Cambridge, UK: Cambridge University Press.

Seidel, Gill. 1992. "The Competing Discourses of HIV/AIDS in Sub-Saharan Africa: Discourses of Right and Empowerment Vs. Discourses of Control and Exclusion." *Social Science and Medicine* 36/3:175–94.

Setel, Philip. 1999. *A Plague of Paradoxes. AIDS, Culture, and Demography in Northern Tanzania.* Chicago: University of Chicago Press.

Shea, Elizabeth. 2001. "The Gene as a Rhetorical Figure: 'Nothing But a Very Applicable Little Word.'" *Science as Culture* 10/4:505–27.

Sherry, Michael S. 1993. "The Language of War in AIDS Discourse," pp. 39–53 in Timothy F. Murphy and Suzanne Poirier (eds.): *Writing AIDS. Gay Literature, Language, and Analysis.* New York: Columbia University Press.

Shilts, Randy. 1987. *And the Band Played On: Politics, People, and the AIDS Epidemic.* New York: St. Martin's Press.

Star, Susan Leigh. 1989. "The Structure of Ill-Structured Solutions: Boundary Objects and Heterogeneous Distributed Problem-Solving," pp. 37–54 in Les Gasser and Michael N. Huhns (eds.): *Distributed Artificial Intelligence,* Vol. 2. London: Pitman.

Star, Susan Leigh, and James R. Griesemer. 1989. "Institutional Ecology, 'Translations' and Boundary Objects: Amateurs and Professionals in

Berkeley's Museum of Vertebrate Zoology, 1907–1939." *Social Studies of Science* 19:387–420.

Stevenson, Michael R. 2001. "Heterosexual Men," pp. 319–21 in Raymond A. Smith (ed.): *Encyclopedia of AIDS. A Social, Political, Cultural, and Scientific Record of the HIV Epidemic.* New York: Penguin.

Stine, Gerald. 1993. *Acquired Immune Deficiency Syndrome. Biological, Medical, Social, and Legal Issues.* Englewood Cliffs, NJ: Prentice Hall.

Strong, Philip, and Virginia Berridge. 1990. "No One Knew Anything: Some Issues in British AIDS Policy," pp. 233–52 in Peter Aggleton (ed.): *AIDS: Individual, Cultural and Policy Dimensions.* London: The Falmer Press.

Stump, David J. 1996. "Afterword: New Directions in the Philosophy of Science Studies," pp. 443–52 in Peter Galison and David J. Stump (eds.): *The Disunity of Science. Boundaries, Contexts, and Power.* Stanford, CA: Stanford University Press.

Sturken, Marita. 1997. *Tangled Memories. The Vietnam War, the AIDS Epidemic, and the Politics of Remembering.* Berkeley: University of California Press.

Swales, John M. 1990. *Genre Analysis. English in Academic and Research Settings.* Cambridge, UK: Cambridge University Press.

Treichler, Paula. 1999. *How to Have Theory in an Epidemic. Cultural Chronicles of AIDS.* Durham, NC: Duke University Press.

Treichler, Paula. 1993. "AIDS Narratives on Television: Whose Story?" pp. 161–99 in Timothy F. Murphy and Suzanne Poirier (eds.): *Writing AIDS. Gay Literature, Language, and Analysis.* New York: Columbia University Press.

Treichler, Paula. 1992. "AIDS, HIV and the Cultural Construction of Reality," pp. 65–100 in Gilbert Herdt and Shirley Lindebaum (eds.): *The Time of AIDS. Social Analysis, Theory and Method.* London: Sage.

Treichler, Paula. 1988a. "AIDS, Gender and Biomedical Discourse: Current Contests for Meaning," pp. 190–266 in Elizabeth Fee and Daniel M. Fox (eds.): *AIDS. The Burdens of History.* Berkeley: University of California Press.

Treichler, Paula. 1988b. "AIDS, Homophobia and Biomedical Discourse. An Epidemic of Significance," pp. 31–70 in Douglas Crimp (ed.): *AIDS: Cultural Analysis/Cultural Activism.* Cambridge, MA: MIT Press.

Tulloch, John, and Simon Chapman. 1992. "Experts in Crisis: The Framing of Radio Debate About the Risk of AIDS to Heterosexuals." *Discourse and Society* 3/4:437–67.

Turner, Stephen. 2003. *Liberal Democracy 3.0: Civil Society in an Age of Experts.* London: Sage.

Turner, Stephen. 1994. *The Social Theory of Practices: Tradition, Tacit Knowledge, and Presuppositions.* Chicago: University of Chicago Press.

Urban, Greg, and Michael Silverstein (eds.). 1996. *Natural Histories of Discourse.* Chicago: University of Chicago Press.

Van Dijk, Teun. 1993. "Principles of Critical Discourse Analysis." *Discourse and Society* 4/2:249–83.

Wermuth, Laurie, Jennifer Ham, and Rebecca L. Robbins. 1992. "Women Don't Wear Condoms. AIDS Risk Among Sexual Partners of IV Drug Users," pp. 72–94 in Joan Huber and Beth Schneider (eds.): *The Social Context of AIDS*. Newbury Park, CA: Sage.

White, Hayden. 1987. *The Content of the Form: Narrative Discourse and Historical Representation*. Baltimore, MD: Johns Hopkins University Press.

White, Hayden. 1985. *Tropics of Discourse: Essays in Cultural Criticism*. Baltimore, MD: Johns Hopkins University Press.

White, Hayden. 1973. *Metahistory: The Historical Imagination in Nineteenth Century Europe*. Baltimore, MD: Johns Hopkins University Press.

Woolgar, Steven. 1988. "Reflexivity is the Ethnographer of the Text," pp. 14–34 in Steve Woolgar (ed.): *Knowledge and Reflexivity. New Frontiers in the Sociology of Knowledge*. London: Sage.

Woolgar, Steven, and Dorothy Pawluch. 1985. "Ontological Gerrymandering: The Anatomy of Social Problems Explanations." *Social Problems* 32/3:214–225.

Wynne, Brian. 1996. "May the Sheep Safely Graze? A Reflexive View on the Expert-Lay Knowledge Divide," pp. 44–83 in Scott Lash, B. Szerszynski, and Brian Wynne (eds.): *Risk, Environment and Modernity*. London: Sage.

Acknowledgment for Quoted Material

(5) Masur, H., Michelis, A., Greene, J. B., et al. 1981. "An Outbreak of Community-Acquired *Pneumocystis Carinii* Penumonia." *New England Journal of Medicine* 305/24, pp. 1431, 1436, 1437. Copyright © 1981, Massachusetts Medical Society. All rights reserved.

(6) Centers for Disease Control and Prevention Task Force on Kaposi's Sarcoma and Opportunistic Infections. 1982. "Epidemiologic Aspects of the Current Outbreak of Kaposi's Sarcoma and Opportunistic Infections." *New England Journal of Medicine* 306/4, p. 252. Copyright © 1982, Massachusetts Medical Society. All rights reserved.

(7) Siegal, F. P., Lopez, C., Hammer, G. S., et al. 1981. "Severe Acquired Immunodeficiency in Male Homosexuals, Manifested by Chronic Perianal Ulcerative Herpes Simplex Lesions." *New England Journal of Medicine* 305/24, pp. 1439, 1441. Copyright © 1981, Massachusetts Medical Society. All rights reserved.

(8) Pape, J. W., Liautaud, B., Thomas, F., et al. 1983. "Characteristics of the Acquired Immunodeficiency Syndrome in Haiti." *New England Journal of Medicine* 309/16, p. 949. Copyright © 1983, Massachusetts Medical Society. All rights reserved.

(9) Desforges, J. F. 1983. "AIDS and Preventive Treatment in Hemophilia." *New England Journal of Medicine* 308/2, p. 94. Copyright © 1983, Massachusetts Medical Society. All rights reserved.

(10) Curran, J. W., Lawrence, D. N., Jaffe, H., et al. 1984. "Acquired Immunodeficiency Syndrome (AIDS) Associated with Transfusions." *New England Journal of Medicine* 310/2, pp. 69, 70. Copyright © 1984, Massachusetts Medical Society. All rights reserved.

(11) Harris, C., Butkens Small, C., Klein, R. S. 1983. "Immunodeficiency in Female Sexual Partners of Men with the Acquired Immunodeficiency Syndrome." *New England Journal of Medicine* 308/20, p. 1181. Copyright © 1983, Massachusetts Medical Society. All rights reserved.

(12) Kreiss, J. K., Koech, D., Plummer, F. A., et al. 1986. "AIDS Virus Infection in Nairobi Prostitutes. Spread of the Epidemic to East Africa." *New England Journal of Medicine* 314/7, p. 417. Copyright © 1986, Massachusetts Medical Society. All rights reserved.

(13) Klein, R. S. 1986. "More on AIDS in Patients on Dialysis." *New England Journal of Medicine* 314/21, p. 1386. Copyright © 1986, Massachusetts Medical Society. All rights reserved.

(14) Gottlieb, M. S., Schroff, R., Schanker, H. M., Weisman, J. D., et al. 1981. "*Pneumocystis carinii* Pneumonia and Mucosal Candidiasis in Previously Healthy Homosexual Men. Evidence of a New Acquired Cellular Immunodeficiency." *New England Journal of Medicine* 305/24, p. 1429. Copyright © 1981, Massachusetts Medical Society. All rights reserved.

(15) Durack, D. T. 1981. "Opportunistic Infections and Kaposi's Sarcoma in Homosexual Men." *New England Journal of Medicine* 305/24, p. 1466. Copyright © 1981, Massachusetts Medical Society. All rights reserved.

(16) Broder, S., and Gallo, R. C. 1984. "A Pathogenic Retrovirus (HTLV-III) Linked to AIDS." *New England Journal of Medicine* 311/20, pp. 1294–5. Copyright © 1984 Massachusetts Medical Society. All rights reserved.

(17) Mellersh, A. R. "AIDS and Authors." Reprinted with permission from Elsevier (*The Lancet*, 1984, II/8393, p. 41).

(18) Hymes, K. B., Cheung, T., Greene, J. B., et al. "Kaposi's Sarcoma in Homosexual Men – A Report of Eight Cases." Reprinted with permission from Elsevier (*The Lancet*, 1981, II/8247, pp. 598–600).

(19) Brennan, R. O., Durack D. T. "Gay Compromise Syndrome." Reprinted with permission from Elsevier (*The Lancet*, 1981, II/8259, p. 1338).

(20) Clumeck, N., Mascart-Lemone, F., de Maubeuge, J., et al. "Acquired Immune Deficiency Syndrome in Black Africans." Reprinted with permission from Elsevier (*The Lancet*, 1983, I/8325, p. 642).

(21) McDonald, M. I., Hamilton, J. D., Durack, D. T. "Hepatitis B Surface Antigen Could Harbour the Infective Agent of AIDS." Reprinted with permission from Elsevier (*The Lancet*, 1983, II/8354, p. 883).

(22) Goedert, J. J., Neuland, C. Y., Wallen, W. C., et al. "Amyl Nitrite May Alter T Lymphocytes in Homosexual Men." Reprinted with permission from Elsevier (*The Lancet*, 1982, I/8269, p. 414).

(23) Teas, J. "Could AIDS Be a New Variant of African Swine Fever Virus?" Reprinted with permission from Elsevier (*The Lancet*, 1983, I/8330, p. 923).

(24) Andreani, T., Modigliani, R., Le Charpentier, Y., et al. "Acquired Immunodeficiency With Intestinal Cryptosporidiosis: Possible Transmission by Haitian Whole Blood." Reprinted with permission from Elsevier (*The Lancet*, 1983, I/8335, pp. 1187, 1190).

(25) Bygbjerg, I. C. "AIDS in a Danish Surgeon (Zaire, 1976)." Reprinted with permission from Elsevier (*The Lancet*, 1983, I/8330, p. 925).

(26) Froebel, K. S., Lowe, G. D., Madhok, R., Forbes, C. D. "AIDS and Hepatitis B." Reprinted with permission from Elsevier (*The Lancet*, 1984, I/8377, p. 632).

(27) Gazzard, B. G., Shangon, D. C., Farthing, C., et al. "Clinical Findings and Serological Evidence of HTLV-III Infection in Homosexual Contacts of Patients with AIDS and Persistent Generalized Lymphadenopathy in London." Reprinted with permission from Elsevier (*The Lancet*, 1984, II/8401, p. 483).

(28) Brun-Vézinet, F., Rouzioux, C., Barré-Sinoussi, F., et al. "Detection of igG Antibodies to Lymphadenopathy-Associated Virus in Patients with AIDS or Lymphadenopathy Syndrome." Reprinted with permission from Elsevier (*The Lancet*, 1984, I/8389, p. 1253).

(29) Goedert, J. J., Sarngadharan, M. G., Biggar, R. J., et al. "Determinants of Retrovirus (HTLV-III) Antibody and Immunodeficiency Conditions in Homosexual Men." Reprinted with permission from Elsevier (*The Lancet*, 1984, II/8405, p. 714).

(30) Ellrodt, A., Barré-Sinoussi, F., le Bras, P., Nugeyre, M. T., et al. "Isolation of Human T-Lymphotropic Retrovirus (LAV) from Zairian Married Couple, One With AIDS, One With Prodromes." Reprinted with permission from Elsevier (*The Lancet*, 1984, I/8391, pp. 1383, 1385).

(31) Francis, D. P., Fiorino, P. M., Broderson, J. R. "Infection of Chimpanzees With Lymphadenopathy-Associated Virus." Reprinted with permission from Elsevier (*The Lancet*, 1984, II/8414, p. 1277).

(32) Moss, A. R., Bacchetti, P., Gorman, M., Dritz, S., et al. "AIDS in the "Gay" Areas of San Francisco." Reprinted with permission from Elsevier (*The Lancet*, 1983, I/8330, p. 924).

(33) Piot, P., Quinn, T. C., Taelman, H. "Acquired Immunodeficiency Syndrome in a Heterosexual Population in Zaire." Reprinted with permission from Elsevier (*The Lancet*, 1984, II/8394, p. 68).

(34) Drew, W. C., Conant, M. A., Huang, E. S., et al. "Cytomegalovirus and Kaposi's Sarcoma in Young Homosexual Men." Reprinted with permission from Elsevier (*The Lancet*, 1982, II/8290, p. 125).

(35) Zakowski, P., Fligiel, S., Berlin, G. W., Johnson, L. R. 1982. "Disseminated *Mycobacterium avium-intracellulare* Infection in Homosexual Men Dying of Acquired Immunodeficiency." *Journal of the American Medical Association* 248/22, p. 2982. Copyright © 1982, American Medical Association. All rights reserved.

(36) Wyckoff, R. F. 1986. "Preventing the Spread of AIDS." *Journal of the American Medical Association* 255/13, p. 1704. Copyright © 1986, American Medical Association. All rights reserved.

(37) Thomas, P. A., Jaffe, H. W., Spira, T. J., et al. 1984. "Unexplained Immunodeficiency in Children. A Surveillance Report." *Journal of the American Medical Association* 252/5, p. 643. Copyright © 1984, American Medical Association. All rights reserved.

(38) Miller, B., Stansfield, S. K., Zack, M. M., et al. 1984. "The Syndrome of Unexplained Generalized Lymphadenopathy in Young Men in New York City. Is It Related to the Acquired Immune Deficiency Syndrome?" *Journal of the American Medical Association* 251/2, pp. 240–1. Copyright © 1984, American Medical Association. All rights reserved.

(39) Mavligit, G. M., Talpaz, M., Hsia, F. T., et al. 1984. "Chronic Immune Stimulation by Sperm Alloantigens. Support for the Hypothesis that Spermatozoa Induce Immune Dysregulation in Homosexual Males." *Journal of the American Medical Association* 251/2, p. 237. Copyright © 1984, American Medical Association. All rights reserved.

(40) Oleske, J., Minnefor, A., Cooper, R. Jr., Thomas, K., et al. 1983. "Immune Deficiency Syndrome in Children." *Journal of the American Medical Association* 249/17, p. 2346. Copyright © 1983, American Medical Association. All rights reserved.

(41) Goedert, J. J., Bigger, R. J., Winn, D. M., Byar, D. P., Strong, D. M., Di Gioia R. A., Grossman, R. J., Sanchez, W. C., Kase, R. G., et al. 1985. "Decreased Helper T-Lymphocytes in Homosexual Men. I. Sexual

Contact in High Incidence Areas for the Acquired Immunodeficiency Syndrome." *American Journal of Epiedmiology* 121/5, p. 629. By permission of the Society for Epidemiologic Research.

(42) Moss, A. R., Osmond, D., Bacchetti, P., Cherman, J. C., Barre-Sinoussi, F., Carlson, J. 1987. "Risk Factors for AIDS and HIV Seropositivity in Homosexual Men." *American Journal of Epidemiology* 125/6, p. 1045. By permission of the Society for Epidemiologic Research.

(43) Miller Riva and Robert Bor. *AIDS. Guide to Clinical Counseling*, p. 43. London, 1989: Science Press. Copyright © 1989, Science Press.

(44) Marx, Jean L. 1982. "New Disease Baffles Medical Community." *Science* 217, p. 619. Copyright © 1982, American Association for the Advancement of Science.

(45) Kalyanaram, V. S., Cabradilla, C. D., Getchell, J. P. 1984. "Antibodies to the Core Protein of Lymphadenopathy-Associated Virus (LAV) in Patients with AIDS." *Science* 225, p. 323. Copyright © 1984, American Association for the Advancement of Science.

(46) Saxinger, W. C., Levine, P. H., Dean, A. G., et al. 1985. "Evidence for Exposure to HTLV-III in Uganda Before 1973." *Science* 227, p. 1038. Copyright © 1985, American Association for the Advancement of Science.

(47) Norman, C. 1985. "Africa and the Origins of AIDS." *Science* 230, p. 1141. Copyright © 1985, American Association for the Advancement of Science.

(48) Kauki, P. J., Alroy, J., Essex, M. 1985. "Isolation of T-Lymphotropic Retrovirus Related to HTLV-III/LAV from Wild-Caught African Green Monkeys." *Science* 230, p. 954. Copyright © 1985, American Association for the Advancement of Science.

(49) Brun-Vézinet, F., Rouzioux, C., Montagnier, L., et al. 1984. "Prevalence of Antibodies to Lymphadenopathy-Associated Retrovirus in African Patients with AIDS." *Science* 226, p. 455. Copyright © 1984, American Association for the Advancement of Science.

Name Index

Subject Index

Milton Keynes UK
Ingram Content Group UK Ltd.
UKHW041519181024
449640UK00003B/14